DETOX your WORLD

Quick and lasting results for a beautiful mind, body and spirit

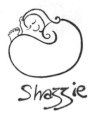

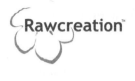

www.shazzie.com

www.rawcreation.com

D0183975

Concept, writing and photography

Shazzie
www.shazzie.com

Editor

David Smith

Design, creation and publication

Rawcreation Ltd
www.rawcreation.com
Tel: +44 (0)8700 113 119

Cover photograph and Shazzie's *after* photographs

Paul Webb

Printing

Printed on chlorine-free fully recyclable and biodegradable paper by Altone Limited, Coton, Cambridge. Set in Times New Roman 10 point.

Note

The information outlined in this book is not intended to be used as a replacement for medical advice. If you are suffering from any health issues, please seek the care of a qualified medical practitioner. When using this book, you must take sole responsibility for all the fantastic things that will happen in your life.

Dedication

To
Steve Merryweather

Thank you for all the love and all the lessons,
I'll treasure them always

Soar high,
beautiful man.

Acknowledgments

Ruth Allen. Your hugs, comforting words and your wisdom stop me in my tracks. Your necessity to dye all your clothes and hats purple, and your strange use of language, make me laugh like nothing else. Don't go ecru!

To all my family, especially Mum, Dad, Jen, Huey, Louie and Dewey. I know I don't need to express how much I love you here, as we all feel it in our hearts — but you've got it anyway! Thank you for all your support and help. You're soooo special and I'm sure the amount of mangoes I owe you is mounting up!

Great thanks also go to the people who supplied testimonials. The proof of your puddings will help the eatings of so many others.

To all who bought this book's older sister, **Detox Delights**. You made me realise there is a big need for this information, which pushed this woman out of bed and onto her computer morning after morning.

To Karen Jessett and Karen Oakley, and to Lisa Currants and Lisa Butcher. Thank you for helping me become all-woman in your own special ways.

To Jatinder, my sweet soul sister. The fire in your eyes, the purity in your heart, and the passion in your soul give me such hope for this beautiful planet of ours.

Special gratitude to David Wolfe for your total commitment for a better world, and the magic you spread through your open-hearted love.

To Joe, for showing me the Best way! José, eres un hombre muy único!

To my editor and friend David Smith. You went above and beyond the call of duty to help me create a book which is already changing lives.

To all my teachers, you shining lights! Bless you all for being around at exactly the right times, proving that time bends to suit, when you want it enough!

And most of all, thanks to you for loving yourself enough to read and use the information within these pages. Bless you.

Contents

The first bits

Foreword by David Wolfe 1

Introduction 3

How to use this book 5

The world of detox

What's all this detox business? 8

What happens when you detox 17

Eating like a human 21

Detoxing to lose weight 27

Detoxing for health 30

After you detox 32

The hat collector 35

Your toxic world

Alcohol 40

Coffee 44

Environmental pollution 46

Skin care 49

The air you breathe 51

Water, water everywhere 56

Household items 60

Mobile phones 62

Smoking 63

System shockers 73

Teeth 79

Detox helpers

Breathing and oxygen 92

Colon cleaning 98

Exercise 102

Laughing 105

Massages and wraps 108

Meditation 111

Natural mind training 115

Reflexology 118

Saunas — the infra-red variety 120

Silver 121

Skin brushing 124

The Tibetan Rejuvenation Rites 127

Vipassana 131

Yoga 133

All about food

What's the best way to eat food? 138

Food for thought 142

Wild and organic food 149

Cooking your food 160

The food you will be eating

Fruit 166

Greens 168

Nuts and seeds 173

Other plant foods 175

Your detox plans

How to detox 178

Making your detox work 181

Turning detox theory into practice 185

Your peaceful three day detox plan 189

Your seven day chakra rejuvenation detox 200

Fasting and juice cleansing 217

Your juice detox 221

Your fast 224

Detox for life 227

Success stories

Arlyn Grant 238

Jatinder Daniels 242

Jay Banks 248

Michele Déradune 250

Tony Thorpe 255

Shazzie 259

The recipes

Food notes 272

Equipment notes 275

Smoothies 277

Juices 279

Drinks 285

Soups 289

Salads 295

Scrummy side dishes 300

Your new dairy 309

Dips, spreads, dressings, sauces and pâtés 312

Very special main meals 318

Special additions 330

Puddings and desserts 333

Entertaining meals 342

Buffet ideas 343

The best meal in the world, ever 344

Resources

Mail order 346

Further support 347

Credits

Thanks 350

References and bibliography 351

The last bits

Recipe index 354

Index 359

Further copies and other products by Shazzie 373

What they say about Detox Your World 374

Foreword by David Wolfe

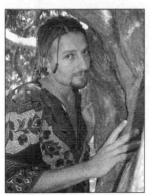

Have you ever walked into someone's home and found stuff everywhere?

Stuff on the counters, stuff on the tables, stuff in the cabinets, stuff in the closets, and loads of stuff in the refrigerator! This is an outward sign that there is too much stuff inside the stomach, intestines, fat cells, and colon!

When there is too much stuff around it is time to Detox Your World.

Shazzie's book, **Detox Your World**, presents an overall strategy for getting rid of excess stuff: excess food, excess toxins, excess chemicals, excess behaviours.

Shazzie shows us how to get all the exits open so that we can comfortably and controllably eliminate all our stuff.

Detox Your World presents a wide variety of health ideas from which to draw upon. In a gentle, attractive way, Shazzie presents us with tools (not rules) with which to transform our health, appearance, and outlook on life. Shazzie includes information as diverse as oxygen therapies, ionic minerals, and raw food nutrition, thus bringing the leading edge to us. She also presents a wonderful array of resources, turning us on to so many new books and health products.

What I found most nourishing about **Detox Your World** was its heightened level of "honesty and realness." This is something that I find innate to the person and is part of the special energy Shazzie brings into the world.

We live in an era where freedom of choice has become the order of the day. When Shazzie decided it was time for her to become happy and healthy, she tapped into all the current sources of health information such as books, the Internet and lectures. The diversity and amount of information from these sources provides us with so many choices never before imagined.

As a natural progression of what Shazzie has experienced and learned, she created this remarkable book containing so much new, up-to-the-minute information that you can experience it all right here, too.

Having been personally nourished by Shazzie's amazing food, I find her recipe section particularly enticing. She has created every different kind of meal — more than one could ever desire. Each recipe is healthy, happy, and cleansing. Shazzie makes it clear that we get to eat great food, and detoxify our bodies at the same time.

Shazzie is, in my opinion, Britain's leading health authority. You may find that this book is the first in a life-long series of transformative books by someone who lives what they teach.

I know that **Detox Your World** will invite many synchronicities into your life and help you experience every day as *The Best Day Ever*!

Enjoy in joy!

David Wolfe
www.davidwolfe.com

Author of **The Sunfood Diet Success System**
Naked Chocolate *(with Shazzie)*
Eating For Beauty

CEO of www.rawfood.com
Director of The Fruit Tree Planting Foundation | www.fruittreefoundation.org

Introduction

When my body started giving up before my life had really begun, I searched endlessly for a way to gain the energy I should have had as a child but somehow missed out. Trying every alternative treatment that came my way, and getting more and more depressed about the state of my mind, body and spirit, I felt this search could go on for years without a solution. I'd seen too many people accept defeat and become victims of their circumstances. It took the realisation that even I, who had been labelled a health freak since the onset of adulthood, had to look outside of the box. That realisation was my treasured key to freedom.

Once I'd discovered that the secret to a fantastic life was to detox my world, I can only describe the subsequent changes I experienced as magical. I became my natural weight, lost all sight of depression, and gained a new outlook and direction in life. For the first time ever in my life I was truly happy, healthy and wise.

It's the wisdom I've uncovered that I want to share with you in this book. Until you begin to live your life in the flow, you may not believe some of the information in this book. If that happens, make notes on how you feel at that time and skip ahead to the next section. Revisit the information a month or two later and see how you feel then. Information only ever resonates fully with you when you are fully ready to receive it. This book will give you the opportunity to go deeper and deeper into lightening your life every time you read it. Very soon, you'll enjoy living all of your life joyfully and in harmony, and that's when you'll truly feel the upward spiraling ever expanding flow.

By following the simple guidelines and suggestions outlined in this book, you can slowly but surely start to detox every part of your life, at the speed and to the extent that you want. It's good to know that more than just unwanted cellulite and colds disappear. When I detoxed, I even moved countries! This book will enable you to alter the course of your life, so you can live the life you were destined to live, and so you can be who you really are. When changes occur with your detox, loving yourself enough to welcome and embrace them will push you to new heights. This is ultimately a discovery of your potential as a human being. How far can you go?

When I realised this wasn't just a physical journey I began to take an interest in yoga, which took me further on my own personal development path than I thought possible. I also discovered a simple set of ancient exercises used by Tibetan Buddhist Monks which really do turn back the clock, and I share those here with you, too.

You have in your hands everything that I've learned about detoxing naturally. A natural detox is important, as it keeps us in an "earth rhythm" that stops us feeling separate and isolated from all around us. Many of today's problems in our society (and increasingly the whole world) stem from feelings of disconnection. Re-establishing that connection with nature gives us more power to live the life we've always wanted, while creating a sustainable and responsible way of living.

During your detox you might feel unsettled, as all around you seems to shift and reform. You simply can't stay in any situation that doesn't serve you when you detox properly. You'll see glimpses of your real life's purpose, which can be awe inspiring or scary! There are suggested methods of dealing with these issues in this book. As you begin to love yourself fully, and realise your magnificence, you may also start to doubt yourself. This is normal, too — just know: above all else, you can do this.

The detox process is just the tip of your transformation iceberg. Your life afterwards can be greatly enhanced by following a few simple guidelines. Very soon, those guidelines just become a natural part of your life, as they make you feel so good, are easy to stick to, and produce such great results. How far to take your post-detox life is always your choice, but you will forever remain changed by your experience. I give you the options to further your transformation, and you decide what's best for you. You can always change your mind later, when you see another glimpse of your magnificence shining through! Detoxing, cleansing and rebuilding never ends: there's no finish line, just greater and greater feelings of freedom and joy. I have found more happiness and health the further I detox my world. I can't see any reason to slow it down, or to revert back to my cheeseburger and chips days. I don't miss that food, or the lifestyle I left behind, and given a little time and patience you won't either.

If you're ready to experience this truly natural, feel-good process and discover the real you, then hold on tight: you are about to **Detox Your World**.

How to use this book

Because you don't live a typical life, I haven't devised a typical detox plan. I've devised several plans and offered many hints and tips to help you detox safely, slowly and permanently. Unless you are seriously ill, please detox at a comfortable pace as it will serve you better in the long run. If you have a serious illness, then it is normally possible to cure it by detoxing and rebuilding. Please do so under the supervision of a qualified holistic or medical practitioner.

Depending on what you want from your detox, you can use this book in several ways:

- If this is your first detox, follow one of the short detox plans first. All recipes and activities are listed, so you don't have to worry that you're not doing it right.

- If you have detoxed before, try the juice cleanse. This will give your body the space to move some older toxins out. I recommend you do this when you have a very light schedule.

- If you have undergone the seven-day detox, and have followed the 75% guide (which you'll learn about soon) for at least another two months, then fasting may be beneficial to you. Please take note of all contraindications regarding fasting as only you can take responsibility for your actions.

- If you want to permanently yet gradually and easily lighten you world, use the *Detox for life* plan. Change one thing at a time, at your own pace, and note your changes, because you'll soon forget the old you, and it's nice to see how far you've travelled.

- If you don't want the rigidity of following any plan, you can simply use the recipes and *Detox helpers*, slowly integrating them into your everyday life. As you absorb and practise the principles of this book, your instincts and intuition will return and you will experiment with other natural recipes and activities — eventually creating your own low-toxin way of living.

- If you get stuck at meal times when you want to create healthy yet satisfying meals, then the 100+ recipes in this book will help. I've also listed some of my other favourite recipe books, so do seek them out to continue creating wonderful, healthy, tasty detox dishes.

With **Detox Your World** as your companion, you can feel great about your lifestyle choices. You can immediately start to eat food which is good for you, and spoil yourself with the *Detox helpers*. This book has been devised so that you never feel like you're missing out, you just soar higher and higher on your new found wings.

5

After you've followed one or more plans, continue to use this book for recipes, activities and inspiration, and periodically clean yourself out using a detox plan. The *Detox for life* plan is flexible and fun, and it will take you to a different level of health and happiness. If you want to devise your own *Detox for life* plan, use the information that you've learned, plus the guidelines in the *Detox for life* section, and customise it by altering the sequence or adding in some extra steps. This is especially useful if you are addicted to drugs such as cigarettes, alcohol, or medication, as I don't cover these in the plan (though I do have some cutting-edge information which just might help you).

Between **Detox Your World** and its sister book **Detox Delights**, there are over 200 recipes to use and adapt for the rest of your life. By always making sure that at least 75% of your food is from my books or other recommended recipe books, you can remain in great condition: for life.

By using this book, you are going to take total responsibility for your life. You may think that going on a detox will be great for your body: losing those few extra pounds, that cellulite and that double chin is a bonus when detoxing. You'll certainly have more energy and look younger. Yet, these physical benefits are just the tip of the iceberg. Many opportunities will open up to you, and your mind will be clearer and able to choose what's right for you, not what you think is best for everyone else in your life.

As you'll see, this book isn't just about food because for good health and happiness you need to take a holistic approach: it's not just what you put in your mouth. This book touches on all aspects of modern life, and helps you work out the best ways to move forward with lightening your load, naturally and effectively.

The world of detox

Let's discover why detox is such a popular word right now. We'll get back to nature and then look at the multi-billion pound industry known as dieting. Once we've done that, we'll have a look at a more sensible, practical and permanent approach to changing your life — for good!

What's all this detox business?

Surely, over the past few years, you've heard enough about detox to last a lifetime? Well, if there's anything new to you in this book, then obviously not. See if you can count how many new concepts you read about — and explore them!

Why detox?

If you've eaten a typical western diet (meat or vegetarian) all your life, you will have taken in more toxins than your body can remove. Eventually, you may start to feel under the weather or ill. The illness can take many forms, such as acne, arthritis, depression, heart disease, lethargy, menstrual pains etc, but the cause remains the same: your body contains too many toxins and is struggling to expel them, because it was never designed to deal with such a high intake on a permanent basis.

By lightening your diet and other toxins that surround you, you allow your body more freedom to remove stored toxins.

Your body will thank you by giving you more energy, healing itself of diseases, and clearing your brain so that it's cobweb-free.

Why "Detox Your World"?

When I say Detox Your World, I really mean it: not only will you find out how to detox yourself via your food intake, you'll discover how your mind, body and spirit fit into the detox puzzle. Because good food is only one key to excellent health, we will constantly look further than your stomach! Your world consists of:

Your body

We all value our lives, often to the extent that we try to secure our physical well-being with money, houses and other forms of accumulated material goods. However, we then abuse our bodies so much that many of us end up sick or dead before we can reap the rewards of many years' hard toil.

Let's start loving our bodies so they really can last a lifetime.

Your immediate environment such as your home and your office

We care for our immediate environments relatively well because they are our "possessions". However, they can be hazardous to our health if we don't take some sensible yet easy steps. This book gives many hints and tips on how to detox your immediate environment, because it all adds up and makes a difference to you. Here's a detox tip to start you off: *The things you own end up owning you.* Less external clutter can often symbolise less internal clutter.

Our miraculous blue and green planet

Our Earth has never been assaulted so disrespectfully by humans before, and right now it's not coping too well. Some of the detox methods in this book automatically make you a better world citizen. If you don't detox your world for yourself, do it for your children. Remember, we've only borrowed the Earth from them, so think about what state you want it to be in when you pass it on.

One side-effect of living so consciously is that you produce less waste. If you have a composter, most of your bin contents will go in there. You can't help but become more environmentally friendly, and we all desperately need to do that.

About toxins

A toxin is a poisonous substance that is capable of causing disease when introduced into your body. This can be a known poison such as mercury, or it could be something subtle such as the cocktail of chemicals created when food is denatured. Probably the most well-known example of this is acrylamide. When scientists discovered that this potentially cancer-causing substance is created when carbohydrate-based food is cooked, crisis meetings were held all over the world! I write more about acrylamide in the *All about food* chapter.

Ingesting too many toxins will impair our health and strain our organs so much that they stop functioning correctly. Eventually they can give up altogether. Too many toxins in the body also overwhelms our defences. As our bodies are busy expelling toxins, we are more susceptible to infections of all kinds. Our immunity drops to very low levels, and our bodies weaken. If we are not genetically strong to start with, we'll also be less able to deal with the symptoms that the toxins cause.

Over months, years and decades of eating food that's toxic to the body, we become weak, susceptible to disease, spiritually bereft and brain-fogged.

The toxin battle

The body, in its infinite wisdom, tries to expel toxins. We might have symptoms such as a runny nose or a cough, but we think we have a cold or the flu so we take drugs to suppress the symptoms. The underlying cause is still there.

> ### Curing the cause
>
> Because of the power of natural detox, you will heal and rejuvenate, not just in a superficial "suppress the symptoms" way, but in a real "cure the cause" way. Because of the huge benefits associated with detox, it is suitable for everyone. When done correctly and sensibly, it is greatly beneficial to every part of you.

The body tries to march the toxins out another way, but we see disease. We take drugs to "cure" that disease, and the toxins remain in the body — alongside many toxic pills and potions. The underlying cause is still there.

If we don't break this "suppress the symptoms" cycle, we find ourselves with serious conditions such as arthritis, cancer, diabetes and heart disease. If we suppress the symptoms of pain at that point, the illness slowly but surely creeps around the body, like ivy strangling a tree. One day, the illness is bigger than we are, and the body, which fought so hard to get the toxins out, just gives out its last breath — it expires. We gave it no other choice.

How we got into this fine mess

When we were born, we had relatively clean and strong bodies (some were cleaner and stronger than others depending on the food and toxins in the mothers' bodies). Decades of eating foods that our body doesn't recognise takes its toll. It just can't push out all the rubbish that it takes in on a modern western diet.

> Though your body is detoxing all the time, the problems start when more rubbish goes in than comes out.

When this happens, your body won't be able to expel as many toxins as it takes in, so it stores them instead. Periodically, it attempts to remove them. Notice that most colds start at the turn of a full moon, new moon, or during a seasonal change. The body detoxifies more at these times, which leads people to believe that there's "a bug going round" because so many people are affected at the same time. I am not saying that bugs don't exist, just that we tend to blame them more than we should.

Though the conventional way of dealing with detox symptoms such as a cold is through suppression with drugs, you will benefit more by not doing this. Letting your body eliminate and rest when it wants to isn't common in our society, but it really is best.

How we live today

Mild symptoms such as headaches, migraines, skin complaints and period pains show that the body is trying to rid itself of harmful toxins. Your body uses its normal elimination organs to metabolise or remove toxins. It is only when you bombard it with unnatural food, distorted eating habits, stressful living and environmental pollutants that you run into problems. Your body was simply not designed to eliminate that much junk.

Your body does the best it can, yet years of toxins being stored in your body take their toll. The toxins are stored in fat cells, they float around the bloodstream, they stick to artery and bowel walls and they lurk inside your organs. Ageing, fatigue, illness and obesity often becomes the everyday reality for most people.

The unlucky ones among us have to deal with asthma, eczema or other diseases which are now becoming "normal" for children. In the USA in 1995, 14.6 million people had asthma. In the UK it was over 3 million: one in seven school children suffering from it. Eczema causes bleeding and itching, and can leave the sufferers in constant agony. I have one very special young friend who switched to a low toxin diet vegan which cured her severe eczema. If she ever eats food that she cannot assimilate, such as bread, her skin starts to hurt, so she does her best to stay away from it. To her, it isn't worth the agony.

If you don't want to suffer like your loved ones,
do something different, today.

As we grow up, allergies, arthritis, cancer, diabetes, heart disease and piles become "normal" for us, too. In the UK, 25% of people suffer from cancer, 15% suffer from arthritis, and 3% of people over 40 suffer from diabetes. Not taking control will make you a statistic. Not taking control will make these numbers continue to rise instead of fall. Not taking control means that it could take your life.

It's a case of knowing that there is a choice, that you don't have to suffer, that there is a better, easier, more pleasant way of living. Then it's just a case of doing it — and that's where you come in...

Living in a detoxed world

Feeling more energetic than you can remember. Going the distance. Losing that bloated feeling. Concentrating and focussing for hours on end. These are some of the first improvements you'll notice when you detox your world.

You don't get so many colds and eventually they stop altogether. I used to have six colds or flu every year which would last for about two weeks, cause me to cough up blood, and leave me feeling very weak. While I was ill I'd manage to eat oven chips and sandwiches "to keep my strength up". Now, if I suffer a cold, it lasts for about three hours and is never more frequent than twice a year (usually around the changes to spring and autumn, which are both very strong cleansing times). That big difference signifies to me that living this way is better for me than living the "normal" way. It signifies to my body that it can concentrate on getting harmful toxins out when it wants, without me blocking all the exits.

> ### Repair and rejuvenation
>
> Once all the harmful toxins are out of the way, the body can really concentrate on rejuvenation and repair — and that's where the real magic starts.

In today's world with all our pollution, we can't remove as many toxins as we would be able to in the natural world. However, we can all make great changes, both inside and out. We can certainly alter enough to prevent ourselves becoming statistics, as those I listed earlier.

Don't you find it crazy that the life-threatening condition known as diabetes is now described as "common"? Do you find it even crazier that there are people who have cured their diabetes through lifestyle changes alone, yet the tablet-touting pharmaceutical industries and doctors won't hear of such "nonsense"? Nature didn't make a great mistake when creating humans — most of us were born with a perfectly working pancreas. The mistake, sadly, was down to us — we just never gave our bodies the correct food to thrive on, time and time again.

However, our bodies are remarkable and can rejuvenate when given the right help.

Let's all start to take control now over
our health and happiness.

After all, nobody else in this world
owes you that responsibility — it's all yours.

The definition of detox

One day I was waiting for a client in a restaurant. I overheard a couple of men aged around 40 discussing their New Year detox diets. My client came in, we hugged and he looked at the menu. "I have to be careful what I order," he said, "I'm on a detox". I should have known.

My client ordered his lunch of char-grilled chicken salad with roast vegetables. It was detox, he explained, because there was no wheat or red meat. He was also off the coffee and tea.

The detoxing men on the other table might have been following a different set of detox guidelines.

That's fine, because it doesn't matter how you detox:
if you take in less toxins than before,
you are officially detoxing.

When you consume the average western diet, so much energy is given to digestion that normal bodily house cleaning has to take second place. Your body simply wasn't designed to have to detox so much stuff in one lifetime! However, as soon as you lighten the load your body can then use its natural cleaning mechanisms to remove old toxins.

Contrary to how most people describe detox,
it isn't what you eat which makes the big difference:
it's what you don't eat.

Because of this startling revelation, you'll be happy to learn that detoxing doesn't mean having to buy lots of pills and potions, and having to eat ghastly green concoctions — unless you want to (I actually really like them)! When detoxing using this book, you'll eat fresh, unadulterated food, organic where possible. You'll do tried and tested *Detox helpers*: you even have the choice to go high-tech, but you don't have to. It works so simply: because these foods are minimal in toxins, and don't cause the immune response and allergic reactions that many everyday foods do, it frees up your body's energy to spend less time on digestion and more time on cleaning, repairing and rejuvenating.

The detox white lie

The detox diets which promise to make a new man or woman of you within three or seven days aren't giving you the whole truth. Maybe because the whole truth is like a horse pill — too big and hard to swallow — at first bite, anyhow. You can't detox many past decades of unhealthy living in a few days, it would be too much of a shock for your body to sustain it! This is why **Detox Your World** works — it offers gradual and simple ways into getting deep down with detox.

The results are on us

98% of your body's cells are renewed within one to two years. All of your body's cells are renewed every seven years. Yet you don't have to wait seven or even two years to see amazing results. Give your body the correct nutrition and activities for a short period of time: it will work hard at correcting itself, and is very forgiving of your sins!

Easy eating

Using **Detox Your World** is easy! There are no complicated potions or supplements, no weighing, measuring, or portion control.

We've gone right back to basics with this detox. We've stopped fighting nature and are now going with its flow.

The beauty of eating this way

When detoxing, you are not denied lovely food. If you like, you can even have pudding for every meal! Eating your favourite fruits, getting massaged, having saunas, swimming, playing and practising yoga sounds more like a pampering health farm than a strict regime, doesn't it?

Eating detox food is certainly not going to make you feel confined to a life sentence of boring food and hard exercise. I will reveal how this simple way of life can provide you with great health benefits as you read through the sections of this chapter. As you eat more food which has a built in feel-good factor, it becomes easier to believe that it's possible for you to step into your magnificence.

Eating this way produces healthy and lasting results.

Who can detox?

As I state several times in this book, if you take in fewer toxins today than you did yesterday, your body is detoxing — it's really that easy. However, if you are pregnant, have an advanced illness, are on "essential" medication or have severe emotional issues, it would be in your interest to consult with a qualified natural medical practitioner first. Your practitioner will guide you in how to safely and effectively detox your way to outstanding health and happiness.

Curing serious illness by detoxing

Many people look to detox plans and lifestyles to cure them of serious illnesses, sometimes as a last resort. While the success rate is high compared to the prognosis, these people are sometimes already damaged beyond repair.

Please don't wait until you become
seriously ill to do something about your health.

Just one century ago, in 1900, only 20% of people in the western society over the age of 40 suffered from degenerative diseases such as arthritis, cancer, diabetes and heart disease. These days that figure stands at around 70%. Please read that again: 70% of people in our society over the age of 40 suffer from crippling and killer diseases such as arthritis, cancer, diabetes and heart disease. These diseases, which were once very rare, are now affecting more people at a younger age. In addition, too many children have arthritis, asthma, cancer, diabetes and eczema. When we detox our world, these diseases stop manifesting so abundantly, especially if we use it as our first resort, rather than our last one.

No retoxing!

Real detoxing is done with the intention not to retox, and that's why this book is so useful. The detox plans fit every occasion, and can be used and adapted over and over. Further, there are over a hundred recipes to use and adapt for the rest of your life.

If, after detoxing, you want to reintroduce food that isn't listed in this book into your diet, remember this. If your intake of non-detox food stays below 25% of your total, you'll be onto a health and happiness winner for the rest of your life!

If you eat more natural food and less unnatural food, you'll retox slower (or not at all) and will feel healthier. Aim to avoid yo-yo detoxing, as that will cause you to deviate from the path of optimal health. I spend a lot of my time creating delicious, varied and satisfying recipes specifically for you to continue your health-giving eating habits long after you've completed your detox plans. I know that if you stay interested in your food choices, you'll be happy to remain eating foods that love your body for all of your life.

If you are ready for health and happiness
it's in your hands right now.

So you see, detoxing isn't just a groovy lifestyle word, it's become a necessity for life due to all our unnatural living. If you want a life free from the common killer diseases, free from aches and pains and free from confusion and lack of clarity, you know what you must do.

Losing weight, cellulite and puffiness
are great benefits of detoxing,
yet the best one of all is gaining
the life you're supposed to have.

What happens when you detox

We've all heard about detox headaches and rashes, and an incomparable high feeling, coupled with bags of energy. Let's delve into the truth behind the headlines.

The benefits of detoxing

Here are some of the benefits you'll feel once you've detoxed. I've split them up into three categories, but in reality you'll just notice a gradual increase towards fantastic health and happiness.

Short term (0 — 6 months)

• Your skin is clearer and smoother, and your hair and nails are stronger.

• Excess mucous in your lungs and nose clears up.

• You have more energy, stamina and flexibility.

• You are more alert and your reflexes are better.

• You lose weight, cellulite start to retreat, and stretch marks begin to fade.

• Your mood becomes lighter, and any mood swings become less noticeable.

• You will sleep better, and wake up ready for the day ahead.

Medium term (6 months — 3 years)

• "Incurable" diseases may start to retreat or disappear. Asthma, arthritis, cancer, adult onset diabetes, eczema, fibromyalgia, heart disease, ME, mental disorders, MS, osteoporosis, ulcerative colitis and many more illnesses have been banished or halted for good by people continuing a detoxed lifestyle. So please believe that with dedication, you can do this, too.

• Other diseases such as bad breath, candida, constipation, cystitis, haemorrhoids, migraines and thrush all start to exit graciously.

• You won't be susceptible to yo-yo weight loss. Your new weight will remain relatively constant. Cellulite can disappear completely, and stretch marks will fade more than ever.

• Your skin colour will even out. You will tan without burning (when sunbathing sensibly and *without* conventional lotion). Wrinkles fade and baggy faces become more taut. Cheekbones become prominent and jowls disappear. You not only feel younger, you look younger, too.

- Your energy levels are at an all-time high. You sleep very well, and wake up feeling clear headed. Your mind is clear, concise and not chattering away in the background all the time.

- Your periods will regulate. There is often less blood loss (sometimes none, yet you still ovulate), less or no pain, and all pre-menstrual symptoms fade or disappear.

- You start to believe that you weren't born to suffer, as life shows you fabulous opportunities which were previously beyond your wildest dreams.

Long term (for life)

- You are at less risk from all major diseases now. Arthritis, all cancers, diabetes, heart disease, and all mental diseases are now much less of a threat.

- You will probably live longer, without senility affecting you so soon, if at all.

- Headaches, colds and all other little aches and pains usually become a thing of the past. Though they may sometimes increase in some people during the initial stages of detox, they gradually wane until they don't exist any more.

- You will be emotionally balanced. If you have deep-rooted emotional issues, they may start to rise to the surface as you detox. Take the opportunity to release them.

- Really, you just become the person you are supposed to be — not one who is malfunctioning due to an excess of artificial material and a lack of reality.

Outside help

Picture that all your emotions are locked away in your cells, and as your cells start to release toxins, they also release emotions.

At any appropriate time, seek counselling or other emotional therapeutic assistance if you feel uncomfortable with the amount of emotions being released.

Side-effects of detox

Your body cleans itself 24/7, taking harmful toxins into the liver and other organs. These elimination organs process the toxins, render them harmless and flush them out in the urine.

However, as most humans think they can eat everything which doesn't immediately kill them, they tend to put more in than the body can take out. The body has to store these toxins in the organs and fat cells.

When you then reduce the amount of toxins going in, your body takes advantage of this and releases the stored toxins to allow them to be processed, rendered harmless and flushed from your body.

As the toxins are released, they can give out one last cry. It's like your body "tastes" the addictive toxin, and wants more. At that moment, you may feel cravings or any of the detox side-effects listed below.

Usually after the third day, the side-effects ease off, and you have a smoother ride from then on.

When you start to detox, you may notice several physical symptoms such as those listed below. At the same time you will feel increased energy, alertness and stamina! It can be a disorienting time because your emotions will also detox. Whenever possible, sit back and enjoy the process.

Remember, you can always control the speed of your detox, and you are not in competition with anyone else.

On a long-term detox you will occasionally notice detox symptoms. They come in waves and might make you feel a bit down or achy for a few days, but once they've passed you'll feel better than you did before they happened. This is your body making a very good job of deep cleaning itself.

Detox side-effects normally don't last very long and are nothing to worry about. If you have any effects which are not mild and continue for more than three days, please seek the help of your preferred practitioner.

Not everyone feels side-effects, and some people only notice one or two for a short time. It can often depend on how healthy you are to start with, what your original diet was like, and how quickly you decided to detox.

My worst side-effect was feeling the cold. This didn't surprise me as it was always something I suffered from before. After about six months my temperature tolerance returned to normal.

Here are some short-term side-effects that you might — or might not — experience:

- Bad breath, bloating, body odour, diarrhoea, dizziness, gas, nausea
- Confusion, emotional imbalance, fatigue, insomnia, the need to rest, tiredness
- Colds, ear infections, headaches, joint aches
- Lack of appetite, temperature intolerance, thirst

- Boils, change in skin texture, itching, rashes, spots
- Irregular or heavier periods

When experiencing these symptoms during a detox, it's known as a healing crisis. I prefer to call it a healing signal, because it really isn't a crisis, it's a good sign that your body is able to remove stored toxins, at long last.

Eating like a human

This could be a book in itself, but I'm putting it all into a large nutshell...

Eating naturally

Here is your first nature lesson in the book. Watch a wildlife documentary that shows animals eating. Really. Then come back to the book.

What did you see?

Did you see a lion wander about, gather some zebra, gazelle and wild grasses, slowly roast it all together to get it all juicy, add flavourings because the cooking made the zebra taste bland, and then sit down with a knife, fork and plate to finally eat the steaming hot fayre? Unlikely.

Did you see a monkey dig up carrots, steam them (because that's more healthy than boiling, isn't it), then gather some fruit, chop it finely and make a fruit salad, topped off with the pasteurised cream it stole from a cow a few days before? Probably not. It's likely that you didn't see an overweight, ill, or depressed lion or monkey, either.

As lions and monkeys have completely different anatomies, they have completely different diets. One eats lots of meat, and the other eats lots of fruit and greens. In the diverse animal kingdom, there isn't one diet that fits all. However, all animals on this earth have something very important in common: if they are truly natural animals, and not kept or fed by humans, they obtain and eat their food very fresh. There's no messing about, no chopping, slicing, dicing, grilling, frying, baking, steaming, sauteeing or adding sauces and salt to try to get some of the flavour they just cooked out.

The lion just grabs and eats.
The monkey just grabs and eats.

OK, the squirrel grabs, stores and eats, but it doesn't pickle, cook or preserve! These animals eat like this because their instinct leads them to it. We eat like we do because our instinct has been replaced by addiction and social conditioning.

Your instinct and you

The recipes and activities in this book will help you rediscover your instinct. When using a detox plan, your food is often simple, and I encourage you to take your snacks as mono meals. A mono meal is made up of one type of food, which is easier for your digestive system to cope with. This means that a snack can be seven oranges, six apples, five bananas, three mangoes, two heads of lettuce or one durian! Eating like this will help you rediscover your long-lost food senses, and it's all very tasty and delicious.

This detox book doesn't endorse weighing, calorie counting, portion control or other counter-intuitive actions. We are into living much more naturally than that.

Within a very short space of time, you will want to season your foods less and less. This natural, clean way of eating will change you at your core, so when you finish a detox plan, you won't retox so readily and end up as frustrated as you might have been before you started. You will want to continue, and try the *Detox for life* plan.

Why do you eat?

Do you eat because:

- You like the taste
- You want the nutrients
- You're addicted to that type of food
- You're tired
- You're awake
- You're sad and need comfort
- You're happy
- It's a party
- Even though you've eaten, you still feel like you're missing something
- Everyone else is eating
- You might not get a chance later

You get the picture! We all eat for more reasons than the only real biological reason to eat — because we are hungry. Because instincts have become lost amongst a whole host of social niceties, traditions and psychological brainwashing, we often eat for every reason other than the fact that we're hungry.

However, when you've detoxed enough, you'll only eat when truly hungry. This is something many of us have never experienced because we have such an abundance of food. You'll also eat a lot more seasonally, just because your instinct is stronger.

Magnetic food

People can have major psychological and physiological attachments to food. Your attachments can be as old as you are. A 30- or 40-year habit is not one that you can break immediately, yet you can do it over time. I broke all my old Yorkshire pudding, roast beef and cheese on toast habits, and I know many others who have done it, too.

I promise to show you how you can do it.

The yellow cheese monster

I remember when nothing comforted me more than cheese. It took me two years from the intention of removing it from my life through action and onto success. Since then, I've learned many tips on how to overcome food addictions, and they are all revealed right here in this book.

> ### Aim high
>
> Keep your sights high, and tell yourself that you are strong enough to make the change. You can become anything you want, simply by being it or acting as if you are it already. It really works like that.

If there is one type of food which is "impossible" to give up, even though you know it's not good for you, think about the emotional reasons behind it.

For me, cheese was a symbol of a loving family life. My dad and I would spend many nights sitting together munching our way through cheese and biscuits, cheese on toast, cream cheese and crackers, and more. My attachment to cheese wasn't just the physical eating, it was to do with the warmth, security and comfort I felt when eating at this special time with the most special man in my life. Try to remember your food memories, and journal them. It's amazing what you find out from your deep stored memories. Understanding them can help to free you from them.

I haven't eaten cheese since I was 18, and I'm very glad from a health and ethical point of view that I was dedicated to breaking the addiction. For two years I repeated in my head "I don't need or eat cheese" and eventually it was true. Now I know of quicker and easier techniques for breaking food addictions, and I share them with you later in this book.

Mood food

Once you study your own eating patterns, you'll see that you eat certain types of foods when you have certain types of moods. When our hormones kick in they can make us feel like we have no control. Have you ever been in a situation where you were resisting the cream cake and resisting the cream cake and resisting the cream cake — and then you just found yourself with half a cream cake in your mouth? Using the detox techniques in this book will break that habit, because there will ultimately be nothing for you to resist. All the food in your home will be so good for you, and you will lose all food cravings, so you will never again find yourself with half a cream cake in your mouth.

Willpower does not come into it.

This isn't about trying to convince yourself of anything, it's about changing yourself radically that you don't see that cream cake as food anymore. This way of living brings out the very best in you!

Remembering that after detoxing you'll need less sleep, all your aches and pains can go away, and you become your natural weight — you'd need willpower to go back to and stick to an average diet, given all the misery it brings!

In the beginning, when your hormones make you do things that your mind has no control over, don't reproach yourself. You aren't on a wagon, so you can't fall off it! You aren't on a diet, so there's no "starting it again tomorrow"! You aren't being told what to do, so there's no-one to deceive — not even yourself. All you are doing is gradually and permanently changing yourself to become the best you possible — now isn't that something you'd love to see?

As you slowly but surely add the best foods to your diet, the bad foods naturally fall away. However, the progress curve isn't straight up, it's like a big dipper, sometimes going up, sometimes going down, but it's always heading skywards when you look at it from a distance, over a period of time.

How toxic is your diet?

The word detox used to be associated with the effects people had when coming off hard drugs, smoking and drinking. Now it's more widely known as a method used to rest the body from so-called normal everyday foods.

Have you thought about why the word detox, which used to represent a drug withdrawal, is also used to represent a "food" withdrawal? True nourishment isn't addictive, and you don't have to take a break from it. False nourishment is addictive and that's why you feel withdrawal symptoms when you detox it. If you need to take time out from bread, coffee, wine, meat, wheat and milk, you also need to question the reintroduction of such foods once the detox plan has ended. If you suffer withdrawal symptoms from removing these items from your diet, yet feel better than normal soon after, it doesn't make sense to start eating them again, does it?

In the *All about food* chapter, I write about the dangers of modern foods, as well as the delights of getting back to eating the foods we were designed to eat. Once you've read that, you can decide for yourself what you want and what you definitely don't want to put in that precious body of yours

When going on the *Detox for life* plan, you will not even need to think about what your normal diet is, or how to alter it. You'll slowly but surely replace your old meals, snacks and drinks with your new ones. As you do it at a slow pace, the toxins from your old diet will come out gently, so hopefully you won't end up with a banging headache or climbing the walls for coffee!

Many people ask me if I think they should change their diet overnight. I always say "No". Going from eating heavily processed foods to fresh foods just makes you suffer from severe physical and psychological cravings. If you have a very toxic diet right now, then please take your detox easy. The aim is always to detox slowly and gradually change your food and lifestyle habits. This will ensure your long term success.

Further information

Books

Intuitive eating is the best feeling ever, and it's such a great place to start improving your food habits because it's so simple. I highly recommend the following books:

Eat Smart Eat Raw
Detox Recipes for a High-Energy Diet
Kate Wood
ISBN: 1904010121

I love this book because the recipes are real, tried and tested and great for families as well as the singleton. Kate has been promoting raw food longer than anyone else in the UK. Her experienced and comforting words endlessly inspire you while detoxing.

You Are What You Eat
The plan that will change your life
Dr Gillian McKeith
ISBN: 0718147650

Gillian's work with this book and her TV series of the same name has altered the face of British supermarkets and the plates on British tables. Her approach to health is fully nutritional, which is very refreshing. Her food plans are easy to follow and give consistently great results for her followers.

Conscious Eating
Gabriel Cousens, MD
ISBN: 1556432852

Don't let the size of this book put you off! It's too big to read in the bath, but makes great bedtime or sunbathing reading. Gabriel covers every aspect of how food affects your body, emotions, mind and spirit. He writes in a holistic manner, exploring the physical, spiritual, and even planetary implications of your diet.

Detoxing to lose weight

Most people in our society are now classed as overweight, and many turn to detox as a dieting aid. That's great, because it works, it's healthy, and it's a fantastic stepping stone to discovering many other detox pleasures. So let's look at the world of diets, and make some sense out of it all.

The word detox is being used more frequently to replace the word diet. After decades of being bombarded with "diets", "detoxing" makes a refreshing change, if nothing else! Yet a detox is so much more profound than any diet can be. It's about lifting the whole of you to greater places, greater experiences, and greater emotions. Diets were never this exciting — or quite as thorough!

Fibre, protein, cabbages and eggs

I grew up surrounded by The F-Plan Diet, Weight Watchers, Slimming Club, The Grapefruit Diet, The Egg Diet, Slim-Fast, The Cambridge Diet and The Cabbage Soup Diet. At any time, at least one member of my family or friends was trying them out. Most of them lost weight. None of them kept the weight off. I quietly observed the yo-yoing of my loved ones, whilst pondering "There must be a better way".

These days we have the Atkins, Zone, South Beach, GI and Blood Type diets. We also have many dieters thinking: "Maybe as the old diets didn't help me keep my weight off, then these new ones will?"

As quickly as one diet is devised, another totally different one knocks it off the number one bestseller slot. However, as they're all so very different, and as we humans are pretty much similar, they can't all be right. Let's have a look at what we know about diets.

When people embark on a weight loss plan, they weigh, measure, skimp, starve and count calories, points and the days until they can stop dieting and go "back to normal". It's clear that if they go back to what they consider their normal habits they will return to the state that made them go on a diet in the first place — and then they'll probably try another diet. This time, the marketing has changed, and they say to their friends, "It's not a diet, it's an eating plan". A plan? They have to plan what they eat? Did the lion in your nature video sit there with his points system working out if he could "afford" an extra leg tonight? What if you fancy something? What if your body is craving something? What if what you planned is tasteless and unsatisfying? Do you stuff it down, with all those negative emotions, whilst trying to think: "It'll make me thin. It's good for me"?

It'$ all about mon£y

It's widely accepted that people in the UK alone spend over £2 billion a year on diet products, yet...

Over 50% of American and British adults are now overweight or obese.

The figures on both sides of the Atlantic are rising at dramatic rates, yet the saddest figure of all is this: only 2% of dieters maintain their weight loss. There is no way to make a 98% failure rate look good, so I have to put my hand on my heart and say that I don't believe any of the traditional and popular diets are successful or safe for the majority of people in the long term.

Diets do not work because they are not natural. They can leave you exhausted, malnourished, and with failed organs. They can also leave you psychologically scarred for life.

Dump the diet, discover detox

The secrets of living a low-toxin lifestyle are all revealed in this book very soon. But briefly, they work in such a simple way it's hardly believable. Take a deep breath...

If you eat food that you are designed to eat, that hasn't been chemically altered via various methods of human intervention, your body has less to deal with when digesting it. It recognises it as food, and digests it quickly and with ease. Then it can get on with doing anything else such as cleaning, repairing, rejuvenating and restructuring without obstruction. Simply by reducing the toxic load going in to your body, you are allowing it to function more efficiently.

When you do this for long enough, you notice that cellulite, double chins, saddle-bags, water retention and extra tummies disappear. If you continue for a while longer, your weight will normalise. Maybe for the first time in your adult life, you become your natural weight. Without calorie, portion or points counting. You can eat any of the recipes in this book in any amount and they will contribute to your weight loss success.

However, the best part is yet to come. When you continue to enjoy eating this way, the weight stays off. You don't have to endure any more diets!

It's easy because it's natural.

When we look at detoxing as the key to vibrant health and natural weight control, we discover that it's not just a "lifestyle" choice or another diet or something to be discussed on daytime television. It's necessary for anyone who wants to regain control, self respect, and vitality — gender or age is irrelevant, so leave a copy of this book lying around on the coffee table of a loved one!

Making friends with the calorie

When detoxing, you don't necessarily reduce your calorific intake. All you do is eat the food that's good for you, so the bad stuff doesn't get a look in.

Where diets are concerned, the general agreement is to take in fewer calories than you use, and lose weight that way. This approach ignores the fact that the body can go into starvation mode and slow the metabolism down so that weight stops being lost. It also ignores the fact that most food has so many of its nutrients stripped out of it that people overeat on more nutrient-deficient food just so they can get some goodness.

Overweight starving people

Have you ever eaten a big meal, felt really stuffed and then opened the fridge door to see what you can have next? That's because you just fed yourself a nutrient-deficient meal. Yes, there may be calories and fibre, but if many of the small yet vital nutrients are missing, then you'll still feel hungry — you haven't been satiated and your body can't do the jobs it wants to without the necessary ingredients. Your body is craving nutrients, but if you've been fed a lifetime of food lies, you won't know what that is. Eventually, you'll find yourself overweight and undernourished.

Because living life the detox way entails eating a fair amount of high-calorie and nutrient-rich, recognisable food, you gain real energy. Then you make friends with the calorie again. About time, too.

Detoxing for health

The miracles

If you maintain a diet low in toxins, you will see apparent miracles occur. This is where many GPs, nutritionists and other "authority" figures will say "that can't be done", or if they witness it, they'll say "that was a fluke". This is where it gets interesting! It's time to leave your preconceptions at the door, because miracles really do happen: just you wait and see.

Are all illnesses due to toxins?

If you have a condition such as fatigue, coldness, hair loss or dry skin, it's likely that a combination of toxins and lack of nutrients are causing this. As most of our food is denatured, we do not receive all the nutrients we need for a healthy mind and body.

However, you can't just take supplements to remedy the lack of nutrients as they don't work in the way we would like. Vitamins and minerals need many other chemicals to make them work. Naturally, these chemicals are found in whole foods. Unnaturally, if the nutrient in question isn't combined with other essential elements, it could cause minerals and other chemicals to be leached out of your body — causing futher imbalance.

As scientists have not yet isolated exactly which chemicals are needed for the safe absorption of each nutrient, the method of megadosing or supplementation can sometimes be useless or even hazardous.

Start to trust the supplementation recommendations
of scientists when they have created
a perfect apple or leaf in the lab!

Scientists are fitting bits of the nutrition puzzle together all the time, but they rarely step back far enough to see the whole picture. Scientists may know a lot more than you and me about chemicals, but they don't know enough. If they did, they could create life just as nature created life. They could spend billions of pounds on creating the nutritional equivalent of apple, yet nature gives us this already in abundance.

I'm with nature all the way here. I see the big picture, and it looks pretty much like an apple, a mango or a kale leaf to me. What does it look like to you?

Having said all that I do believe some supplementation is useful, even if it's just for a short period of time so that your body can recover quicker after decades of eating less than optimal food. It's also true that even our organic food isn't as nutritious as wild food, and our soils are becoming more depleted each day. Intelligent supplementation will fill in any gaps you find you may have, and we are all different in that way because our weaknesses are all different.

Recovering your instincts

The beauty of detoxing naturally is that you get your instincts back. You become so much more real, and you then get in touch with your inner wisdom. It was there all along, it was just a little fogged.

In no time, you will know when you need certain nutrients because you'll feel the need for certain foods. Then, after eating them until full, you'll feel satisfied. You'll also feel the need to eat more seasonally (which works out cheaper for you!), as nature created foods at certain times of the year for a reason. As an example, I can often be seen loading up on nature's vitamin C during the autumn. Just before the cold of the winter sets in, beautiful jewel-like gigantic rosehips beckon me to eat their sweet tomato-like flesh.

Finally, as your body will have real food that it can get to work on, you'll have so much more energy to do the things you always wanted to but couldn't fit in. At last — you will feel balanced.

This is the time when you take off your dieting/illness/suffering/nutritional handcuffs. You are finally free!

In the *Success stories*, you'll see time and again how real people detoxed for health. I know of thousands of people who have triumphed over medication and prognoses of death after detoxing. Every story is a miracle. I personally couldn't do all I do if I ate an average western diet. Being healthy to me simply means that I have a real life that I enjoy fully because my body and mind can keep up with my wishes!

After your detox

Some people believe that if they do a really good detox, they can then follow it with the worst eating, drinking and drug-taking habits ever. Their reasoning is that as the body has had a holiday, it's stronger and more capable of processing the new toxins it's ingesting. This isn't untrue, but it can't be used as a reason. When you've detoxed, you'll notice so many health benefits, and you'll feel so good, why on earth would you then want to go back to how you felt before? It doesn't make sense to detox a load of horrible chemicals one month (which, let's be honest, shouldn't have been put into your body in the first place) if you're going to reintroduce them again the next month.

It's potentially hazardous to continue detoxing and retoxing — it shocks your body and might leave you in a worse state than before. Please detox with the intention of remaining detoxed, and maybe even go further than just physical body cleansing. **Detox Your World** shows you how, and gently guides you all the way.

When you have health, you are rich to pursue the things in life which you are passionate about.

How to remain detoxed

A tried and tested method of remaining detoxed is to eat at least 75% of your food unprocessed, uncooked and natural. But this doesn't mean that 25% of your diet should consist of chip butties, washed down with cola! If you eat unnatural food, you can buffer the effects by having a green salad beforehand. In addition, make sure at least two meals a day are highly unadulterated. If it sounds a bit extreme right now, I promise that you'll find this easier to think about once you have completed a detox plan and experienced some of my tasty recipes!

Staying balanced

If you choose to eat less than 75% natural foods, there is a high chance that your health and happiness will not be as good as it potentially could be. No detox plans can save you if you continually retox. The detox plans which promise to totally clean you out in a few days, when you have decades of crud in your system, are selling something that doesn't exist. There are quick results, but no quick fixes if you don't permanently pursue a healthier way of living. Personally, I think it's worth the effort because without health you really have nothing.

However, as ultimate health is not the only objective in life, weigh up all your necessities and priorities. If you feel that you don't even want to eat 75% natural food as part of your total daily intake, then that's fine. Just make sure your choices are informed, and that you eat consciously. It is better to eat slightly worse and have a happy outlook, than to have a perfect diet and stress yourself out at everything that happens to you.

There are no rules in this book, just suggested guidelines and tried and tested results. Discover what works for you, but keep pushing yourself a little bit, as an uphill struggle is more pleasant than a downhill tumble!

You are like a butterfly

After you've detoxed, you'll feel like a butterfly who's spent far too long being a caterpillar. Along with all the physical benefits, you will feel lighter in your mind — you won't have the weight of the world on your shoulders any more. Decisions will be easier to make, and your life's dreams will start to come true.

How does this happen, just by altering your food intake? It's all to do with natural and universal laws. There are some great books which explain this. Browse the Internet or go to a book shop to see what you're drawn to — that'll be the book with the answers you need right now.

One trilogy which answered many questions for me was **Conversations With God** by Neale Donald Walsch. I'm not religious at all, so if the title is putting you off, don't let it. Imagine that you're asking your deep subconscious for the answers to life — that's what this book is like.

As your perceptions on life alter, you realise that a whole new world is waiting for you. It's amazing what's out there — have fun finding it!

Beyond detoxing

Once you've followed one of the detox plans outlined here, or if you simply eat only from the recipes in the book, you may feel motivated enough to continue beyond the detox zone.

If you are happy to eat more than 75% of your food as uncooked, plant-based and organic food, you will witness more than excellent results.

Go as high as you can,
because you won't want to come down!

Eating 100% uncooked, plant-based, organic food is the jackpot that you win if you dare to gamble away the safety of the existence that you currently know. This is taking the red pill! This is where I am at, and nobody can pull me down. I've found Eden, and I'm staying here. I might just rename myself Eve! This is paradisiacal eating at its best, food as nature intended, natural nutrition. You are very blessed to have allowed this information into your life, and I know it will make enough of an impact for you to pursue the promises that are unfolding in front of your eyes this very second!

You are more than you thought you were

So you know that it's possible to cure yourself of disease, that you can become your natural weight, and that your mind starts to behave itself, but what if you don't have any illnesses? What will happen to you after you've been detoxing for a while? That's a very interesting question.

What happens is that your human potential gets an airing. You become the greatest you can be. Little broken things like the inability to multiply, read maps or put names to faces get fixed.

You step into your magnificence.

New opportunities are shown to you, and you revel in your choices rather than recoil from them. You get a taste of life and you are ready for more...

The hat collector

With the help of a lovely lady called Betty, you can now build up a mental picture of how and why you detox.

Who is Betty?

Betty is a hoarder who can't stop buying hats. She buys them mail order, and gets deliveries all day long. Because the postman is always knocking, and she's always taking in new boxes, she doesn't have time to clean her house, and she is fast running out of space for her ever-growing collection.

Betty is running out of space

It's not long before Betty has so many hats that her wardrobe is bursting, so she puts her new hats in her cupboard. One day the cupboard gets to bursting point, too. By this point, Betty is so addicted to the thrill of hat buying that she does it compulsively and without thought. She just loves it when the postman knocks, and it makes her feel loved, warm and cozy when she's opening the boxes.

Betty eventually starts storing the boxes under her bed, but soon her bed runs out of space. Betty is drowning in hats, but won't stop buying them as she loves them so much, and she would feel lonely without them.

In the end, Betty just scatters her new hats all over her bedroom floor. Everything is a mess but she loves her hats too much to part with them: she depends on them for company, they cheer up her otherwise sad and lonely existence.

Are you running out of space?

Now think about when you eat. You are excited about eating because it fills an emotional hole. You eat food which you know makes you overweight and unhealthy, because you are mentally and physically addicted to it. Your body is so busy trying to digest the food (store the hats) that it doesn't have time to clean itself out as it normally would. Betty's wardrobe, cupboard and bed could be your heart, liver and kidneys. Think of the floor as your skin, a large organ which can only take so much before it breaks out.

Betty cleans up her act

One day, Betty decides enough is enough. Many "coincidental" things trigger her to clean her house. Maybe, like you, she holds a book in her hands which explains how messy the whole hat collection business is! With a sentimental tear in her eye, Betty

35

gathers her precious hats from the floor and takes them out of the house. In the same way, your toxins will be purged from your fat cells and taken out of your body.

Betty is blue about losing her collection, but feels a great lift of spirits, knowing that her bedroom will soon be how it used to be — all clean and sparkly. She also feels a little tired at all the hard work she's been doing, but knows that in a few days she will feel better than she can remember. In the beginning, you may need to sleep more than normal as your body decides to take advantage of the extra cleaning it is doing.

With her new cleared floor, Betty remembers with fondness how she loved the rosy carpet. As your skin is cleared, you gain the rosy, blemish-free cheeks of childhood.

Continuing the purge

Because Betty is determined to clear her whole room, she continues purging. She knows she can't do it all in one day, so she spreads the purging over a few weeks. To get the hats from under the bed, Betty has to stack them on the new clean floor for a short time. Similarly, sometimes toxins will come out through your skin as deeper and deeper layers of stored toxins are eventually released. Very soon, Betty will have a lovely clean room, and will begin to appreciate the beauty of the shoes hidden at the bottom of her cupboard, because she'd forgotten what they looked like. You'll also gaze down at your lump-free legs, your slim ankles and your beautiful feet — with no tummy obstructing the view!

No going back

If Betty goes back to her old ways, she'll suffer the same problems as before. She needs to like the change so much that she won't go back. To ensure she remembers the nightmare of hats, she takes lots of photos and writes down how the clutter made her feel.

> Journal your changes, because you will change
> so much that you soon won't remember
> how you used to look, act and feel.

As time goes by, you might forget what you looked and felt like before, so when you detox, make notes of the changes you notice in yourself, and take some photos of how you were.

Think about answering some of these questions in a journal:

- Do you have less sleep in your eyes when you wake up?
- Are you less bloated?
- Do you have more energy?
- Do people keep asking you what you've done differently?
- Do you feel all glowy?
- Do you feel more confident and ready to face new challenges?

Jotting down a few simple bullet points, or even writing an essay, taking photos or making a chart with stars will ensure you remember how you were, thus keeping you lovely and clean, just like Betty's shiny happy bedroom.

Your toxic world

We live in a highly unnatural world — a world that your body hasn't been designed for. In this chapter we're going to look at some of the major non-food toxic loads which might be affecting your body, and how to reduce or eliminate them. Please stick with this chapter, it's not as light-hearted as the others, but it could just save your life.

Toxins aren't only in the food we eat. They're in our air, our clothing, household materials, computers, cars and books. In fact, if you're in contact with anything that isn't natural (and by natural, I mean made by nature in its original form), then you are placing extra burden on your body.

Thankfully, you don't have to become The Person In The Plastic Bubble. I'm going to show you how you can make positive changes and still have a life. If you first change the things that are easy or necessary for you to change, you'll find other changes easier to make as time goes on.

Alcohol

Most people in our society drink at social occasions and don't consider the amount they drink to be hazardous. However, the truth about alcohol is similar to the truth about all other drugs: no-one really knows exactly how much causes irreversible harm, and even a small amount affects us negatively.

> ## Buzzy bees
>
> Bees drink sap from lime trees. Sometimes this ferments, the bees get drunk and they can't fly straight. If they make it back to the hive, the bouncer bees don't let them in until they've sobered up. If they persist in getting drunk, the bouncer bees bite their legs off. They literally become legless!

For example, the UK guidelines state that women should have 2-3 units of alcohol or less, and men should have 3-4 units or less, per day. This adds up to about two pints of normal beer for a man each day and three small glasses of wine for a woman. I perceive that as a large amount of toxins to be regularly putting in your body. The guidelines state that if you regularly drink more than the suggested amounts, it could lead to problems. I always take these kinds of guidelines with a pinch of sea salt, because they change too often to believe these people know what they're talking about.

Even though the UK Department of Health states that there are no significant risks to health at the recommended levels, we need only to glance at our drinking culture to see that not many people are even following those guidelines. According to a recent study, people in the UK drink more for "I want to forget about my life" reasons than anyone else in Europe. If you're one of them, then it might be a bumpy road to "I love my life so much I wouldn't ever want to forget about it", yet it's very possible.

The guidelines in the UK also conflict with the guidelines in the USA. The US Guidelines on Alcohol Consumption, 2000 state: "Even one drink per day can slightly raise the risk of breast cancer". So now we're seeing that smaller amounts than the maximum recommended doses can increase cancer risks. Isn't it interesting how these "authorities" can give out differing information around the world? Without significant racial differences between us and our American friends there's no reason for this mismatch — unless these guidelines are arbitrary in the first place.

Alcohol isn't only bad for your health. It's antisocial and can cause your mood to be altered, which in turn can lead to violence. Quite often, toxic depressed thoughts raise their head, and leave you feeling less than light and life-loving.

Alcohol and your body

When you have a drink, it's quickly absorbed from your stomach and alimentary tract into your bloodstream, and then spreads throughout your body and brain. As blood alcohol levels rise, your judgement is gradually impaired, and you lose some co-ordination. As the alcohol passes through your liver, the liver metabolises and detoxifies it and turns it into energy for the body. Women metabolise alcohol slower than men, and that, combined with the fact that women are usually smaller than men and have a higher fat ratio (alcohol can't penetrate fat), accounts for the difference in recommended daily units.

When we drink in "excess", there are links to breast cancer in women, as well as to mouth, liver and lung cancer in both genders. If you also smoke, alcohol-related cancer risks increase.

Although some studies have concluded that drinking a small amount of alcohol can protect against coronary heart disease amongst the most at-risk groups by raising the levels of good cholesterol, I believe that the best way to stop arteries hardening and being lined is to alter your diet and lifestyle over the long term. Using a known toxin to counteract the effects of other toxins is not a truly effective way to go about reclaiming your health.

Liver damage

Depending on the strength of your constitution, the potential killer disease called liver cirrhosis can affect you either sooner, later or not at all. In some cases, alcohol users can drink as little as three or four units a day for only a few years before they start to show symptoms. In other cases, people can drink heavily for years and never develop signs of the disease.

A lifetime of heavy drinking makes the liver become fatty. This fat inhibits the blood supply which delivers oxygen and other nutrients to liver cells. When malnourished, the liver cells die, and scar tissue takes their place. This is the condition known as cirrhosis.

When drinkers suffer from cirrhosis, they don't have enough liver cells to metabolise the alcohol, which results in an increasing intolerance to it.

Because we can't live without a liver, it's advisable not to risk getting into this potentially lethal situation.

The brain

Women really do pull the short straw with alcohol damage, as it affects their brains, livers and hearts more than men. Brain "shrinkage" is common amongst long-time heavy drinkers of both sexes, but alcoholic women also fare worse than alcoholic men, averaging an 11% smaller brain volume than healthy women. The results of brain shrinkage may make women and men more susceptible to cognitive decline and dementia in later life.

For a long time, alcoholism has been linked to dementia, but it's only just been discovered that women are more at risk. The great news is that the brain can recover in many ways when the person stops drinking alcohol. Tests have shown that the shrunken brain fills out again and damaged nerves repair themselves, though dead nerves can't be replaced. I like that kind of news because it's encouraging to people who want to give up alcohol — they know that they can regenerate a part of them which has been lost.

Monkey madness

A troop of monkeys on the Caribbean island of St Kitts have discovered a taste for alcohol from the leftovers of the sugar cane harvest each year. They now go to great lengths to steal from bars on the beach. Most monkeys drink in moderation; 12% are classed as steady drinkers; and 5% are heavy drinkers. And some monkeys are teetotal: if they taste alcohol in a drink, they'll leave it and steal another. Guess what? Most humans drink in moderation; 12% are steady drinkers; and 5% are heavy drinkers. And the same percentage of humans and monkeys are teetotal.

Family history

There is a strong link between relatives suffering from excessive alcohol use. If your family before you were heavy alcohol users, be extra cautious that the habit doesn't sneak up on you. The best way to manage that is to just not drink alcohol.

Alcohol and babies

If a woman drinks alcohol during pregnancy her child might suffer from Foetal Alcohol Syndrome. The child can grow up with learning difficulties, behavioural problems, or even brain damage, deformities and stunted growth.

To prevent the possibility of alcohol damaging your child for life, please don't drink at all during pregnancy.

When you think about what alcohol can do to a developing baby, when you think how it can lead to dementia, how it can make you lose your liver, and how it could kill you, do you still have enough of a reason to continue?

To summarise

If you drink alone to mask problems, or just so you can function during the day, please seek professional help and invest in an InnerTalk CD on alcohol — you'll read more about InnerTalk later.

If you drink one or two glasses of wine a month, then you are not likely to cause yourself major damage. If you regularly drink alcohol, don't expect to achieve vibrant health, glowing skin and endless energy. Ultimately, alcohol suppresses and depresses you.

Decide how you want to live your life, and only put things into your body which will help you get there.

Further information

Web sites

alcoholism.about.com — A short overview on alcohol.

www.acad.org.uk — Advice and counselling on alcohol and drugs (because even though it is legal, alcohol is a drug).

Book

Alcohol
How to Give It Up and Be Glad You Did
Philip Tate
ISBN: 1884365108

This practical guide has helped many overcome alcohol over-use and abuse. Written in an easy-to-read self-help format, Dr Tate explains how to take control of your actions and emotions.

CD

Freedom from Alcohol
InnerTalk

This uses thought modification technology which is clinically tested and proven by doctors, scientists and medical researchers. The programme is based on the Alcoholics Anonymous 12-step formula to help you address your attitude towards alcohol in a positive manner that enables abstention.

Coffee

It's a lovely feeling, holding your hands round a hot cup of coffee, gently taking in its aroma and then sipping the bitter-sweet dark liquid. As more and more coffee shops spring up around the UK, it's overtaking tea as being the drink of choice. However, there is a darker side to coffee, and I don't just mean caffeine — though that features, too! Diabetes, cancer and heart disease have all been linked to coffee drinking, so let's see what it's all about.

Caffeine

Caffeine is a stimulant drug, alongside cocaine and amphetamines. Because caffeine is legal and the other two aren't, it's widely accepted, yet is still harmful.

If you drink about two cups of strong coffee, you are receiving the stimulant dose of 200mg of caffeine. If you drink more than that, it's likely that you will suffer withdrawal symptoms when you stop drinking. 29% of coffee drinkers declare that they couldn't do without coffee, because of its physical and psychological addictive qualities.

Some tests have shown that caffeine increases aggression as well as the risk of diabetes. In addition, if you drink large amounts of coffee during pregnancy, there may be a higher risk of your baby developing late or being small. I have to stress that these tests and observations are not conclusive, but I personally wouldn't take the risk, especially if it involved the life of another who was borrowing my womb! In addition to this, more than 163mg of caffeine per day (less than two cups) can increase the risk of miscarriage.

The cholesterol connection

Ground (instant) coffee has been shown to raise cholesterol levels by up to 10%. Because cholesterol is linked to heart disease, you can understand why people theorise about the coffee and heart disease connection.

The other chemicals

Caffeine receives most of the limelight, yet there are about 800 chemicals in coffee. Only 21 have been tested for carcinogenic properties, and 16 of those have tested positive.

Is coffee starting to leave a bad taste in your mouth?

Quitting coffee

The slow approach is best here. Withdrawal symptoms aren't nice and so should be avoided as much as possible. If you drink one or two cups per day, you could come straight off coffee and probably not feel any symptoms. If you drink more than two cups a day, gradually cut down. For example, you could have one cup fewer per day for a week, and each subsequent week reduce the amount again by one cupful per day. Alternatively, try having the same number of cups per day but only fill your cup three-quarters full. Gradually make it half full, and then substitute one coffee-time fix for a glass of water or some herbal tea. This might work better for you as it keeps you in the same drink ritual as you're used to. I love drinking a blend of pau d'Arco with goji berries and olive leaf, brewed up in a caffetier and sweetened with a little raw agave nectar. It gives me the feeling of coffee and I get massive anti-viral, anti-parasitical, antioxidant and anti-fungal health benefits.

If you withdraw from coffee too quickly you could feel the normal detox symptoms, including headaches, sickness, depression, fatigue, anxiety, and aches and pains. This is enough evidence in itself that coffee is just another addictive drug, which doesn't make you feel the best you can feel.

If you don't want to cut out coffee totally (yet!), then use the above method to cut down to no more than two cups per day.

Further information

Book

The World of Caffeine
The Science and Culture of the World's Most Popular Drug
Bennett Alan Weinberg and Bonnie Bealer
ISBN: 0415927226

With lots of medical facts about caffeine, this book has proved to be a great companion to those wishing to be released from caffeine's clutches. The book also describes caffeine's relationship with art, religion, society, politics and literature. A really thorough and interesting book.

Environmental pollution

Sexless animals and infertility

More and more river animals are becoming asexual — that is, they are born without a specific gender, and are unable to reproduce.

You can see this in action in Georgia, USA, where environmentalists claim that a pulp mill has released heavy doses of dioxins into Rice Creek. Biologists are now finding sterile largemouth bass and alligators. Onlookers note sexless animals, female fish with male genitals and deformed fish with lesions.

Dioxins disrupt the building blocks of life, leaving hormones in a mess, and immune systems shot.

Now let's take a look at humans. Today in the USA one in three people have fertility problems. In the UK, we're not far behind at one in four.

If you don't think twice when you buy toxic ingredients or products, when you flush the loo, or when you don't recycle or compost, then you are not much different to the big companies with toxic waste who don't think twice when they dump into rivers. The actions of millions of people add up. What you do makes a big difference to our planet.

The deformities and suffering of river animals are a warning sign for us. Please produce as little toxic waste as possible, so our world can go on creating with infinite beauty.

Living a low-toxin life naturally leaves you with fewer toxins to dump. Most of your food waste goes on your compost, your clothes can be unbleached and made of natural materials, packaging is minimal and you no longer pour poisons down your sink. You'll find that you won't have to consciously do much about pollution when you detox your world, because it happens automatically.

Bodies are intelligent — they will rarely allow a heavily toxic or sick woman to carry another life because both lives would become at risk. Once your body is clean, then the ability to conceive could increase.

Asthma, eczema and other childhood diseases

Another direct result of environmental pollution is the early onset of childhood diseases. As more and more children suffer from these illnesses, the reasons why are becoming clearer. Toxins in the home, toxins in the food, toxins in the schools and toxins on the streets are all big contributors to these diseases.

If you have a child who suffers with a disease, then detoxing their world will really help.

Do it gradually, and don't take them off their medication without medical supervision.

- Put them in natural organic clothes
- Place lots of plants in their bedroom
- Give them as much raw organic food as possible and supplement with MSM
- Buy them a therapeutic ioniser
- Take them off wheat and milk products

Then sit back and wait for the results. This may take a few weeks, and they might show detox signals as the toxins come out, but you should see some healing signs before long.

As your child starts to recover, detox their world more by following many of the suggestions in this book. Be aware that their nutritional needs are different to ours, and adjust any plans accordingly. Please don't fast a child or put the child on a restricted diet without medical supervision.

Living in a town with no trees, no greenery and no fresh air is very detrimental to all of us on every level, and it can easily manifest as common childhood diseases. Take your child to the countryside as much as possible, and if moving there is an option, do it for their sake, as well as yours.

Adults in danger

Just as we are responsible for bringing our children up in cleaner environments, we have to do the same for ourselves.

I personally have an Elanra Therapeutic Ioniser in my bedroom. I have organic cotton bedding. My walls are painted with Ecos paint, the purest paint on the planet. I sleep on a magnetic bed. I drink ionised alkalised water. I think you get the point I'm making! It's the little things that we do in our houses that make the big difference. I changed one thing at a time in my house until I was happy with it. I make sure I do the same for the environment at large, too. Making one small change after another makes detoxing your world seem effortless.

Further information

Book

Natural Mothering
A Guide to Holistic Therapies for Pregnancy, Birth, and Early Childhood
Nicky Wesson
ISBN: 089281733X

Magazine

The Mother Magazine — This is a bi-monthly British publication (sold internationally) which offers holistic advice and support to parents from all walks of life. To subscribe, you can visit www.themothermagazine.co.uk

CD

I Can: build a child's esteem
InnerTalk

As some children can become disfigured by their illnesses, this CD will help boost their belief in themselves. This is an important part of detoxing and healing, as they will gradually let go of negative emotions about themselves.

Skin care

I used to write a regular column about natural beauty, and uncovered information which could make your hair curl — or turn luminous green and fall out. However, there is far too much information to list here. All I'd like to point out to you is that most commercial body products, make-up and toiletries are toxic to your body — even most of the ones that say "natural" or "organic". As you are detoxing yourself holistically, make yourself aware of exactly what you are putting on your skin.

Common toxins in toiletries

Toxic babies
22% of babies born in America today are medically diagnosed as having toxaemia, because their mothers have been so poisoned by their food and environment.

Toxins such as Sodium Lauryl Sulphate (SLS) and Propylene Glycol (PG) are in most everyday toiletries, make up, and baby products. Jointly, they've been linked to rashes, hair loss, flaking skin, mouth ulceration, eye damage, cancer, kidney damage and liver damage.

Talc is in baby powders, face powders, body powders and condoms. It's a major cause of ovarian cancer when used in the genital area. It can also harm lungs if inhaled. You can use white clay or simple conrflour instead of talc if you feel you need to use something.

You'll soon read about the highly toxic fluoride in much detail. But here's a taster for you. When you next brush your teeth, consider this real message which is put on tubes of toothpaste in various countries: "Warning: Keep out of the reach of children under six years of age. In case of accidental overdose, seek professional assistance or contact a poison control centre immediately." Since less than a tube of toothpaste is considered a toxic dose for a child, it makes you wonder why you are told to put it in your mouth twice a day, every single day of your life!

Alternatives to commercial toiletries

As you become more pure, don't be surprised that your lovely expensive cosmetics no longer feel good on your skin. I remember giving away over £200 worth of products to a friend after I'd detoxed for only a few months. Now I can't believe I used to put all that stuff on my skin every day! When this happens to you, just be happy that you're lightening your load. It soon becomes obvious that you didn't need them anyway, as skin becomes as smooth as silk, wrinkles fade, and blotches disappear.

Because our skin is absorbent, the saying "if you can't eat it, don't put it on your skin" holds true. So as a stress-buster, there's nothing more relaxing than creating your own natural cosmetics in your spare time. Experiment with your friends and loved ones by making and using natural cosmetics for and on each other. Try using clays, mineral salts, blended fruits, nuts, algaes, MSM and cold pressed oils.

If you don't have the time or inclination to make your own body products, then there are some less-than-really-naughty products out there. Check out your local herbalists, health-food stores or even market stalls. Lush's Fresh range is one of the best commercial natural toiletries that I've used.

Further information

Books

Clear Skin
Karen Jessett
ISBN 0954740505

Karen believes that your food and lifestyle affect your skin. If you suffer from acne or breakouts, or even if you just want an energy boost, then this lovely book is for you.

Recipes For Natural Beauty
Neal's Yard Remedies
ISBN: 1902463668

Neal's Yard Remedies are renowned for creating natural and often organic products. Now you can make your own lovely Neal's Yard-style products.

Natural Beauty for All Seasons
More Than 250 Simple Recipes and Gift-Giving Ideas for Year-Round Beauty
Janice Cox
ISBN: 0805046550

Create natural products for your body and face, to keep or to give away. If you are in a giving mood, there are even gift and packaging ideas for all occasions.

Web sites

www.healthrecipes.com/beauty.htm and **www.fatfreekitchen.com/beauty.html** both offer natural beauty recipes for you to experiment and treat yourself with.

The air you breathe

We'll delve deep into oxygen later in the book, but for now let's talk about the other stuff in our air.

Some of the worst offenders in your home are:

Benzene — found in tobacco smoke, petrol, synthetic fibres, plastics, inks, oils, detergents.

Carbon monoxide — this silent killer is in all our homes in small amounts. Sometimes faulty equipment can cause lethal doses to seep out into the rooms of the unsuspecting.

Formaldehyde — that toxin found in a whole host of furnishings. Your MDF has lots of this, as do carpets, clothes, paper goods and household goods, including some so-called air fresheners!

Trichloroethlene — is a smelly and potentially very dangerous pollutant found in adhesives, dry-cleaning fluids (and dry-cleaned clothes), lacquers, paints and varnishes.

Xylene — is a sweet-smelling gas used as a cleaning agent and paint thinner. It's also found in paints, varnishes, petrol and cigarette smoke.

People use air fresheners to make their homes smell more pleasant, but they can often contribute to more toxic build up. Many of them contain artificial musk (often just called perfume on the ingredients) which disturbs hormones.

The lighter way to live is to remove the items causing a bad odour in the first place. Also, by filling your home with plants, they will naturally filter the air for you.

Plant power

Because plants absorb the toxins in your home, it makes sense to live with as many as possible. Making your indoor home a jungle, and turning your outdoors into another room is a great way to become light on toxins. Plants filter carbon dioxide, carbon monoxide, hydrogen, methane, alcohol, ammonia, formaldehyde and benzene.

To remove many toxins from your home, take a look at these miraculous and essential plants, then go out and buy some today:

Areca palm removes formaldehyde and xylene

Azalea removes formaldehyde

Bamboo removes formaldehyde

Boston fern removes formaldehyde, and is the number one plant for doing so

Chrysanthemum removes formaldehyde, benzene and trichloroethlene

Corn Palm removes formaldehyde

Dracaena Marginata removes benzene and trichloroethlene

English ivy removes benzene and formaldehyde

Gerbera daisy removes benzene and trichloroethlene

Golden pathos removes formaldehyde

Mother-in-law's tongue removes formaldehyde

Peace lily removes trichloroethlene

Poinsettia removes formaldehyde

Spider plant removes formaldehyde, xylene and carbon monoxide

Striped dracaena removes formaldehyde and trichloroethlene

Just one spider plant can remove about 96% of the carbon monoxide in a small room.

Plants in bedrooms

I've always wondered why people say "don't put plants in bedrooms as they absorb oxygen at night and give out carbon monoxide." When looking at the natural model, we see that all animals sleep in the presence of thousands of plants. Therefore, I sleep with plants in my bedroom!

For those who still have an aversion to sleeping with "normal" plants, pop an orchid or aloe beside your pillow and all will be well. These plants do the opposite to other plants, releasing oxygen at night. As with other plants, they also work to remove toxins in the air, so now there's no excuse. Surround yourself with plants to be healthy and happy.

What do plants do with all the toxins?

It's clever how this symbiosis works. You provide the toxins for the plant to filter out, and it absorbs them, recycles them as food and then uses them to grow. When they've grown bigger, they can remove more toxins from your world than before. Don't you just love the pattern of nature?

Ionisers

Remove dust with an ioniser
The US Department of Agriculture discovered 52% less dust and 95% less bacteria were present in a room which was ionised.

Just before a thunderstorm many people feel sad and destructive. However, during or just after a storm, we often feel happy and bouncy. Have you also noticed that we feel refreshed when we're near waterfalls or by the sea, yet we feel irritated and uncomfortable when we're in enclosed areas — especially ones where there are lots of unnatural objects. This is all down to the action of positive and negative ions.

If you'd like to feel like you're strolling by the sea more often, the answer is easy — invest in an ioniser. Ionisers take positive ions out of the atmosphere in your home and office, and deliver negative ions. Negative ions are prolific in the atmosphere after a thunderstorm, and even when you are taking a shower (which is why you sing in the shower!). Ionisers also remove dust, smoke, stale smells and other baddies from the air, which is very beneficial to all of us, and life-changing to those who have sensitivities. People with asthma, hay fever, catarrh, sinusitis, bronchitis, migraines, and more have found massive relief of their symptoms just by adding ionisers to their rooms.

Dust particles from man-made carpets and fabrics, alongside dust mite poo, swirl into our air because they are electrically charged. The use of an ioniser will reduce these particles.

Ionisers work in the same way as a thunderstorm, by emitting streams of negative ions into the surrounding air, which cause it to become negatively charged. This causes the particles to be attracted to one another, they become heavy, and fall to the ground, leaving the air cleaner. If you have a HEPA filter on your vacuum, you can happily suck them up, knowing you're not going to redistribute them into the air.

With about 1 in 9 children now suffering from asthma, it's important to make your atmosphere as naturally clean as possible. If you can reduce suffering by simply adding air purifiers and ionisers to your home, it's a really small price to pay.

Extra special ionisers

You can now buy therapeutic ionisers, which do more than the average ioniser. Medical and complementary practitioners recommend the therapeutic ioniser due to its great powers. Other ionisers generate larger negative ions, which clean the air. The therapeutic ioniser generates tiny negative ions of oxygen which are then inhaled, enter the bloodstream, and give you all the benefits of an oxygen-rich body.

If you are going to invest in an ioniser, I recommend you choose a therapeutic one.

Let some air in

We are all aware of external pollution such as cars, but the real danger lies in the home. The US Environmental Protection Agency states that indoor air is two to ten times more dangerous than outdoor air. This is partly due to the way we've sealed ourselves in. Most of our homes are so energy efficient that nothing escapes — not even the poisonous gas from your furniture. Studies suggest that these newer sealed homes contain 200% more allergens than older houses.

Keep your windows open as much as possible, use a HEPA filter on your vacuum, get ionisers and switch to very gentle environmentally friendly household cleaning fluids. Buy non-toxic carpets and furniture.

Cats get everywhere

Cat dander is the number one human allergy trigger. A study in Philadelphia, USA entailed the testing of random houses for this irritant. Amazingly, 100% were found to contain cat dander, even though there were no cats living in many of the houses tested.

If you are suffering from cat-allergy type symptoms, fitting ionisers and air filters and using HEPA filters is sure to help you.

One study discovered that as a result of carpets outgassing, moulds, mildews, fungi, dust mites etc, a baby crawling on the floor inhales a toxic equivalent of four cigarettes per day. I hope that puts this issue into enough perspective to take action.

In the car

You can now buy in-car ionisers, which I recommend if you spend more than a few minutes a day in your room on wheels.

Clothes

Beautiful and practical though some man-made fibres are, they do not do your health any favours. As well as giving off positive electrical charges which can contribute to allergic reactions and affect moods, they often inhibit the breathing of the skin.

As with everything, take the sensible approach to reclaiming your vitality, and just make sure that when you buy new clothes, they're all-natural, such as cotton, hemp, ramie, linen and so on. Organic and unbleached are the very best clothes for you, so do look out for them. They make you feel so serene when wearing them!

I don't recommend wool because it contains lanolin which is a known human-skin irritant. It's also a bit of an ugly thought to know that about one-third of wool in the UK comes from slaughtered sheep, and I personally try to keep my affiliation with the slaughter house as distant as possible. Nature made wool to keep sheep warm, not humans.

Further information

Book

My House Is Killing Me!
The Home Guide for Families With Allergies and Asthma
Jeffrey C May
ISBN: 089281733X

Home Safe Home
Non-toxic, Natural and Earthwise
Debra Lynn Dadd
ISBN: 087477859X

This useful book provides more than four hundred tips so you can remove harmful substances from your home. There are also tips on purchasing natural food, clothing, and cosmetics.

Water, water everywhere

...and not a drop to drink. Though we have tap water on, well, on tap, I don't recommend anyone drinks it unless they're really really thirsty.

Chlorine

Amongst other toxins, chlorine is present in most public water. It's used because it kills harmful bacteria and other water-borne, disease-causing organisms. However, chlorine may also seriously affect your health when absorbed over a long period.

We can be affected by chlorine by ingesting, absorption through the skin or by breathing it in. When in a hot shower, we breathe it in and it's transferred directly into the bloodstream where it disrupts the functioning of your cells. Because of this cell disruption, chlorine and its by-products have been linked to bladder, colon, liver, rectal and stomach cancers, as well as allergic reactions, anaemia, atherosclerosis, and heart disease. Chlorine can destroy protein in your body and have adverse effects on skin and hair.

We have no option but to have chlorine in our tap water, so we need to take action once it's left the tap, before it goes anywhere near us.

The best way to remove this inorganic compound from your world — as well as radon gas and heavy metals such as lead and aluminium — is to fit filters to your taps. You can get special ones for kitchen, shower and bath outlets, and I'd advise the use of all of them. If you can't filter your bath water, use a product called The Crystal Ball, which promises to filter out 100% of chlorine from your bath. It's a ball which you place in the bath as you're running the water, and it just bobs about, filtering as it goes.

Once you've installed your filters, you will notice that dry and itchy skin is replaced by smoother, itch-free skin. Dry hair becomes smoother as it rinses cleaner, and any green tinges disappear, too! If you suffer from eye irritation, that also can disappear.

What to drink

We're often told by nutritionists to drink about eight glasses of water a day. That's about 1.5-2 litres. Most people cook most of their food most of the time. When food is cooked, about 80% of its water content can be lost. Because of this unnatural yet widely practised act, the food becomes water-deficient, and then the same happens to you. If you don't cook your food, you need less additional water.

Dehydrating food also causes a lot of the water content to be lost. I keep dehydrated recipes to a minimum in my books and in my life. They're great for a bit of variety, or to show off to friends, but I would never eat or recommend them every day. Take a look at a sundried tomato and then rehydrate it. It doesn't become a nice juicy plump tomato like it originally was, it remains dark red, concentrated and strongly flavoured. Foods like this are useful in transitioning to a detoxed life, and great for the odd treat, but because they've lost their water, they shouldn't be used as dietary staples.

In nature, our close primate relatives drink small amounts of water from holes in trees and other convenient places. They don't constantly have a glass or sports bottle by their side, or measure their daily intake. However, for now, you might have to. One of the major reasons we can feel so bad is because we're dehydrated through years of extracting the water from our food before eating it. Don't try to mimic nature yet with this one — make sure you get enough water to help rehydrate your body because you need to after years of dehydrating it.

Dr. Batmanghelidj, the author of the fantastic must-read book **Your Body's Many Cries For Water** states: "Chronic and persistently increasing dehydration is the root cause of almost all currently encountered major diseases of the human body." If you take a look at X-rays of people with diseases, there are often dark patches inside the body which indicate lack of moisture in those parts. Dr. Batmanghelidj says that allergies, asthma, arthritis, back pain, diabetes, high cholesterol, high blood pressure, heart problems, migraines, obesity, peptic ulcers and water retention are all a result of too little water in the body. I would say that it's not quite that simple, as humans have removed more than water from their diet, but it's certainly a great start to give your body the liquid it needs.

Adding more water to your daily life is so easy and cheap, you can start right now.

Attempting to replace your lost water with hot or fizzy drinks will not rehydrate you properly. Your body needs good clean, easy-to-recognise water. Mineral water, distilled water, pure rain water and water from the source are all much better than tap water. Let's look at some other great water sources...

Magic watermelons

Eat a watermelon and notice what happens. You appear to wee out more than you ate! Why? Well, it has a high vitamin C and potassium content which causes it to act as a diuretic. Natural diuretics such as watermelon don't just remove water from your body, they help march out the toxins, too. I think that sipping on some blended watermelon is one of the loveliest detox treats in the world!

Live water

If you've ever heard of people putting crystals, leaves, fruit or other life-giving objects in their drinking water and thought they were a bit odd, think again. Water can lose its structure and not be as effective in the body. By adding any of these items to water, you can "restructure" it, and voilà, you have a liquid that the body recognises and can use. Try it for a while, you will probably notice the difference. Feel the water going into your cells instead of pooling in your stomach — that's the beauty of restructured water, it gets to where it needs to go quicker! I also add a dash of MSM powder to my water, as it's a great cell food, detoxifier and water enhancer.

Young coconut water

Coconut water has long been held in high regard by anyone who knows its secrets. Scientists recently latched onto this and have come up with a way of preserving it without losing its nutrients. They filter 'it through porcelain, which renders it sterile enough to have a shelf life. This is great news for us in the UK, as I've never seen an organic fresh young coconut here. The raw packaged version comes under the brand of Dr Martin's Coco Drink or Milk, and tastes very close to fresh coconut.

However, if organic young coconuts became available, I would always go for those. There's something very satisfying about cutting open a coconut, drinking the juice and then scooping the flesh out with your fingers. An average 6-9 month-young coconut has about 750ml of water in it. In a Chinese shop, you can pick a non-organic one up for about £1 or £2 — what great value for the best drink on earth! Many people are attracted to young coconuts because of their taste and the way it makes them feel. Technically, it has the same level of electrolytic balance as we have in our blood, and it has even been used for blood transfusions. It is nature's first isotonic drink, and when mixed with celery juice, gives you an extremely nutritious sports drink.

Are you thirsty?

Most people suffer from dehydration because their bodies haven't been given enough liquid, or enough of the right liquid. If you feel extreme thirst, are unable to drink, appear flushed, and your skin is warm and dry, you might be dehydrated. Dizziness and cramping are also common symptoms. If you feel like this when detoxing, it might be that your body is releasing toxins quicker than it's removing them. Drink live water with MSM if you can. See a doctor if you can't drink or if symptoms get worse or persist.

Further information

Books

Your Body's Many Cries For Water
A Revolutionary Natural Way to Prevent Illness and Restore Good Health
Dr F Batmanghelidj
ISBN: 095309216X

People who have followed the good doctor's advice have reported many illnesses disappearing. It's a very powerful book, and I highly recommend it to you.

Messages From Water
Dr Masaru Emoto
ISBN: 4939098001

One of the most beautiful books in the world, Dr Emoto displays photographs of water reacting to messages such as prayer, thoughts and music.It offers real evidence about your impact on your world.

Household items

There are too many household toxins to discuss in detail, so here is a small taster, with a selection of good sources of further information.

Toxic fumes and your inner world

Cleaning fluids, bleaches, paints, carpets and upholstery can all give off toxic fumes. Leaning over the bath when scrubbing with your average household cleaning fluid, without using gloves and inhaling isn't conducive to detoxing your inner world.

Buy "earth-friendly" products for your home whenever you can. For cleaning your house, go back to grandmother-type recipes — there are some great books available even if Grandma isn't. Lemon juice, vinegar and soda crystals can replace most of your house cleaning needs. I know people who throw half a lemon into their washing machine with their clothes — so they never use washing powder.

Many products now use the cleansing power of orange peel extract, which is a natural turpentine and grease remover.

Eating utensils

Toxins are in so many items, so the more natural we make our home, the better. Our dishes, plates, knives and forks shouldn't be plastic. Scratched or worn items can leak dangerous chemicals directly into food, which are then passed into your body. Use ceramic, metal and wood items instead.

Paint

Paint tins give health warnings for a good reason, yet we merrily and frequently plaster our walls with new paint. Where modern products such as paint are required, look out for the least hazardous brands around. Always paint with the windows wide open, don't sleep in a newly painted room, and add lots of plants to help absorb the toxins.

Further information

Books

The New Natural House Book
Creating a Healthy, Harmonious and Ecologically Sound Home
David Pearson
ISBN: 0684847337

This is a classic in eco-house creation. It's been around since 1989, but has been completely revised. It promises to enhance your environment and your well-being by bringing you hundreds of energy-saving and money-saving tips. A great all-round book for those planning on making big house changes.

Folk Wisdom for a Natural Home
by Beverly Pagram
ISBN: 1570760780

This very practical, knowledgeable and environmentally sound book offers hints and tips for every home problem. If you want to clean or repair anything in your home the non-toxic way, this is your book.

The Cure For All Cancers
Including over 100 Case Histories of Persons Cured
Dr Hulda Clark
ISBN: 1890035009

This book was one of the first health books I read, and I'll always be grateful to Dr Clarke for sharing this controversial information. Clarke suggests that certain common household products play a large part in causing cancer. By eliminating these products, the cancer can also be eliminated or reduced. If you are suffering from a major toxic overload, then you need to read this book and decide for yourself if you want to act upon her advice.

Web site

www.greenbrands.co.uk — this is a natural products web site which offers a Home Detox Kit. This kit contains all the products necessary to clean your house a friendlier way.

www.ecospaints.com — I painted my whole house with Ecos paints, and there was absolutely no smell. Ecos claim that their paints are about 7000 times purer than their closest competitor. All their products are vegan, too.

Mobile phones

Walking around any city these days is like something out of a futuristic film. Everybody is either texting or talking on mobile phones. Spending time outside with friends is peppered with beep-beeps or ring-rings, and it seems that nobody gets the chance to be in peace any more. This alone is stressful and therefore toxic to us. Of course mobile phones are useful, but to use them so constantly as many of us do can be detrimental to your health in several ways.

The cancer link

I mention cancer so many times in this book simply because our highly toxic lifestyle is a major contribution to ill-health. By slowly but surely reducing our exposure to unnatural products, we do indeed start detoxing our world.

Tests to determine microwave radiation in mobile phones have concluded that former claims of mobile phones being safe are not true.

Depending on how close the mobile phone antenna is held to the head, up to 60% of the microwave radiation penetrates the head. Some microwaves reach up to 4cm into the brain.

The increase in oral cancer happened at the same time as the emergence of the mobile generation. Though televisions, computers and cars are all toxic to us, it's the mobile phone that gets held up close to our face.

My advice

If you have a mobile phone, then turn it off when you don't need it. You do not have to be disturbed and stressed every hour of the day. Just let your friends know that you have decided to make more of your free time than talking on the phone or texting.

Buy some of the good mobile phone protection products, and use them immediately. I use the Tachyon device, and noticed the difference as soon as I put it on my phone. If you're not cooking your food so much, it makes sense to not fry your brain!

Smoking

Even if you don't smoke, please read this. There is some valuable information in here that you may be able to pass on to a loved one who smokes.

Most adults smoke because they are now addicted after being subjected to childhood peer-pressure. When I lived in Spain, most of the adults smoked. As with Brits, they knew that smoking caused cancer, but that knowledge was hidden under thoughts of "let's go out and party, hang round and look cool with our mates, and ask groovy guys or girls for a light". However, all across Europe, more cancer deaths can be attributed to smoking tobacco than to any other single risk factor.

Starting smoking

In the UK more young girls than ever smoke because the anti-smoking messages aren't as effective as peer-pressure and subliminal pro-smoking messages. I've never smoked, thanks to my melodramatic nature. You see, at the ripe old age of 12, I was hanging out with my friend, and she suddenly produced a packet of cigarettes. I don't know where she got them from, but we each lit one up and started smoking — right there in the street. Prepared to feel sick and disgusted like the publicity showed, I actually liked the taste and the sensation and thought it was going to be a great new interesting and cool hobby. After three drags on the cigarette I studied the red burning lit end causing everything to turn to ash. Then I looked at the filter. It was no longer that beautiful white fluffy-toy type material, it was now yellowy-brown. It hadn't filtered the bad stuff out at all! I threw the cigarette on the floor and stamped on it. "I'm not smoking that!", I exclaimed. "I'll get cancer." Thank heavens for my sense of observation, it saved me a lot of future health problems, and a massive amount of money.

So, just as I didn't listen to the anti-smoking messages, and tried a cigarette, other young people who take up smoking also don't get why it's bad. I was lucky that something else guided me. I've never really been subject to peer-pressure, and I'm sure that helped. If you have children, know that they are influenced by your behaviour the most. Bring them up to respect themselves, to believe in themselves and to always want to create the best possible situation for themselves — this might just make a difference to the choices they make around their peers. And if that doesn't work, let them read this:

Watching a smoker die

When I originally wrote this chapter, I lived in the same house as a smoker. He was 78, and so was doing well when you compare him to most British men who only live to an average age of 75 (it's 80 for women). But I knew that the end to his life wouldn't be graceful, pleasant or pain-free. You see, the doctors thought he had lung cancer. Every night, he coughed the most painful cough. Remember when you last had a cold with a cough? You cough and cough for three days in a row, and you think "I can't take any more of this, my throat is red raw". Imagine the three days turning into three weeks, into three months, and imagine the pain multiplying at the same rate. Then imagine vomiting every meal up, as this man did. Your stomach is wretched and your body is saying "no more", yet every last ounce of instinct has been squeezed out of you, so you just reach for a cigarette. At least you can keep that down. Imagine, too, waking up with blood on your pillow every morning, not knowing anything about it until you see it. Imagine it getting worse, not better, because you won't give up smoking and the hospital says you're a lost cause.

If you smoke, you have have a 50% chance of not having to imagine — it's heads or tails that it happens to you.

Why do so many turn a blind eye?

People in our culture still seem so blind to cancer, though it hits one in three of us at some time in our lives and kills one in four of us. Lung cancer is by far the biggest killer, taking 22% of cancer victims to their grave. The second biggest killer, colon cancer, trails at a lowly 11%. In fact, there are over 200 types of cancer, but the big four — lung, breast, colon and prostate — account for over 50% of all new cases.

About 50% of smokers will die of lung cancer or other smoking-related diseases such as heart disease and chronic lung disease. About 50% of those die before middle age. So if you smoke, you have a 25% chance of a very early death.

Imagine not living to see your children grow up, not collecting the pension you dutifully paid every month and leaving your soul mate behind.

Each year in the UK, 120,000 people are killed by lung cancer, and yet it's the single most preventable cause of early death in the world. It's also not confined to just smokers. If you don't smoke, but you live, work or play with smokers, then you're at risk too. Passive smoking is responsible for several hundred deaths in the UK each year. If you have cigarette smoke in your daily life, such as at work, home, pubs or clubs, take steps now to alter the situation by sourcing smoke-free environments. Your health is your only wealth, don't let other people compromise that for you.

Let's look at these facts:

- Death from lung cancer is the most common cause of cancer death in the UK.

- Smoking causes nine out of ten cases of lung cancer.

- Smoking is also a risk factor for cancer of the bladder, kidney, cervix, throat (pharynx and larynx), mouth, oesophagus, pancreas and stomach as well as for some types of leukaemia (cancer of the blood).

- Smoking causes about a third of all cancer deaths.

- Lung cancer kills one person every 15 minutes in the UK.

- Passive smoking is particularly harmful to babies and children whose parents smoke in the home and may cause or contribute to: miscarriage, premature birth, low birth weight, stillbirth, cot death, glue ear, asthma and other respiratory problems.

The toxins in smoke

Cigarette smoke contains about 4000 chemicals, many of which are toxic and can cause cellular damage. Some are carcinogenic. The main ingredients of cigarette smoke are:

Nicotine

This doesn't cause cancer but it is a highly addictive and very fast-acting drug. Once inhaled, nicotine reaches the brain in less than 15 seconds. Most smokers are addicted to nicotine and crave cigarettes to feed their addiction. This is the key ingredient that keeps people buying cigarettes and keeps the tobacco companies in business.

Carbon monoxide

This is a tasteless, odourless and poisonous gas. Remember the carbon monoxide public awareness adverts? At the same time as the government were telling you to get your boiler checked because carbon monoxide is lethal, they were still profiting from cigarettes. When you smoke, carbon monoxide is taken up by your bloodstream quickly and impairs your breathing. Inhaling too much carbon monoxide causes coma and death by asphyxiation. How much of a toxin is too much? We know that toxins taken in small amounts might not kill immediately, but they do have a long-term effect on your body which has to try to expel or at least store them.

Tar

This isn't one chemical like the others listed, but rather a combination of chemicals. Many of these are known to cause cancer. Around 70% of the tar in cigarettes is deposited in the smoker's lungs.

Acetone

This is the strong smelling ingredient in nail polish remover. That guardian of health and truth, the US Environmental Protection Agency, has specifically listed acetone as one of the few solvents that is not a Hazardous Air Pollutant and does not cause cancer, or other very serious illnesses. It's interesting to note, then, that when animals are exposed to acetone over a long period of time the damage includes kidney, liver, and nerve damage, increased birth defects, and lowered ability to reproduce in males. I don't cite animal studies in this book, as they go against the gentle and ethical way of living which I pursue, but you can guarantee that if animals suffer the above effects, then humans will also suffer some of them to some degree.

Small amounts of inhaled acetone are broken down by the liver into non-harmful chemicals, but breathing moderate-to-high levels of acetone for short periods of time can cause nose, throat, lung, and eye irritation, headaches, dizziness, confusion, increased pulse rate, sickness, unconsciousness and maybe even coma. Swallowing very high levels of acetone can result in unconsciousness and damage to the skin in your mouth. Skin contact can result in irritation and damage to your skin.

Ammonia

Exposure to high concentrations of ammonia in the air may cause severe burns to your skin, eyes, throat, and lungs. It can also cause high blood pressure. In extreme cases, blindness, lung damage, heart attack, or death could occur. Breathing lower concentrations will cause coughing and nose and throat irritation.

If you swallow ammonia, you could burn your mouth, throat, and stomach. Concentrated ammonia spilled on the skin will cause burns, irritation to the nose and lungs, lung damage, increased heart rate, and high blood pressure. Scientists don't yet know whether ammonia can cause cancer and so the US Department of Health and Human Services (DHHS), the International Agency for Research on Cancer (IARC), and the EPA haven't classified ammonia for carcinogenicity.

Arsenic

Arsenic cannot be destroyed in the environment, but it does change its form. If you breathe high levels of arsenic, you can expect a sore throat or irritated lungs. If you ingest high levels of arsenic you could die. Even if you're exposed to lower levels of arsenic, you could experience sickness, decreased production of both red and white blood cells, and an abnormal heart beat.

If you ingest or breathe low levels of arsenic over a period of time, your skin may darken and you could get small small warts on your palms, soles and torso. Though organic arsenic compounds are less toxic than inorganic arsenic compounds, exposure to high levels may result in similar effects.

Arsenic can increase the risk of lung cancer, skin cancer, bladder cancer, liver cancer, kidney cancer, and prostate cancer. The World Health Organisation (WHO), the DHHS, and the EPA have all determined that inorganic arsenic is a human carcinogen.

Benzene

Benzene is a natural part of crude oil, petrol and cigarette smoke.

Outdoor air contains low levels of benzene from tobacco smoke, service stations, car exhaust fumes, and industrial emissions. Indoor air often contains higher levels of benzene from products such as glues, paints, furniture wax, and detergents.

If you breathe in high levels of benzene, you could become drowsy and dizzy, while your heart rate increases, you get tremors and you become unconscious. Very high levels can result in death. Irregular periods and a decrease in the size of ovaries has been reported by some women who breathed in high levels of benzene for several months.

If you ingest high levels of benzene via food or drink, you may vomit, become dizzy and sleepy and have convulsions and a rapid heart rate. Again, death may result.

Your blood is affected by long term (over a year) exposure to benzene. It is harmful to your bone marrow and can cause your red blood cells to decrease. Long-term exposure to high levels of benzene can cause leukaemia. The DHHS states that benzene is a known human carcinogen.

Cadmium

Cadmium is a natural element in the earth's crust. Fish, plants and animals take up cadmium from the environment. Cadmium can build up in your body from many years of exposure to low levels. When you smoke, you breathe in cadmium.

If you breathe in high levels of cadmium your lungs can be severely damaged and death could result. Even if you are exposed to lower levels of cadmium in your air, food, or water over a period of time, it will build up in your kidneys and could cause kidney disease, lung damage or fragile bones.

The DHHS says that cadmium and cadmium compounds "may reasonably be anticipated to be carcinogens".

Formaldehyde

Also known as methanol, methylene oxide, oxymethyline, methylaldehyde and oxomethane, formaldehyde is a colourless and flammable gas that has a distinct smell.

Formaldehyde dissolves easily. Most formaldehyde in the air breaks down into formic acid and carbon monoxide. Smog is a major source of formaldehyde, as are cigarettes, gas cookers, and open fireplaces.

Your eyes, nose, throat and skin can be irritated by low levels of formaldehyde. People with asthma may be more sensitive to the effects of formaldehyde when inhaled.

Drinking large amounts of formaldehyde can cause severe pain, vomiting, coma, and possible death.

The DHHS says that formaldehyde may reasonably be anticipated to be a carcinogen.

More chemicals than you can shake your cigarette at

The above-mentioned chemicals all combine together to become even more deadly. When reading the list, it's easy to realise how the death and cancer statistics can be so high. Remember:

Lung cancer kills one person every 15 minutes in the UK

The smoking trends

Fewer men are smoking in the UK than ever before. They are also kicking the habit at a faster rate than anyone else in the world. At the peak in the late 1940s, 8 in 10 men smoked, yet it's now only 3 in 10. As a result, fewer men are dying from lung cancer. Women started smoking later than men, and have been slower to quit, so the lung cancer rates for women have not yet started to reduce. However, at this time, more men still die from lung cancer than women.

Young adults present a different story. 40% of 20-24 year olds are smokers. The UK's 15-24 year age group has one of the highest smoking rates in Europe. Amongst 15 year-olds, 21% of boys and 25% of girls smoke.

Manual workers are more than twice as likely to smoke compared to non-manual workers. Further, people living in "deprived" areas are at greater risk of dying from 10 out of the 20 major cancers. These 10 cancers are all smoking-related.

The risks of smoking

Tobacco smoking has no safe level of use. Please read that again.

Tobacco smoking has **no** safe level of use

It is the only consumer product that kills a high proportion of those who use it in the way intended by the manufacturers. We know all this, yet it is still legal.

The risk of getting lung cancer from smoking is directly related to the number of cigarettes smoked. The higher the consumption, the higher the risk.

Cutting the risks by quitting

Smokers who stop before the age of 35 have a life expectancy not significantly different from lifelong non-smokers. Even stopping in middle age has great benefits. The longer you don't smoke, the more you lower your risk. Your risks are halved by staying off cigarettes for ten years.

It is never too late to quit smoking. The sooner you quit, the greater the long-term benefits for your health.

How to quit

You will gain instant benefits from quitting smoking: improvements in your breathing, sighs of relief from those around you, your taste and smell improving, your clothes and breath not smelling like an ash tray, skin problems clearing up, and your bank balance rising. Remember that as you've been ingesting these toxins, you body has been trying to expel them because they are dangerous to you. When trying to get toxins out, your skin might be the organ of choice for expulsion. When the toxins are no longer introduced into your body, your skin and other organs get a much-needed holiday.

In 2000, 72% of smokers said that they wanted to give up, and nine out of ten of those cited at least one health-related motivation behind this.

But how do most people give up? Well, there are hundreds of ways, which include smoker's support groups (support groups work very well, but can end up being an emotional crutch for many months), hypnotism, nicotine patches, etc, but my favourite is this...

Success speaker Anthony Robbins states in his fantastic book, **Unlimited Power**, that the "switch" method is the best of all when retraining the mind to think about what it puts in the body. This technique not only applies to smoking, you can use it for changing any habit. Here's how it works: You reach for a cigarette for many reasons. If you do something else instead which you really really hate, the mind is very quickly tricked into associating that horrible action with smoking, and you don't crave smoking anymore! I know of one person who carried lemons round with him. Every time he wanted a cigarette, he cut a lemon in half and squirted it in his mouth. Very soon he was free from his cigarette addiction — for good. Try it with something you don't like, today!

Withdrawal effects

When using standard quitting techniques, the physical craving for a cigarette can disappear as soon as one week after giving up. But the psychological cravings may last for much longer. Help is available to improve your chance of quitting successfully – read the further information section for ideas, but also be creative. Read books on addiction, health, and lung cancer. Visit a cancer ward in your local hospital. Look for cancer information on the Internet. If you can only scare yourself into giving up, then do that. It's worth it.

How to make giving up easy

It's a little known fact that smokers are searching for a more alkaline state of being. They are generally quite acidic, and smoking temporarily gives the illusion that this is being neutralised. If you neutralise your acid state of being, then one physical reason for smoking immediately goes out of the window. Alkalise yourself today by drinking a green juice every morning and every night, and having alakliser drops in your water.

Nicotine replacement products have helped many people give up. This is how my parents finally kicked the habit after trying everything from cigarette holders to hypnotism. My sister, on the other hand, gave up without the need for anything, though she had a good motive: she discovered she was pregnant.

Use the resources below to widen your knowledge about the harm smoking does to you and those you smoke around, then take action. My friend Joe gave up smoking using Allen Carr's techniques, as have millions of other people in the world. His method is so successful that his books have been translated into over 20 languages.

It's your responsibility

Everything you do is your responsibility. Don't blame anyone else if you smoke, because that's just a lame excuse not to quit. Smoking is not only personally irresponsible, it's socially and environmentally irresponsible. How can you think you're doing your bit for the environment if you are polluting your personal environment? Get some self respect, and kill this habit before it kills you.

Remember the poisonous effects of the chemicals inhaled by smokers and their loved ones? It's legal for companies to produce something that causes death, cancer, heart disease, etc when used to their specifications. Ask yourself "Why is it legal?" When the society and government that is supposed to look after you condones your slow and torturous death, you need to take responsibility.

Listen to your inner voice, and if that doesn't work, listen to a sick and dying man coughing his guts up.

Further information

Web sites

www.cancer.org.uk
www.lungcanceronline.org
www.givingupsmoking.co.uk
www.quitsmoking.com

Books

You Can Stop Smoking
Jacquelyn Rogers
ISBN: 0671523031

Jacquelyn Rogers finally found cigarette freedom after arming herself with the facts about her physical addiction and psychological dependence. She created a programme which not only helped herself, it's helped over 1 million others to quit within 4 weeks.

Allen Carr's Easy Way to Stop Smoking
Allen Carr
(books and DVDs)

Allen Carr promises that his techniques will turn you into a happy non-smoker immediately and permanently, and without using willpower, suffering withdrawal symptoms or putting on weight.

CD
Stop smoking
InnerTalk

If you smoke and would like to stop, this is the time to invest in InnerTalk's fantastic **Stop Smoking** from the *Habits and Addictions* range. Combine this CD with reading one of the above books, and you are onto a winner.

Other
Contact Quitline (UK) on 0800 002200 or talk to your doctor.

Research
Look up lung cancer photos on the web. Check out more statistics for smoking and cancer and think about how those statistics apply to you. For example, if half of all smokers get lung cancer, and you and your brother smoke, statistically either you or your brother will die from lung cancer. Who would you rather it be? Think about the statistics for cancer, think about what you want in your life, for yourself and your loved ones, then give up smoking. With these wonderful resources, of course you can do it!

System shockers

Alarm clocks

You're on a tropical island and a handsome waiter passes you a freshly mixed coconut and pineapple shake. He is wearing a grass skirt, and winks at you. You feel like you're in heaven — the sun is tanning your skin, while the sea laps at your toes. Then... BRI-I-I-I-I-NG! BRI-I-I-I-I-NG! BRI-I-I-I-I-NG! Your alarm clock wakes you with a start. It's 7am on Monday morning and reality strikes you like lightning.

Think about how you feel when that alarm clock goes off. Are you gently woken from your dream, brought round in a loving, peaceful manner and able to start the day calmly? Probably not.

The beauty about detoxing your world is that you can make tiny changes, such as obtaining a gentle wake up clock, and it will make a massive difference to your life. The idea behind it is so simple, it amazes me that they are not standard. The difference in these clocks is that they switch on very quietly and gradually get louder and louder until they're at the level you set. You really do get woken gently, just as if it was a loving tender kiss on your cheek.

You can also buy sunrise clocks, which gently create natural full spectrum light in your room. This causes your body to start producing its wake up hormones. These clocks are great for anyone who switches their alarm clock off 15 times before eventually conceding that there's no escaping the Monday morning rat race.

More people in the western world die on a Monday morning than at any other time, simply due to stress. Don't let your alarm clock exacerbate the situation — invest in a gentle clock today, or change your life so you can wake up when you want!

Cold floors

I once read about a man who constantly suffered from colds in the winter. He went to see a complementary therapist who asked him what he did in the mornings, when getting out of bed. He explained that he got up, went to the toilet, and then went to the kitchen to make a cup of tea, taking the tea back to bed. The therapist asked him what the kitchen floor was made of, and did he wear socks or slippers. The patient said the flooring was lino, and he was barefoot. Without offering any herbal concoctions, the therapist solved the mystery of this otherwise healthy man. "Wear slippers". The theory is simple — your feet are warm and cozy for about 8 hours, then you subject them to ten minutes of tea-making coldness. As the walls of the nose are directly affected by the feet, they contract which causes the glands to stop functioning. This is a perfect opportunity for nasty air-borne germs to enter the body and wreak havoc.

I included the above story for you because even if you don't have cold floors, things might be happening to you as a result of some minor shock that you persistently give your body. Just be aware of your habits for a week and see what you can pick up. Making a small change such as wearing slippers or not sitting on a cold toilet seat (my pet hate!) can make a big difference to your body's defences.

Sense pollution

> ### Set yourself free
>
> Your quality of life is very important. Would you rather have 100 years in a prison or one day of freedom? If you'd like the one day of freedom, then start taking risks. As my favourite saying goes "leap and the safety net will appear".

Increasing numbers of people are becoming ultra-sensitive to noise. At the worst point in my life the fridge downstairs, which was in a room with the door closed, kept me awake. The little red standby light on the stereo in the bedroom pierced my closed eyes. On the window I had a pair of curtains, blackout curtains and a blind, yet the morning light still gave me migraines. I could never sleep with a clock or a watch in the room as the ticking drove me mad, and the children next door to me woke me up running up and down their stairs getting ready for school —and that was when I had a pillow wrapped round my head to keep the noise of the fridge and the light of the sun out!

Normal noise pollution is bad enough — noisy neighbours, cars and motorbikes zooming past and honking their horns, televisions and stereos booming through walls and people in your house screaming at each other. But when you're in such a toxic state that your body is in the first stages of giving up, it can be as bad or worse than the experience I described.

To overcome sense pollution, you can employ various methods. Be creative here. If you can soundproof rooms, double or triple glaze your windows, add carpets, curtains and cloth wall hangings — then do it.

However, be aware that blocking the noise out also blocks the light and life out. Be careful when taking these anti-noise steps that you don't do other parts of yourself harm. If noise is that bad where you live, consider moving, you might not even have to change jobs. I'm a great believer in tele-working. The days of getting to an office easily are long gone for most, so tele-working is a great option. Self motivation is a key factor, but if your employer is willing to offer several or all days working from home, why not move out of the city and get fresh in the country?

After I detoxed my world, my sensitivity to noise and light went away. I no longer feel like I'm being penetrated by everything around me! If you have noise-sensitivity, then I've got my fingers crossed that this will work for you.

Television

> ### Exercise for couch potatoes
>
> If you live with a couch potato, hide the remote control. They'll burn up lots of calories looking for their battery-operated pet!

Where do I start with this one? Watch people in a room when they are watching the television. Watch the way they eat, barely conscious that food is going in their mouths. Watch when one of them talks and the other one says "Shhhh". Watch when the phone rings and they tut because they've been interrupted. This all happens because most of the content on television is sucking their brains dry! Some studies have shown that when people watch the television, their brains display less activity than when they're asleep. Being a couch potato isn't likely to leave you feeling fulfilled and joyous, but rather scared and with a distorted view of the world.

Television can be addictive, can represent a world which isn't true due to biased media coverage, and can also be bad for your health. Not many people exercise when watching the television, and those using video games are at added risk of repetitive strain injury (RSI).

Why don't you?

If you watch more than two or three hours of television a week, think about how to cut it down. Decide what's really worth watching. If you don't live in the Queen Vic, you don't need to know what's going on in it. If you use the television for escapism, that's a big sign that you need to change your life so you want to live it to the full, not run from it. If you use the television for company, do the old clichéd but workable alternative and get out and join an evening class or club. Record any programmes that you really want to watch, and then watch them when you want, not when you're being programmed to!

Some people watch the television to wind down after a hard day's work, but a change is really as good as a rest, and so doing something pleasant and creative is a much healthier way of winding down. A lot of people prepare food, partake in hobbies, play with loved ones or do exercise. There are so many more constructive ways to live.

Even if your television is on in another room, you will be affected by it. If you have a partner who watches a lot of television, and you don't, then come to an agreement that it is off for at least half the time you are both at home. That is the real meaning of equality, isn't it? Please don't feel guilty asking for this either, no one person should dominate communal living space, so have your say today!

I remember having a plant near a big television in my home, and all the leaves fell off the side which faced the television. This is interesting considering that radiation levels have been kept in check since 1968, and are not now considered harmful. If it can destroy a plant, then what is it doing to a human who sits close to it, day in, day out for years? I eventually had to move my plant, but would have much preferred to throw away the big black mind-sucking box!

Vaccinations

Whole books have been written on the risks of vaccinations. However, as much as it has been "proved" that they don't work and are dangerous, it has also been "proved" that they do work, and their benefits seriously outweigh their risks. This method of proving can go on until the cows come home, as it will never be agreed upon by all sides. There is a lot of money involved in the vaccination industry, and so the authorities which receive money when vaccines are sold will go on endorsing their use for a long while yet. I know people who have been crippled or killed by vaccines. Having seen the worst side of vaccinations, I personally could never impose it on my child or myself.

Sadly, you can't un-vaccinate yourself. If you suffer alleged vaccine-related symptoms, such as autism, arthritis, Crohn's disease, diabetes, ME, meningitis etc, then you can strengthen your body naturally to fight these diseases. Take in lots of wild and organic greens, either blended or juiced, and make the most of coriander and zeolites. Use some of the *Detox helpers* in this book and contact a natural practitioner who will be able to safely guide you into boosting your body's ability to fight the effects of vaccinations. Read Jatinder's tale in *Success stories*, which shows you how she and her family overcame terrible illnesses which they believe were caused by vaccinations.

Tuberculosis slammer

On 29th January 2001, health researcher Jock Doubleday offered a reward of $20,000 to anyone in the US licensed medical world who would drink the contents of an empty vaccine. To date nobody has taken up this offer. To clarify, he offered to pay someone to drink a mixture of standard vaccine additive ingredients, an "empty vaccine" — one without bacteria or viruses in it. It sounds safe enough for an adult to drink a mixture that is routinely injected into babies all over the world, so why has nobody stepped forward to claim the money and take the drink? Maybe it has something to do with the common ingredients listed as additives to a vaccination. If you don't fancy having thimerosal (derived from mercury), ethylene glycol (antifreeze), phenol (a disinfectant dye), benzethonium chloride (disinfectant), human diploid cells (from human aborted foetal tissue) and aluminium roaming around inside your body — think twice before you do it to your children.

If you need to go to a country and vaccinations are required, you can probably find a homeopath who can treat and certify you, which is much less toxic.

If you are faced with the decision of whether to vaccinate yourself or your children, I highly recommend that you read as much as you can on this subject before you make up your mind. If you become educated by both sides, you can make a much better decision than relying on government leaflets which are sponsored by the pharmaceutical industry.

Further information

Books

Vaccination Bible
Lynne McTaggart
ISBN: 0953473406

This health writer has created another brilliant and useful book here. She will give you the other side of the argument in clear English, which helps you make your mind up on such an important subject.

The Vaccination Dilemma
A Natural Approach
Christine Murphy
ISBN: 1930051107

Murphy states that children are expected to have 37 doses of eleven different vaccines within their first five years of life. She looks at the risks and diseases associated with vaccinations, and explains how natural immunity works. A book full of resources, this should be on every parent's bookshelf.

Magazines

The Mother Magazine

If all parenting magazines seem a little disconnected for your liking, then pick up a copy of **The Mother Magazine**. Edited by my good friend Veronika, it offers a refreshingly different view on all aspects of parenthood, and frequently discusses vaccination and how to deal with your doctors.

For more information, visit **www.themothermagazine.co.uk**.

Teeth

Natural animals, living the low-toxin lifestyle, don't get the holes, cracks and breaks in their teeth that we get. This is fortunate, as lions probably don't have the temperament to endure a session of root canal therapy!

When you look at the teeth of "undeveloped" societies, you usually see straight, strong and bright teeth. These people don't have braces, fillings, crowns, veneers or reconstruction, yet their teeth are infinitely more beautiful than ours. This isn't a fluke. When being formed in the womb, we are exposed to whatever toxins the mother has in her body that her placenta can't filter out. This, along with the quality of nutrients we receive, has a great effect on our development — and one noticeable feature for many of us westerners is that our faces aren't as symmetrical as they should be. You can also notice it in animals that are fed by humans, such as domestic cats and dogs. Because there are only two factors which play a part, it's easy to reverse the effects in subsequent generations. By simply becoming less toxic and improving nutritional intake as a life-long habit, our future children's teeth and everything else can become more perfect than ours. Surely all mothers would want this for their children.

I know of people who have reversed holes in their teeth by constantly chewing on wild greens. I know of people who have reversed transparent teeth by having massive quantities of green juices. If you have tooth or gum disease, you can easily improve them with masses of green foods, so long as you're consistent.

Cleaning teeth

It isn't natural to put toxic substances into your mouth two or three times a day, scrub really hard and then rinse with another toxic substance — yet that's what happens to most of us when we brush our teeth. The levels of toxins are low, but multiply this by the number of times you've ever brushed your teeth, and you get more than a minimal amount of toxic exposure. If you think that governments, dentists and doctors wouldn't allow us to use toxic substances, think again. It's not in their interests to prevent tooth decay, as it doesn't make financial sense to them. 95% of all Americans have mercury fillings — if we prevented tooth decay, their dentists wouldn't have much of a job left.

Fluoride is a toxic by-product from aluminium production. "Silver" fillings contain more mercury than any other metal, yet are called "silver" when marketed to the public, because the public knows mercury is a deadly poison. I don't know where the lies and deception end, but when armed with the truth we can make newer, more intelligent choices.

A big toxin lurks inside most toothpastes — it's called fluoride

Nuclear energy produces nuclear waste as a by-product, cheese produces whey as a by-product, and so on. By-products can be a large percentage of the crude matter, and a waste of money if not sold on to another market. Thus, companies put whey in fabric conditioner and washing up liquid and call it a softener, but no-one wants nuclear waste so it becomes a bit of a nuisance to dispose of. When aluminium is produced, sodium fluoride is created as a by-product. Originally, the producers sold it as rat poison and insecticide, but they were always on the look out for other, bigger, markets.

Fluoride causes disease and kills people

In the USA, about 10,000 cancer deaths per year are linked to water fluoridation.

As little as 0.2ppm of fluoride reduces the migration rate of human white blood cells and causes further reductions as its volume increases. White blood cells are the body's soldiers that fight toxins: if their production is suppressed, your total well-being is compromised.

Fluoride interferes with collagen formation and results in the body's inability to decide which tissues should be mineralised and which tissues should not. This means that mineralisation of tissues such as bone (which should be mineralised) is disrupted while tendons, ligaments, muscles and other soft tissues (which should not be mineralised) start to become mineralised. This effect, known as skeletal fluorosis, has been linked with causing or triggering arthritis, arteriosclerosis, brittle bones, wrinkled skin, osteoporosis, scleroderma, muscular dystrophy, rheumatoid arthritis and lupus.

Fluoride has also been linked with diseases such as neurological impairment, enzyme inhibition, Alzheimer's disease and dementia.

Because dangerous chemicals are used in items such as toothpaste, many animals suffer cruel and unnecessary experiments. I'm sure you don't want that on your conscience, especially when there are viable alternatives.

Even though it's acknowledged by toothpaste manufacturers that a family-sized tube of toothpaste (containing 199 milligrams of fluoride) can kill a 25lb child, there are no current plans to ban fluoride from your toothpaste or tap water. You have to make that decision yourself. Ban it from your house today.

Fluoride doesn't prevent tooth decay

Although original tests seemed to indicate that sodium fluoride prevented tooth decay, they've since been re-examined, and it's been noted that about 40-70% of the children tested developed fluorosis as a result of the added fluoride.

Further, the authorities in Toronto, Canada, have been adding fluoride to water for around 40 years, yet Vancouver has never done this. Vancouver has a considerably lower cavity rate than Toronto.

Why is fluoride allowed, if it's so dangerous and doesn't even prevent tooth decay?

The only way we can ensure that we're protected from harmful chemicals these days is to educate ourselves as much as possible.

> Governments won't do it for you, it's not on their agenda: so you have to put it on yours.

My fluoride story

At the age of 16, I was somehow guided away from using products with added fluoride. Though my instincts were weak, thankfully they sometimes served me well. I stopped drinking tap water, and began using a non-fluoride toothpaste, though I had read nothing of its dangers at that time.

So, 22 years later, now I've had more years of no fluoride than added fluoride — what's the result? Do I have rotten, weak, sensitive teeth for lack of fluoride? Have I got more cavities, more fillings and root canals? No, I have very strong teeth, which aren't sensitive, and I haven't developed a cavity since well before the age of 16. In addition, I've been a vegan for 20 of those years, and the lack of calcium from cow's milk hasn't adversely affected me at all.

After I had my mercury fillings removed, I had my teeth cleaned by a dental hygienist. She was amazed at how clean and plaqueless my teeth were. Dental hygienists push an object like a mini nail file in between the teeth, to remove built-up plaque. They also use a metal scraper to go round the back and sides of the teeth, chipping away at the plaque. My hygienist said that there was barely anything there, even though I had not had my teeth scraped for about 12 years prior to this.

She asked me what my diet was, and I told her. At that time I'd had a low-toxin diet for about a year, but I'd never been interested in fizzy drinks or sweets as an adult. All I have as a reminder of a childhood with a bad diet are my molars which are filled as far as the eye can see. I never even had big cavities as a child, so we'll find out why the fillings are so big in a minute.

My hygienist told me to carry on doing what I was doing, and said she wished all her clients were as conscious of what they put in their mouths as I was.

Some other toothpaste tales

It's been reported that sodium lauryl sulphate, which is present in many tooth cleaning products, contributes to dental holes. Other reports claim that dental decay doesn't happen because of what is put on the teeth, it happens on the inside. In other words, it's not necessarily the acid in your fruit juice, but the acidity of your body that contributes to dental decay. Even further reports claim that decay is caused by nanobacteria that's transferred via dental equipment, kissing or food sharing.

How to keep teeth clean, naturally

Now I've hopefully dissuaded you from using toothpaste containing fluoride, here's some advice on the best way to clean your teeth.

Because our teeth are not spaced out correctly (due to malformation as babes-in-wombs), we do need to take care in brushing to remove food and plaque. A soft toothbrush is best for the job, and you can choose to add a bit of sea salt, some strawberries or some of the less toxic toothpastes available. I use Mint Toothpaste by The Green People Company Ltd, or the Desert Essence range which are available in health food shops and on the Internet. Look for toothpaste made with natural organic ingredients, and without fluoride. Only brush your teeth when you feel the need, and don't over-brush. If you brush a tooth for 30 seconds a day, that adds up to over 90 hours over the course of 30 years. There's only so much enamel on your teeth, so take care not to brush it away.

Tooth enemies

You may have gathered by now that the idea of this book is to eat as much natural food and as little unnatural food as possible. This is to the advantage of all parts of your body, as you are a whole entity, and not lots of separate parts, needing individual treatment.

However, anything which is processed will adversely affect your teeth. The more natural fresh, raw and ripe food that you eat, the less processed, artificial, chemical-ladened food you'll eat. Ripe fruit is important for your digestion, but essential for your teeth. Unripe fruit contains more acid than your teeth like. If you are eating fruit which makes your teeth hurt, it's probably not ripe.

Most oranges tend to be more acidic than our teeth can safely handle. If you want to consume oranges (and you should, as they are really great for you!), then juice them and suck through a straw. If you eat them whole, clean your teeth about 20 minutes afterwards, either with a soft brush, or by chewing some dark green leaves.

Just for the waste of it

Colas and other fizzy sugary drinks are tooth dissolvers. All refined sugar will affect your teeth, and considering that the average American manages to eat his or her own weight in refined sugar each year, there's no wonder that dentists are so rich.

Tooth friends

Natural, unprocessed foods and foods high in minerals are tooth friends. Organic green juices or superfoods supply an abundance of minerals to help your teeth stay strong.

We have a natural sweet tooth because we are frugivores (mainly fruit-eating) by design. However, much commercial fruit is picked under-ripe and still acidic or starchy, instead of sweet. When we don't get the sugar we instinctively need and want from our natural sources, we reach for cakes, biscuits, fizzy drinks etc. This sugar isn't what our body wanted but it tastes "right" to us, and our body makes some use of it, so we accept it.

The damage these foods do to the whole body is well-documented, and there are great addictions associated with these foods. If you have a sweet tooth, and reach for bad foods time and time again, start reaching for tooth-friendly ripe organic fruit instead. Eat the fruit on its own (mono-eating) until you are full, or make puddings and smoothies following the recipes in this book and its companion recipe book, **Detox Delights**. Experiment with your own sweet favourites. These foods won't harm your teeth or body like their man-made poor substitutes do, so remove all guilty feelings about eating sweet food. However, be aware that some modern fruits don't have the amount of minerals that you need, and so it's very important to do as suggested above, and take your greens seriously. Tooth demineralisation from lack of greens does occur, and isn't pleasant with symptoms ranging from transparency and holes, to chips. So please take responsibility, and go green as often as you go multi-coloured.

Do you want rotting and painful teeth or beautiful and strong teeth? The choice is yours — make it today.

Tooth decay

From what I've already written, it's clear why humans suffer from tooth decay so much more than our wild animal friends. But what happens to us when we get cavities?

I'd like a mouthful of metal, please

- 95% of all Americans have mercury in their mouth.

- Amalgam fillings are a mixture of about 50% mercury, with varying levels of silver, tin, copper and zinc, and were first created about 160 years ago.

- Fillings give our bodies 3-4 times more mercury than we would ever get from all other environmental sources put together.

Mercury fillings require the removal of healthy tooth material

The filling material itself is weak and can't be used in a thin layer. The dentist must drill deeply into the softer dentine area of the tooth and drill undercuts into the healthy tooth where there is no disease. This approach was developed in 1908 by GV Black. As a result of this kind of filling, the tooth becomes weakened by 75%. This is why my molar fillings were so big. Before I knew how dentists applied fillings, I was always so confused by this as I didn't remember seeing massive holes in my teeth as a child.

Root canal, anyone?

Mercury fillings also expand after being placed in the tooth. The bigger the filling the more they expand. If any moisture gets into the filling they expand rapidly. Temperature can also cause expansion. All this expansion within the tooth eventually results in fracture.

Once broken, the tooth may require a root canal, crown or extraction. Often the fracture is so severe that in spite of all efforts the tooth is lost.

And then it gets scary

Once in the mouth, and for the duration, mercury vapour constantly leaches out of this mixture and into your tooth, jaw, body, breath, blood and brain.

When you consume hot food and drinks the rate at which mercury vapour leaves the filling and enters the mouth, lungs, gastrointestinal tract, bloodstream, brain and tissues, increases. As your shiny mercury amalgam fillings start to corrode, ionic mercury is released and travels through your teeth, jaw, blood and gastrointestinal tract. It is known that mercury is poisonous as both metallic vapour and as mercuric ions.

Dentists still use mercury amalgam because it's inexpensive and easy to work with.

As mad as a hatter

Remember the saying "Mad as a hatter"? It comes from a time when hatters used to go insane due to working with large amounts of mercury. Now ponder this: Medical doctors always used to have the highest drug addiction and suicide rate amongst professionals in the USA. As it's now been superseded by dentists, who have a relatively easy time of it compared to doctors, you have to wonder what caused this shift. I believe that mercury poisoning has had a direct result on the mental health and well-being of our dentists.

"But mercury isn't toxic"

Although the above statement would appear to contradict this, many dentists and authorities still insist that mercury is not toxic. How strange, then, that dentists discourage pregnant women from having their mercury fillings removed, as it might harm the baby. How strange, then, that dentists are warned about touching or breathing in mercury vapour. How strange, then, that dentists suffer from an increased number of lymphocytes in the blood, which indicates continuing stress on the immunological system, which is usually associated with an acute or chronic "infection".

And how strange that dentists seem to be going mad.

In addition, dentists are warned about toxic effects when working with amalgam, and yet this information isn't passed on to the patient — if you have had amalgam fillings, do you remember being given any warnings?

You know that authorities have something to hide when they tell practising dentists that they can't openly announce that mercury fillings are toxic or even tell their clients what percentage of mercury is in the filling. Yet this is a fact in one of the biggest countries in the world — guess which one?

You know the authorities have something to hide when they name a filling by one of its minor, more attractive components, rather than its main component.

Mercury fillings are promoted as "silver fillings" because that's easier for consumers to swallow.

Is it?

So if amalgam is a cheap and safe material for keeping your teeth healthy, and the mercury it contains is no hazard to your health, or to the health of dentists and their employees, why do some experts say...

Mercury is a toxin

Mercury-amalgam has never been scientifically proven to be safe for use in this way on humans. Its history is so old, that it started around the same time as mercury pills were prescribed for the treatment of syphilis. Now many dental authorities use its history as a way of saying it's safe. Wasn't smoking promoted as good for the lungs once?

Many experts say that mercury leaks from fillings and exposes the body to a continuous low dose of it. As it's well known for being a highly toxic heavy metal, experts say that this leakage is a big threat to anyone exposed to mercury and has caused mercury poisoning.

Think back to the aluminium story, where fluoride is a by-product. Well, mercury waste is treated more like nuclear waste: it's collected for deposition in special rock shelters because it's that hazardous.

Effects of mercury poisoning and amalgam fillings

If sufficient doses of mercury get into river water, all the life dies or future generations are seriously affected and mutated.

In 1988, some of the world's most prominent mercury researchers declared that mercury from amalgam fillings can permanently damage the brain, kidneys and immune function of children. Please read the above again.

Mercury causes brain damage in children. Children are still being filled with mercury.

Mercury has also been linked to gastrointestinal problems, sleep disturbance, concentration problems, memory disturbance, apathy, restlessness, bleeding gums and other mouth disorders in large-scale studies.

After one researcher completed his experiments, which linked Alzheimer's disease with mercury vapour, he declared that he would be getting his fillings out as soon as possible, and would be asking the same of his wife.

Mercury released from fillings builds up in the brain, kidneys, liver, pituitary, adrenals, and other parts of the body.

Mercury from amalgam fillings has been implicated as a possible contributory factor in some cases of multiple sclerosis, Parkinson's disease, IBS, reproductive disorders, allergies, and a variety of other illnesses.

Mercury from fillings in pregnant women has been shown to cause mercury accumulation in the brain, kidneys and liver of human foetuses. Studies have shown that mercury can be passed to infants via breast milk.

Even pro-mercury experts admit that new techniques demonstrate that mercury is released from amalgam fillings, yet they insist that just because there have been few actual direct proofs of mercury-associated disease, that all the accumulative health problems which people suffer are not mercury-related. This isn't enough of a justification to keep a known toxin in the mouths of millions.

Alternatives to toxic mercury fillings

The best material around today to fill teeth is white glass ionomer. It looks like part of the tooth, instead of ugly faded metal. It forms true chemical bonds to the tooth material. This prevents microleakage of food particles and so doesn't allow for rot to set in under the filling which is a major source of new decay with amalgams. In addition, the chemical bond makes the restoration an integral part of the tooth itself, so through tensile strength and adhesion, it actually restores the tooth to a single entity. All past materials without chemical bonding ability leaves the patient with a hollow shell of a tooth and a hard lump of filling material sitting in a hole, disconnected to that shell.

My story

Some dentists will tell you that mercury amalgam is not dangerous, or it's more dangerous to "disturb it" by removing it. I feel differently.

When I had my amalgam out, I opted for it to be done on two separate days, so that my mouth wouldn't be numb all over from the injections. I chose a composite material, and asked for a dental dam to be used. This is a big piece of rubber which goes inside the mouth, and is cut where the tooth is. It's sealed by clips and it ensures that no mercury can drip down the throat. I asked the dentist if I should hold my breath while drilling, and he said that it wasn't necessary. I didn't believe that, so I held my breath. I'm glad I had been practising yogic breathing for a while before this, as it meant I didn't need to breathe at all while he drilled. If you can't hold your breath for what sometimes seems like ages, ask for a nasal hood, so you can breathe clean air whilst the dentist is drilling. After I had the first batch out, I felt like I had heavy cold symptoms for about a week. My head was very heavy, my eyes were puffy and I couldn't concentrate. I'm a highly sensitive person, so I knew I'd be affected. The second lot was a bit different, the dam didn't fit properly and some mercury leaked down — I could taste it as it was going down my throat. I knew it was only a tiny bit but I wanted it out, not in me! After that session, I felt the same symptoms as before but for a bit longer.

Then something amazing happened. For the first time in my life I felt switched-on, connected, real. I started getting a sense of direction — my internal compass was working again! The metal in my mouth was short-circuiting me, and causing much of the confusion I'd previously felt. That experience alone made it all worth it!

Please take action today

First of all, don't panic by what you've just read! Your body is doing everything it can to protect you from toxins all the time, so just knowing that you have poison in your mouth will make no difference. If you have mercury fillings, please get them out. Even if you have to get one replaced every two months for financial reasons, it's worth it.

If you can't have them replaced (maybe you're pregnant), then be aware that any chewing, grinding of teeth, computer terminal exposure, hot food, tooth brushing and braces cause the release of significantly increased amounts of mercury from the fillings. Minimise these activities, and have the fillings replaced as soon as is possible.

If you're scared of the dentist, then please use some relaxation techniques to make your experience easier. Some dentists will be able to help you with this. I have a great dislike of needles, and ask for the anaesthetic gel (which used to just be for children) to be used before I let a needle go anywhere near me. I also use my voice of reason, as I know that mercury is so bad for me, this temporary trauma is worth it a million times over.

Some people with diseases ranging from rheumatoid arthritis and food sensitivities to depression and lupus have "miraculously" recovered after having their mercury fillings removed. Some people who had fillings at a young age never remember feeling well, yet as soon as the fillings came out they felt better than they could ever remember.

A recent survey in Sweden showed that of 268 patients who had amalgam fillings removed, 80% showed permanent health improvement. Three quarters of those improved within six months. There were no signs of the positive effects disappearing as might be expected with a placebo effect.

There have been some exaggerated claims by people who profit from amalgam removal, but I'm glad that this hasn't distracted from the real message. Mercury doesn't belong in your mouth. I personally wouldn't spend time on expensive allergy or vapour tests. It's quicker and cheaper to just have the mercury removed.

Although removing your mercury may cure you of existing illnesses, or at least relieve the symptoms to some degree, there is also a chance that it might not. If you are ill, please don't pin all your hopes of recovery just on mercury removal. It's wise to embark on a more holistic, balanced approach to living well.

Future fillings

The future is bright! When our friend medical ozone is blasted onto cavities, it kills the bacteria streptococcus mutans, which has to be present for our teeth to rot. This allows the tooth enamel to naturally rebuild, and no fillings are needed. In the UK, this treatment is starting to be rolled out across the country as I write this book.

If you can't get this treatment, then composite filling materials are the next best solution. As well as strengthening the tooth, composite is less dangerous, more attractive and lasts longer than amalgam. Most initial composite fillings require only minimal natural tooth removal. As well as restoring decayed areas, they can seal up weak spots so decay can't penetrate further.

Let's recap

Now you have this information, there is no need for your future children or grandchildren to face the risks of lots of cavities and mercury fillings. Encourage them to eat well, to brush kindly, and take them for dental fissures if you think it will help.

Further Information

Web sites

www.toxicteeth.org — If you need further convincing about amalgam.

www.dentalfearcentral.org — Helps with any dentist aversions you may have.

www.the-o-zone.cc — All about ozone dentistry.

www.integratedhealthpractice.com — A UK dentist, John Roberts, who takes the holistic approach. I had the great pleasure of meeting him, and I would trust this man 100% with my mouth and health. Over several months, he helped restore the health of a friend who was told by her doctor that she was going to die. She is now leaping around with more energy than she knows what to do with — she really did detox her world! Based in Huddersfield, you can make an appointment with John on +44 (0)1484 514451.

Books

Uninformed Consent
The Hidden Dangers in Dental Care
Hal A. Huggins and Thomas E. Levy
ISBN: 1-57174-117-8

This book details how many diseases are preventable by reducing the toxins in our bodies. With emphasis on the toxins in modern dentistry, Uninformed Consent details how immune systems become depressed, and how illnesses occur after dentist treatment. The book will educate you enough to make an informed choice when you next visit the man in the mask.

Whole-Body Dentistry
Discover The Missing Piece To Better Health
Mark A. Breiner DDS
ISBN: 0967844304

Looking at dentistry from a holistic point of view isn't common, but is very worthwhile. This book explains that the health of the mouth is a reflection of the rest of the body, and discusses the effect of dental treatment on the rest of the body. Nutrition, meridians, homeopathy, etc are all covered in relevant ways. You also get the chance to read patients' stories on how they discovered what was wrong with them.

Product

Seagreens food capsules

In January 2001, **Seagreens Food Capsules** were endorsed by the British Society for Mercury-Free Dentistry for post-operative detoxification in amalgam extraction: Daily two capsules morning and one capsule evening for three weeks, then normal daily intake of one or two capsules as required.

Zeolites are minerals formed when molten lava contacts lake or sea water. Clinoptilolite is a type of zeolite that has a honeycomb-like structure which can trap and bind toxins, heavy metals (uranium, aluminum, lead, mercury, arsenic and cadmium), viral particles, and other impurities. They are then removed from the body. It's been used for over 800 years by real practitioners.

Detox helpers

We concentrate on food so much in this book as it's most people's weakest link. However, there are other, non-food related activities which will help you detox. Here is an extensive yet not conclusive list of them. They're actually a selection of my favourites, so I know they work well! You don't have to try all of them, just pick those that appeal to you. Note that these helpers all give you a great sense of well being, make you feel happy and relaxed. Who said detox had to be hard?

Breathing and oxygen

There is less oxygen in our atmosphere now than ever before. Around 200 years ago, our air would have contained about 38% oxygen. These days, the average is 21% and plummeting. Even if we live a relatively healthy lifestyle, our oxygen intake can be boosted for the greatest possible health. Exercise is a fantastic way to do this, and here are a couple of my favourite non-exercise methods.

Conscious breathing

Most adults breathe very shallowly, which causes their bodies to function less than optimally. We only notice how bad our breathing is when we go up some stairs and quickly become breathless. We just need to do a few simple exercises to prevent this happening, to activate our lymph system and to let more life in.

Yogis and yoginis know the importance of good breathing — it's what their practice is based on. Though the western world is now waking up to yoga, breathing is sometimes still not given the importance that it deserves.

Pranayama — mastering your life force

The word pranayama comes from prana, meaning life force, and anyama, meaning control. So pranayama means mastering our life force. The use of pranayama breathing techniques allows you to control the flow of prana in your body. If you ever felt depleted, then these simple yet highly effective exercises are for you.

As an added bonus to our physical wellness, we know that when we have mastered our life force, we become fully present (in the moment), and can continue our daily practices with conscious mindfulness.

A very popular type of pranayama is called nadi shodhana, or the sweet breath. When you practise this, your blood receives more oxygen than with other types of pranayama. I love it for its simplicity, and because it's suitable for most people. It entails breathing through alternate nostrils at a slow and steady pace. Nadi means channel, which refers to the energy pathways through which prana flows. Shodhana means cleansing. This is great for detox, because nadi shodhana literally means channel or nerve cleaning.

The advantages of practising the sweet breath are far reaching. Your mind will become calmer and clearer, and stress will be reduced. It's also a great way to warm up your body and gain resistance to diseases.

This is an excellent stress-busting technique.
Expect to feel tranquil and serene as you practise, and
for a good while afterwards.

How to practise the sweet breath

Sit in any comfortable posture, preferably on the floor in the lotus position or with your legs crossed. If you can't sit like this, sit against a wall with your legs straight out in front of you. Remember to keep your spine straight and your head upright.

Relax your body and close your eyes.

Curl your index and middle fingers inwards towards your palm. Put your thumb next to your right nostril and your third and little fingers by your left nostril.

Gently press against your left nostril to close it with the fingers in position, and inhale through your right nostril. This breath should be slow, steady and full. Feel the breath coming into all parts of your lungs, filling your tummy area, as well as your chest.

Once you have inhaled, gently press the right nostril with your thumb to close it, and remove your fingers to open your left nostril. Exhale fully, in the same slow and steady manner.

Then repeat the exercise, but inhale through your left nostril, and exhale through your right one.

You have just completed one round of the sweet breath. Practise four more, and then relax. Slowly build this up every day to 10 or 20 rounds, and you will soon love the far-reaching effects this practice has on your total well-being.

Taking it further

Because of the sensitive nature of pranayama, it is best to learn different techniques direct from a teacher. Many yoga teachers are qualified in teaching pranayama and would be happy to give you private tuition so you can learn some basic techniques. You can also buy very reasonably priced pranayama lessons from www.pranayama.org. They sell lessons based on very specific breathing exercises, which can help with creativity, weight loss and bliss, among many other subjects.

If you don't want to learn specific breathing techniques, try making a promise to yourself that you will stand outside in the fresh air once an hour and take ten deep and mindful breaths. This will ensure that you get a good dose of oxygen into your body to help your detox.

Ozone therapy — the high-tech detox helper

Though we are wanting to get back to a more natural state, we must also recognise that the average toxic body needs a lot of help to recover from years of unnatural living. For this reason, I let my clients know about various high-tech treatments. Ozone therapy is a very quick and effective method to help you get a foot up on the health ladder. As with all my suggestions, they are not alternatives to living a healthy life, they are assistants in that quest.

Ozone therapy is one of the best high-tech helpers I know of. It's been used successfully for decades throughout Europe. Nowadays, it's more widely available throughout the world. Its uptake within the medical profession is slow, and in some cases inhibited. Because no drug company can patent ozone, their resistance to anything which will not make money for them (regardless of the benefits it has on people) is quite apparent. This is why you are more likely to find ozone treatment from an "alternative" therapist.

Ever since ozone was used in World War I to treat illnesses such as mustard gas burns, therapists have paid close attention to this simple treatment. These days, the ozone used is called medical ozone. It's pure and concentrated, so differs from atmospheric ozone. Medical ozone generators deliver pure ozone-oxygen mixtures in the required dose.

Ozone therapy is used for a wide variety of conditions. Practitioners have had success with many diseases, including: allergies, arthritis, cancer, candida, childhood hearing loss, Crohn's disease, CNS disorders, colitis, glaucoma, heart disease, hepatitis, herpes, HIV/AIDS, IBS, MS and parasites.

Practitioners also administer ozone to people who are apparently symptomless, and they experience positive effects. Athletes' performances increase by around 10%, the elderly don't contract yearly flu and most people report euphoria alongside their bodies functioning better after the treatment.

While having ozone treatment, I asked my doctor whether many of his clients used this treatment as a preventative method. He replied that quite a few patients, especially the older ones, have ozone as a preventative measure before the winter sets in. They make an appointment for a course of ten, taking two a week. They then don't suffer any of the adverse winter effects which can creep up on most of us when winter strikes.

The methods of administration vary:

* Autohaemotherapy (AHT), is a doctor-administered technique. Blood is extracted, mixed with ozone and replaced.

* The steam sauna method is very relaxing. Your whole body (except for your head) is encased in an ozone-delivering steam sauna.

* Insufflation is used for localised topical problems, as a bag of ozone is gently released around the affected area.

Researchers have reported that ozone breaks up fats and rejuvenates cells to keep you looking younger for longer. The more I read about ozone therapy, the more I believe that it has a positive effect on every part of the body. This may be in part because people are oxygen-deficient these days, due to our diets, indoor lifestyles, and the atmosphere. Though the other oxygen-enhancing activities in this section can help give you boundless energy and joy over time, a course of ozone treatments can quickly transport you to a place where it's easier to enjoy a healthy lifestyle.

How it works

Ozone treatment stimulates the white blood cells, which enables them to fight any existing infection. It prompts the body to produce interferon and other anti-cancer agents at a higher rate than normal. As it increases the amount of oxygen in the blood, and helps deliver oxygen to all of the cells in the body, pathogens such as viruses, bacteria, fungi and yeasts die. This is because these pathogens are anaerobic — they can't survive in an oxygen-rich environment. It also lightens the body's toxic load by dissolving and eliminating petrochemicals, which are various toxins introduced into the body via food and environmental factors.

What it does

Let's look at some of the major benefits of ozone and its by-product, hydrogen peroxide:

* Tumours are inhibited because it is anti-neoplastic (kills abnormal tissue mass).

* Bacteria, fungi, viruses and yeasts are killed.

* Blood flows more freely which helps heart patients.

* Levels of interferon, interleuken-2 and other anti-cancer agents increase.

* The antioxidant enzyme system, which scavenges free radicals in the body, increases.

* The metabolism is stimulated so proteins, carbohydrates and fats are broken down and used as energy.

As it's so destructive to pathogens, you may be wondering why it doesn't destroy your good cells. This is because our cells have a membrane which ozone can't penetrate. Pathogens don't have this membrane, so the ozone molecule combines with it and oxidises it. Once the pathogen is oxidised into a safe product, your body disposes of it through the normal elimination channels.

My experience

When I tried the AHT treatment, I felt a variety of great effects. I felt super-strong, needed even less sleep, felt very happy, had less of an appetite, was mega-creative and productive and generally high, yet grounded. I put this down to the fact that my body wasn't having to fight so many pathogens, so could redirect its resources to assist me in my daily life. As much as I don't like to interfere with nature, the evidence I felt with my own body, combined with the astounding testimonials from others, has convinced me that ozone therapy is a great high-tech detox helper.

Further information

Books

The Yoga of Breath
A Step-by-step Guide to Pranayama
Richard Rosen
ISBN: 1570628890

This lovely book offers step-by-step descriptions and illustrations, so you know how to practise correctly. There are many tips, as well as the philosophy of pranayama to read up on.

Oxygen Healing Therapies
For Optimum Health and Vitality
Nathaniel Altman
ISBN: 0892817933

Described as an unpretentious, valuable guide to ozone and hydrogen peroxide therapies, this book really delivers. Demystifying and explaining many terms, this book speaks to you in a language you understand. This is a must for anyone interested in optimum health and longevity.

Flood Your Body With Oxygen
Therapy For Our Polluted World
Ed McCabe
ISBN: 0962052728

Ed stands out as a shining beacon in the world of true therapies. Each page of this book contains startling revelations about how you can heal yourselves, your animals and your plants. He discusses the history, politics and future of oxygen therapies in a passionate and very real manner.

Video

Breath of Yoga
Sophie Alexander and Lynda Hills

This video has its roots in traditional routines yet is adapted for people with busy lives to be able to open up to yoga. Correct breathing is emphasised throughout, and part 4 of the video is all about breath control.

Web sites

www.pranayama.org — here you can buy very inexpensive breathing technique courses for all areas of your life.

www.deepsloweasy.com/html/intro.htm — an online interactive set of breathing exercises, to help you breathe correctly.

www.ozonetherapy.co.uk — Ozone therapy information and practitioners for the UK.

www.oxygenhealingtherapies.com — USA-based, this web site also offers information and therapists.

www.williamhittcenter.com — Based just across the US border in Mexico, this doctor is your ozone miracle man, dealing with immunology, addiction and allergies.

www.medichina.com — This is the medical centre where I experienced my AHT ozone therapy. If you can't find AHT in the UK, a cheap flight to Spain may be perfect for you.

Colon cleaning

From the purity of air to the stagnation of faeces in one step... What you are about to read isn't for the faint-hearted or easily disgusted, but it is very interesting.

Your skin and your colon

Within the world of complementary therapies the relationship between the skin and our internal organs has long been recognised. There is a strong connection between the skin and the colon. A skilled practitioner can easily detect colon malfunction by looking at the client's skin. In other words, it's easy to "spot" if someone's colon is clogged, just by looking at their face. When you clean your colon, your skin will normally thank you for it, by becoming smooth and sparkling.

Colonic irrigation

Your colon is about five feet long — it eliminates waste and regulates your body's water content. Your colon is also home to countless bacteria which synthesise there, such as vitamin K and some B vitamins.

> Your colon really is like a hotel
> and you are a walking planet.

Because of the impossibly silly things we have eaten over the years, and the lack of exercise, our colons are probably not in the best of shape. Lingering waste material such as impacted faeces, dead cellular tissue, accumulated mucous, parasites and worms, are the hooligans from out of town, wrecking your colon-hotel. In turn, this makes your body-planet suffer and not be as productive or happy as it could be. When cleaning up our act, we need to find a way to re-establish harmony by gently asking our visitors to leave — or by hosing them out of town.

Waste material is quite toxic and some experts claim that these toxins can re-enter your bloodstream, making you feel ill or tired. You can also feel under the weather because impacted material impairs your colon's ability to assimilate some minerals and vitamins, so you become deficient in nutrients that you are actually eating. Also, when the colon is toxic, the muscular action known as peristalsis, which feels like a mild cramping and results in you doing your business, is slowed down and can cause a colon traffic jam.

Because of our lifestyles, we in the UK hold the trophy for the world's worst colons.

This is nothing to be proud of, as it can lead to colon cancer and death if we allow it to fester. If you suffer from backaches, bad breath, bloating and gas, body odour, confusion, constipation, diarrhoea, fatigue, headaches, irritability or skin problems, then the chances are that you are backed up. When you remove the toxins, your body will become more capable of functioning correctly. One in three people consulting GPs have a bowel problem such as irritable bowel syndrome, colitis and crohn's disease. Bowel disease has a knock on effect on the body and can manifest as other illnesses.

Sometimes you might need a little help with your regularity, especially in the first months of changing your life. Toilet habits become irregular, and it's not uncommon to swing from going ten times a day to three times a week, but you do soon become much more regular, and it all comes out easier, too.

If you feel you need added assistance until your sporadic toilet visits regulate, a colonic or enema will help you get it all out. The experience of having a colonic is unique. I found my first one to be pleasant, and I was intrigued at what came out. I passed a lot of "silt" as the therapist called it — old stuff that had been trapped for a long while.

A colonic (or colonic hydrotherapy to give it its proper name) should only be administered by a trained therapist. The therapist gently inserts a tube into your bottom (it's greased so there's no pain) and then slowly introduces water. The therapist rubs your tummy to help circulate the water, and then it's drained out along with the bowel contents. This is repeated several times, and each time the water goes further until all five feet of your colon is empty. Sometimes a herbal solution is used which can encourage impacted faecal matter to be released from the colon walls. Also, probiotics can be implanted at the end of the treatment.

If you have a healthy colon it often follows that you have a healthy body.

Interestingly colonics were recorded even around the time of Jesus:

"Seek, therefore, a large trailing gourd, having a stalk the length of a man; take out its inwards and fill it with water from the river which the sun has warmed. ...suffer the end of the stalk of the trailing gourd to enter your hinder parts, that the water may flow through all your bowels. ...Then let the water run out from your body, that it may carry away from within it all the unclean and evil-smelling things of Satan. And you shall see with your eyes and smell with your nose all the abominations, and uncleannesses which defiled the temple of your body; even all the sins which abode in your body, tormenting you with all manner of pains." Extracted from the wonderful book **The Essene Gospel of Peace**, Book One, translated and edited by Edmond Szekely.

Although colonics are as old as the hills, some argue that they do not clear out impacted faecal matter, that they cause good bacteria to be lost and that you can ruin the whole ecosystem in your colon hotel. On the other hand, colonic hydrotherapists state that the washing out of putrefied material increases the good intestinal flora because good bacteria can only breed in a clean environment which is free of putrefaction and its accompanying harmful bacteria. They also state that valuable nutrients can better be absorbed in a clean environment than in a putrefied one. I feel that if you've ever treated your body more like a landfill site than a temple, a colonic could help you feel better, cleaner and happier.

Work it

As well as cleansing the colon, colonics exercise the colon muscles. Healthy people can feel this action naturally, but people who are eating a standard western diet (which leaves them without enough fibre or water) don't feel it. Instead of the colon actively pushing the waste matter out, the colon is so full that the waste matter pushes itself out! If you don't feel peristalsis naturally, then a course of colonics could be just the type of internal aerobics you need to get you going. In addition, the colon gradually re-shapes itself, so deformed pockets, twists and other problems can disappear.

Enemas

Enemas are used to empty the rectum, which is the lowest 8 to 12 inches of the colon. They come into their own when you are suffering from constipation, which can sometimes happen with sudden diet changes, when fasting or when on juice cleanses. Constipation is so uncomfortable, that I totally endorse the relief that enemas can give. However, if you are constantly constipated you must see a specialist, as it's obvious something isn't working right in your body. Please do not rely on enemas or colonics for regular means of emptying out.

Enemas are also for cleansing your body with herbs, coffee, MSM and spirulina.

Making a date with the toilet

You know when your colon is healthy, because your toilet habits regulate. The healthy transit time of food through our bodies should be less than 24 hours. The average UK transit time is 60 hours for men and 70 hours for women. Healthy animals and people who live more natural lives, such as the Aboriginal people, empty their bowels soon after each meal. The actual poo itself (or stool, if we're going to get into words which no one actually says in real conversation) should come out quickly and easily, with no straining, and should begin to break apart in the toilet. If you only go once a day or even less, or if you squeeze and strain or if your result is more like a log, your colon has some serious exercising and cleansing to do.

Start off by increasing your water or fresh juice intake, and make sure your diet is full of natural fibre (the sort you find in fresh fruit and vegetables, not the stuff which is sprinkled on your cereal). Then, make a series of appointments with a colon hydrotherapist, to accelerate your healing and cleansing.

It smells of roses!

After eating this way for so long, your poo will not stink, it will actually start to smell attractive. I still can't believe the stench when I go into public toilets, because of all the putrid rotting flesh being expelled from people. I am so glad that doesn't come out of me.

Further information

Book

Colon Health, The Key to Vibrant Life
Dr Norman Walker
ISBN: 0890190690

This author is one of the most amazing people in the world. He lived to well over 100, and even has a juicer named after him. Dr Walker details how to do colon cleanses to ensure you remain in the best of health. I recommend this book to everyone interested in having a fully functioning body.

Web site

www.colonic-association.com — You can find many therapists and lots of information here.

Exercise

I cannot overemphasise how important exercise is. Look back to your nature video and see what animals do to keep fit. They certainly don't spend hours at a computer, and then further hours slumped in front of a television, all the time thinking "I'll do something tomorrow". So why do we humans seem to be so inherently lazy and unmotivated?

Becoming motivated

Much of our lack of motivation is created by our lifeless food, which causes us to be lifeless. We are what we eat, after all. We also have social conditioning and energy conservation issues to overcome when changing the way we respond towards exercise. No other animals think that they must exercise, they do it because it's intrinsic to their lifestyle, unlike us. However, we can change things.

I've successfully used InnerTalk technology with my clients to get them over the exercise hurdle. It's shown that even the biggest couch potatoes turn into shoestring fries! Have a look at the section called *Natural mind training* for more information.

also, when you start to eat food that's alive, you feel alive. You won't be able to slump for hours on end when you have eaten food that gives you real energy.

Once you are exercising regularly you are more likely to continue, as it becomes habitual. There is nothing more satisfying than looking back at old photos of yourself complete with spongy legs, and then looking down at your smooth toned pins, so do remember to take a few pictures to enable you to make this smug comparison.

Though all forms of exercise are valid and great for you, the one I'm focussing on here is rebounding, because it reaches every part of you and doesn't cause stress to your joints. Swimming would also be in my top five recommended exercises. My number one exercise is playing. Most adults who rediscover their ability to play, find that their bodies move as they were designed to and life seems so much easier. If you feel far too grown up to play, do the next best thing and go out dancing. Dancing is a top activity for making you feel happy, so now you can justify those late nights out, so long as you catch up on your sleep soon afterwards!

What is a rebounder?

A rebounder is a little trampoline, and when used properly is very safe. Some fold in half which saves on storage space. You can use it indoors as most ceilings are high enough for you not to hit them! If you only want to take up one form of exercise to assist with your detoxing, then go for the rebounder. It's an all-round workout, which is fun, quick, cheap, space-saving and easy. People of all ages can rebound. Children love the thrill of it, older people love the gentleness of it.

How do I use it?

I recommend rebounding above most other exercises because you can notice a big difference in a small amount of time. This is really the busy person's exercise. If you only have 10 minutes a day to spare, this is the exercise for you. The makers of the rebounder claim that 10 minutes rebounding produces the same results as 30 minutes jogging, and because you aren't pounding on a hard surface, your body doesn't get shocked.

To get started, just jumping up and down will give you results. I like to rebound to music, and do all silly arm and leg movements and it actually improves co-ordination. You can do situps on a rebounder, which is really comfortable. If you're not sure what else to do, you can buy an accompanying specialist rebounding video.

Who is it good for?

Everybody! People of all ages benefit from this form of exercise.

If you suffer from arthritis, cystic fibrosis, heart problems, MS, Parkinson's disease, varicose veins etc, you could well notice an improvement in your symptoms. As rebounding affects every single cell, muscle and organ all at the same time, your body quickly undergoes noticeable positive changes.

NASA states "Rebound exercise is the most efficient and effective form of exercise yet devised by man."

Rebounding and your lymph

Because the lymph system doesn't have a pump of its own (unlike the blood system which relies on the heart to move it around), we need to do something to move our lymph. If we don't move it, trapped toxins start building up and turning nasty. Luckily, it's easy to move it — just move yourself! By moving yourself, you breathe more, and this causes the lymph to move, which in turn helps to remove toxins.

Rebounding is a great way to get your lymph going, and it's so much fun.

What does it do?

Other benefits to you when rebounding include:

* Improved co-ordination
* Faster reflexes
* Better circulation
* Increased mobility
* Higher energy levels
* Loss of excess weight
* Reduced pain
* Reduced stress
* Reduced tension
* Improved muscle tone
* Boosted immune functions

Further information

CDs

InnerTalk's *Excellence In Sport* covers body building, golf, judo, tennis and many more activities. However, for most people I would recommend **Joy of exercise and being fit**, which will quickly change your way of thinking so that you love exercising, without you having to procrastinate for years first. I remember the first time I played this CD, I suddenly found myself in my exercise clothes, running up and down the stairs, not knowing what had got into me!

Video

Cardio-bounce plus video
Margaret Hawkins

A great video to inspire you when atop your rebounder.

Web site

www.keepingfit.co.uk — this has a great section on which types of exercises you might want to take up. There's even a discussion forum, so you can keep super-motivated with other like-minded people.

Laughing

Laughter therapy, also called humour therapy, has been known to cure people of cancer. As cancer is a symptom of an extremely toxic body, then it's clear that we can use laughter as a detoxification tool.

Originally used alongside medical procedures, some people now opt to try laughter as a cure on its own before considering going under the knife — and it has worked. Laughter increases the number and activity level of natural killer cells that attack viral-infected cells and some types of cancer and tumour cells. So you can literally laugh toxins out of your body!

What it does

Laughter has been proven to:

- Relieve pain and increase tolerance to pain, by releasing the body's natural painkillers — endorphins.

- Relax, as stress hormones such as epinephrine, cortisol, dopac and growth hormones are lowered.

- Reduce emotional stress, by reducing stress hormones.

- Boost the immune system as it activates the fighting T-cells and disease-fighting proteins known as Gamma-interferon and disease destroying antibodies called B-cells.

- Lower blood pressure, especially in women.

- Increase muscle flexion.

- Give your body an internal massage.

How it works

When you laugh, you breathe much more, taking in and using more oxygen. Your heart rate increases, which stimulates the circulatory system. As we know from the sections on breathing and exercise, these actions prompt the body to detox faster and more efficiently. As stated above, it also releases and inhibits a cocktail of hormones and cells which benefit your body.

How it can help you

When on the detox plans, we can make use of this information. If you ever feel a strong period of emotional detox, put on your favourite comedy video and start laughing. This doesn't suppress the emotions coming out, but it will boost your feel–good hormones, so you can continue living your life easier.

If you find yourself detoxing through your lungs, you can increase their strength by laughing. The antibody IgA (immunoglobulin A) is released when laughing, and fights upper respiratory tract diseases.

The beneficial effects of laughing can last all day, so it could be worth trying ten minutes of laughter in the morning. If you journey to work, buy yourself a comedy tape or CD and play it in your car or on your headphones in the mornings. You will be much healthier for the rest of the day.

> The best effect of all is that laughter can inspire you to try something new, to think differently, and can change your beliefs.

When you spend a significant amount of time laughing, it's as if a door in your mind opens, and as you walk through it, you have a whole new room of possibilities open to you. This side-effect of laughing complements exactly how you will feel with your other detox techniques, so do get serious about laughing.

Further information

Book

The Healing Power of Humor
Techniques for Getting Through Loss, Setbacks, Upsets, Disappointments, Difficulties, Trials, Tribulations, and All That
Allen Klein
ISBN: 0874775191

Web sites

www.laughteryoga.org

A web site featuring "The Giggling Guru", the man who has developed the new concept of Laughter Yoga by combining ancient yoga techniques with the science of laughter for health, happiness and world peace. It lists all current European laughter workshops and a comprehensive list of American laughter clubs.

www.worldlaughtertour.com

Valuable life-enhancing information, such as "Sense of humour is the #1 romantically attractive trait".

Things to do

- Find a laughter workshop in your area, and treat yourself to some fun time away.
- Rent or buy a video of your favourite comedian or comedy film. Watch it with friends for a bigger laugh.
- Have a pillow fight and bounce up and down on your bed!
- The secret of comedy is in the timing. When you know you're pre-menstrual, make sure you have a laughter source close at hand (with some raw chocolates close to the other hand).

Massages and wraps

This has to be the most luxurious part of detox. Most people in the world love to receive massages, and if you're one of them, you're in for a treat. It's great to know that massages don't just make you feel good — they perform a really important function. As well as positively affecting your physical health, massages provide one of our basic needs — touch. I have a book on hugging that says you need at least four hugs a day just to function! It's the same with massages, life is so much easier with massage in it.

Massage

Good massages will move toxins which are stuck in the lymph nodes and get them into the bloodstream, where the body can deal with them. You've probably heard of lymphatic drainage massage, where the therapist works on moving toxins towards the lymph and stimulating the body to release trapped toxins. There are a whole host of other massage techniques, and all of them are valuable when detoxing.

Researchers have made connections with impacted colons and breast cancer, due to the backing up of lymph fluid. This is why we have to look at our health from a distance, not close up to the problem area. Once we clean all of the body, overall immune and absorption functions increase, which in turn gives you a perfect working machine.

Aromatherapy massage uses essential flower and plant oils in conjunction with touch. Some of these oils assist in the detox process. Ask your therapist for a detoxifying massage, and she or he will create the most suitable blend for you. If you are self-massaging, try blends using some of the following: bergamot, black pepper, eucalyptus, fennel, frankincense, ginger, grapefruit, juniper, rosemary or sandalwood. Please be aware that some essential oils should not be used during pregnancy, so refer to an aromatherapy book for usage instructions.

Wraps

If you've ever had a mud wrap, you'll probably recall the luxurious feeling of silky smooth skin, more skin tone, and feeling thinner. This isn't just down to the tight bandages! Mud wraps do draw toxins out of the skin, because they act like dirt magnets.

I've been told that if you surround an egg with clay and leave it for a day or two, when you crack it open, there would be nothing in the egg. Not being one to do such things to eggs, I can't confirm it, but it does make sense as clay absorbs stuff so readily. When we think about wrapping ourselves in clay, we can now understand how it works.

I used to use red Spanish clay straight from my garden to do mud wraps, but in the UK, that's not so possible! Luckily, the experience is great, no matter which type of mud you use. If you can't visit a salon for this lovely treatment, you can buy clay from many natural health and beauty companies. You can also create a body wrap out of other products, such as algae, oil, salt, ginger or lime.

Types of clay

Green clay acts fast to absorb oils and toxins. Use this if you are short of time, or if your skin is oily.

White clay is very gentle. Use this if your skin is sensitive, mature or very dry. It will purify, soften and exfoliate your skin.

Fuller's earth absorbs bacteria and toxins. Used as a body or face mask, the slightly gritty texture is great for exfoliating. If you accidentally ingest a poison, eat some Fuller's earth. It will absorb some of the poison, and stop you being so ill.

What happens when you are wrapped

You are in a warm environment, and your therapist paints or rubs mud or another absorbing product all over you. You are then wrapped in plastic wrap, bandages or foil, and then wrapped up in very warm blankets. A while later, you are unwrapped and you shower to remove the product. Your skin glows, you feel great, and the effects remain for several days. If you want to treat yourself while on your detox, this is the one!

Benefits

As well as drawing out toxins from the skin, mud wraps remove the dead layer of skin and make you feel smooth and silky all over. On a deeper level, mud wraps can offer relief from joint and rheumatic pain, even out the skin tone and scars and improve the complexion. As clay can absorb excess radiation, cancer patients undergoing radiation therapy can find relief to skin burns by using clay between treatments.

Eating your mud

This isn't just something pregnant ladies do! Many wild animals will eat mud, especially the vegetarian animals. Clay is such a great absorber, that it can neutralise gas, toxins and pathogens from your insides when eaten. Even peat is eaten by some, and has been noted to boost the immune system and enhance the production of cancer-killing cells. If you are interested in investigating this subject further, talk to your local herbalist or natural health practitioner.

Further information

Books

KISS Guide to Massage
Clare Maxwell-Hudson
ISBN: 0751334375

This book is in the "Keep It Simple" series, and is a great introduction to many forms of massage. Detailing techniques, and giving information about oils and equipment, this book makes an excellent starting place for anyone wanting to know more about massage.

A Place to Spa
Eloise Napier
ISBN: 1840912731

If you're going to treat yourself in style, this book will help you choose where to splash your cash. There are details on some of the world's best spas ranging from holistic sanctuaries to island resorts. This is the book to buy if you really believe you deserve the best. Just remember to take me with you!

Web site

www.massageresource.com — A wonderfully easy-to-navigate web site, which tells you about all the different types of massage, and provides a resource for finding a therapist near you.

Things to do

- If money is tight, get together with a friend and do a massage swap. Massage each other on different days, otherwise you'll lose out on the magical post-massage effect.

- Buy a mud wrap treatment from a natural cosmetics store, and pamper yourself for a day. Ask a friend or partner to help, as it feels so much better when you experience the touch of someone else.

- Book a special massage at a local salon, and ask someone to drive you there and back, so you can make the most of your relaxing time.

- Make sure you hug your loved ones every time you greet them.

Meditation

Thankfully, this wise practice is slowly trickling into our skeptical western society and is being accepted as a means of lowering stress, building immunity and assisting in the quest for joy and a quiet mind.

What is meditation?

Meditation can be something to practise which relieves the symptoms of western living, it can be used in religious practices, and it can also be used as a way of feeling your connection with the universe. It doesn't have to take any particular form, so you don't have to sit in lotus position with a candle in front of you, unless you want to! It really just means contemplative practice, as that is all you do when you meditate.

Recently, scientists have started to study the effects and benefits of meditation, which is great for those who need "proof" of something before they'll try it. However, many people in many societies throughout the world have known of its benefits for millennia.

Going inward

When we spend most of our waking life "thinking" or diverting our attention on other outward things such as watching the television, we lose a large part of our natural selves. Remember your wildlife video? Chances are, you saw some of the animals spending a great deal of time appearing to meditate. If you have any animals, you'll also see them do it, too. They are living a more present life than we allow ourselves.

To stop the madness, and detox our minds, we need to turn our focus from the outside to the inside. This is where meditation comes in — we can meditate to re-establish what we want and need in life.

> As soon as we stop thinking and doing
> we become human *beings*.

As we slowly get in touch with what we are, and remember the grand plan life has to offer us, we can then begin to live our lives in a clear and crisp way. Maybe you don't yet believe this but we all have a calling, something special to achieve or be in our lives. Meditation releases that distant memory to us, so we can become the best example of who we really are. Ultimately, as we learn to meditate through our daily lives, we return to a state we were born to be in: Bliss. Each animal on your wildlife video has bliss in its eyes. Each enlightened person you might have encountered radiates bliss. You can also rediscover where you left your bliss, and go back and fetch it. Once you are in a blissful state, you have ultimate freedom, regardless of your physical circumstances. You make things happen, you are your creator.

How to meditate

I've given some meditation ideas using mantras (words) in *Your seven day chakra detox*, and there are many more ways to meditate. Always make sure your telephones are turned off, and that nobody can disturb you. This is "me" time! An easy way to start is to sit comfortably with your spine straight. If you need to support your spine or even lie down, that's fine. Place your palms upwards.

Have a beautiful object in front of you and concentrate on it for 10 or 15 minutes. If your thoughts start coming in, repeat one word over and over, slowly and purposefully. You can do this either out loud or in your head. Another easy way to remove your thoughts is to concentrate on your breathing. Count in for four and count out for four.

If something happens, if you feel an itch or an achy leg, just observe it without judgement. Do the same for thoughts, observe and don't judge.

Once you have finished, go for a walk in the fresh air, light an incense stick, take a shower, read a meaningful book or poem, or write in your journal.

Try to practise once a day. If you have the time, aim for a practice of half an hour to an hour a day. If you don't have that amount of time, just do what you can. Even five minutes of sitting and repeating a word will benefit you enormously.

If you are really pushed for time, repeat a mantra whilst doing your daily chores. This is moving meditation and is just as effective.

Over a short amount of time, you will find yourself able to meditate for longer periods without your mind jumping in.

Very quickly you will notice that you are more relaxed and more consciously aware.

Once you are used to sitting still for this amount of time, you will be able to go into deep meditative states, where you can literally discover anything. This doesn't happen overnight, and sometimes requires the love and guidance of a guru.

Benefits of meditation

You will become wise. As you start to see yourself remain calm all the time, and realise the importance or unimportance of certain situations, you will feel an equilibrium that you never felt before. Old feelings of hate, anger, fear, jealousy and even pain will all melt away.

You will begin to know yourself and others more. As you make the connection that everything is one, and therefore you are everything, you will realise that you can, have, do and be anything you want or need, because it is all within you already. What's even more fantastic is that you will always begin to want what's best for your higher self. You will notice your relationships improve as you find expression and love more easy.

You will become more intuitive. This happens whenever you lighten your life, so if you develop your meditation practice alongside lightening your food choices and practising yoga, you will know so much more than you thought possible! You'll soon see how your old life restricted the real you, and you'll gravitate towards the things, events and people which serve you the best.

You will become less stressful, more relaxed, blood pressure will drop, your immunity will be boosted, even diseases can disappear as your mind and body begin to work in harmony with each other.

Further information

Book

Journey of Awakening
A Meditator's Guidebook
Ram Dass
ISBN: 0553285726

The author explores mantra, prayer, singing and visualisation within meditation, and offers suggestions on which method would be most suitable for you. There are many beautiful teachings and words in this book, which assist you on your journey.

CDs

Meditation & Visualisation
Medwyn Goodall

This beautiful music relaxes you and enables you to visualise or meditate easier. It will leave you feeling harmonious and tranquil. It is also excellent if you have difficulty sleeping.

Contact Meditation
InnerTalk

Many people now use meditation for bio-feedback purposes, stress management, pain control and the search for spiritual knowledge/experience. This programme facilitates deep reflective meditation that is often called contact meditation. At these deep inner levels, many things are possible.

Things to do

- Make a room in your house very peaceful and conducive to meditation. If you live in a noisy place, add some nature background music or an indoor waterfall.

- Create your own altar, where you place photos, feathers that you find on walks, stones and fresh flowers. Also place your hopes and aspirations on the altar, and watch them come to fruition as you concentrate on your special items.

- Join a local meditation group or go on a weekend intensive meditation course. It's a great way to meditate and you get to meet so many people similar to you.

Natural mind training

There are several ways of training your mind to co-operate with what you think you want, and I've never experienced anything quite so amazing, effortless and instant as the InnerTalk CD collection.

Most InnerTalk programmes feature a choice of music or nature sounds. Personally, I prefer the nature sounds as the music is pseudo-classical, which I'm not keen on. The only other sounds you hear are some dim and distant voices, which you can't understand, and shouldn't try to. They are actually speaking powerful, life-changing affirmations which your subconscious mind picks up on, even though you can't understand them.

What do you do?

Just play your chosen CD in the background, and carry on with your normal life — you don't need to listen to it, or to concentrate. This is because InnerTalk programmes tap into our natural human ability to absorb information even when we're not thinking about it. You can even play them when you are watching the television (and yes, there is a CD which will obliterate television addiction). There is also a set of affirmations in each CD, and it's recommended that you read these just once a week.

The makers of InnerTalk claim that you need to play the CD for 30 days to really change the way you behave. However, I noticed differences in myself after just three days, which apparently isn't uncommon.

There are InnerTalk CDs for all occasions, and I highly recommend that you check out their product list for one which suits you.

InnerTalk technology is backed by independent studies at leading universities, and proven effective by the hundreds of thousands of satisfied users around the world. In the UK, four out of five customers are so impressed by InnerTalk that they buy a second CD within a month!

How it works

Your left brain is naturally resistant to positive messages. Regardless of how many times we tell ourselves what we want to be like, only a limited amount of change can occur. This is why we often feel like we have the devil on one shoulder and an angel on the other! All those statements that you grew up with, such as "You're lazy, fat, not good enough, ugly, stupid" are in no hurry to leave you.

However, InnerTalk sidesteps the rational thoughts of your left brain and forces positive, permissive thoughts into your mind. Indirect messages such as "It's okay to succeed" enter the right side of your brain. If the messages were direct, your left brain would jump in and say "I've never succeeded at anything. What makes this time any different?", but InnerTalk sneaks the statement right past it!

The right side of your brain is known as the spatial brain and is associated with emotional and subconscious learning as well as creativity. It's less discriminating and absorbs information without question or analysis. Your right brain stores all those old negative words that we might have heard as a child. "You're ugly" and "You're no good" are buried deep within this part of the brain.

When we use affirmations and positive thinking, we are relying on our left, conscious, brain. However, our emotional imprint is too deep to reach, so regardless of our efforts, many negative beliefs will stay.

InnerTalk gets in to your deep subconscious brain. Its authoritative statements such as "I am beautiful" and "I succeed in everything I do" float gently into your brain and counteract all of those years of negative programming.

I like to call this positive brainwashing!

Because your analytical left brain can't argue with the permissive statement and the non-analytical right hemisphere simply accepts the authoritarian statement, your brain simply changes its mind about things!

Further information

Web site

www.detoxyourworld.com — We stock all of the CD titles on the **Detox Your World** web site. Here is a selection of the most popular amongst life-lighteners:

Accelerated healing and wellbeing	Sleep soundly
Powerful immune system	Freedom from junk food
Clear skin	Freedom from stress
Relax now	Weight loss now
Joy of exercise and being fit	Quantum younging
Fit and athletic	Up from depression
Healing the past	Energetic

Accepting change	Soaring self-confidence
Bliss: coherent emotion	Forgiving and letting go
Contact meditation	Centering
Love, light and life	Ending self-destructive patterns
Manifesting your vision	Self disciplined and determined
End procrastination	Personal power
Visualisation	Stop self-sabotage
Stop smoking	Freedom from substance abuse
Impulse control	Freedom from alcohol
Freedom from sugar	Natural breast enlargement*

I've added **Natural breast enlargement** to this section because I would rather someone tried this CD before even thinking about having a dangerous (not to mention bank-breaking) breast enlargement operation. So, although it's not technically a detox-related CD, it can help improve body image thoughts and offers a very safe alternative to the surgeon's knife and jelly-bags! I actually used this one, and went up a cup size. I then went up two further cup sizes when I had my baby! I went from A to D with no surgery!

Things to do

- Buy the InnerTalk CD which you think will help you the most, and play it for at least an hour each day for 30 days. As you don't have to listen to it, you can just go about your daily life! If you can't play it during the day, put it on repeat at night while you sleep — it will work perfectly.

- About 80% of people who buy an InnerTalk CD are so impressed with their positive changes that they buy another one in the same month! If you start to fall in love with the positive changes InnerTalk offers, then have a look at some of the spiritual titles to see what else life has to offer you.

Reflexology

This non-invasive foot pressure therapy has become increasingly popular over the last few years. We can use it to help us when detoxing, as it releases areas that are stagnant or imbalanced. Reflexology has been noted in ancient Egypt, China and India. Inside an Egyptian pyramid there are drawings of people having their hands and feet worked. In the ancient texts of China and India, reference is made to working areas of the feet.

How does it work?

Practitioners say that there are reflexes in the feet and hands which correspond to all of the body's organs and systems. When pressure is applied to those reflexes, balance is restored.

What happens during a session

On your first visit, you'll have a health consultation, so it will take a little longer. The therapist will wash or bathe your feet (this relaxes you and it's more pleasant for the therapist!).

Then the therapist will work your feet (sometimes the hands and ears, too) for about 45-60 minutes. Western reflexology practitioners generally only use their fingers and hands, and it feels like a hard foot massage.

When the practitioner finds a "crystally" area, you may feel slight pain or discomfort, or a grinding feeling under the skin. Generally, it's a very pleasant treatment, and most of the time you feel extremely relaxed and may fall asleep.

Because of the detoxification that occurs with reflexology, you may notice that you urinate more afterwards. This is due to stimulation of the kidneys. You should also notice that your other toilet habits are better, and even your circulation.

What reflexology can do

I've had excellent experiences with reflexology. Before I changed my entire way of living, I was extremely stressed. Many things in my body had stopped functioning correctly, as my hormones were way off balance. I had a course of reflexology by a lovely therapist called Kelli. During the first one she told me that she could feel a lump in my womb area. Years later, after detoxing my whole body, a lump of skin did come out of my womb! It is amazing what a reflexologist can "read" in your body. She also told me that my hormones were way off, and that my neck was tense, that I didn't digest food very well, and all the other things that I knew were wrong with me! But aside from the useful diagnosis, she slowly started to unravel this tense ball of wool that I'd become. Over the weeks, I noticed less pain in my body, I was happier, I felt less "stuck" in my life. It gave me enough of a boost to be able to look for other things to continue the good work that Kelli had started. Therapists often recommend a course of ten reflexology treatments to anyone who feels this imbalanced. That combined with some of the other detox helpers will really help the new you break through.

Further information

Book

The Complete Illustrated Guide to Reflexology
Inge Dougans
ISBN: 0007131119

This beautiful full-colour book explains how stress can be relieved and health can be promoted. The history and holistic importance of reflexology is explained. You also get a guide on how to treat yourself and a massive resource section.

Video

Reflexology
A Practical Guide
Carol Gilbey

This video is useful if you're interested in setting up a practice or just want to see the basic techniques used. It's extremely practical and easy to follow with its step-by-step approach.

Web site

www.aor.org.uk

UK association for Reflexologists. Find your nearest therapist, and more information on this fascinating subject.

Saunas — the infra-red variety

Saunas have been used by many cultures for cleansing, relaxing and rejuvenating purposes. We are probably all familiar with the hot coal saunas, so let's take a look at the infra-red saunas.

What is an infra-red sauna?

A conventional sauna heats the air, which in turn heats us and all other objects within it. An infra-red sauna does the opposite: it heats objects, and not the air. Infra-red heat penetrates about three to four centimetres below your skin which causes your body to sweat at a temperature of 43-49 degrees celsius.

Is it safe?

Hospitals have been using them for more than 30 years for premature babies, so they're safe for old and new alike.

What can the sauna do for me?

You can lose weight in an infra-red sauna. It helps your body eliminate excess moisture, salt and subcutaneous fat. In addition, sweating increases the heart rate which consumes additional energy. This sounds like a rather easy and pleasant way to detox, doesn't it?

At just above 43 degrees celsius fat becomes water soluble and can be expelled by sweating. One infra-red sauna session could burn as many calories as a 30 minute jogging session!

Toxins such as nicotine, alcohol, cholesterol and heavy metals can be removed by sweating.

There is also a pain relief effect from using these saunas, as your muscles relax and more healing oxygen is delivered to them.

Can everyone use it?

If you are on medication or are pregnant, you should contact your doctor first. Otherwise, enjoy!

Further information

Ask at your local health centre, beauty salon or gym if they are going to install an infra-red sauna.

Silver

It might seem strange to you, to use silver as a detox tool, but stick with me for a while!

First, I want to let you know about the difference between the silvers available. You may have heard of colloidal silver, but the best type is ionic silver. Ionic (angstrom-sized) silver is water soluble, and very very tiny, so it can go straight to work. For those of you into numbers: an angstrom is 1/10,000th of a micron. This makes it equal to one hundred millionth of a centimetre. The tiny size enables it to penetrate the cell membrane and it is then assimilated by the cell. Colloidal particles can't do this, as they're just too big. Colloidal silver is large in comparison and can get stuck between the cells. It actually caused one man in the USA to turn blue, because he'd taken so much! People came up to him and ask "Are you dead?" or "Are you a smurf?" I've been using ionic silver for years now, and there is no sign of blueness in me!

Silver is known as nature's most powerful antibiotic, yet unlike medical antibiotics, it only kills the bad, anaerobic bacteria. It also kills viruses, fungi and other non-aerobic pathogens. It is so strong that it can kill over 650 pathogens in your body. Further, there is no recorded case of resistant strains of viruses developing.

Over half of the world's airlines use silver to purify the drinking water aboard their aircraft. NASA uses a silver system for the water in its space shuttles.

Minerals are essential to our health, yet because of modern farming and eating methods, we are becoming increasingly deficient in them. If you detox your body without reminer-alising it, you may not receive the full benefits of this way of life. 99% of Americans are deficient in minerals. When someone is greatly deficient in even one of the major minerals, disease occurs. Minerals are so important because they are the foundations of health. All nutrients such as vitamins, enzymes, amino acids, sugars and fats need minerals to work. Minerals combine with enzymes into alkaline detoxing agents which neutralise the acid by-products of cells. Though I have experienced fantastic results on a combined ionic mineral plan, I have to say that silver stands out head and shoulders above all others when detoxing.

The history of silver

An old USA law required hospitals to bathe newborn babies' eyes in a silver solution. This was to make sure they wouldn't go blind if the mother had gonorrhea. As the solution was dark, it made all the babies have panda eyes for several days afterwards!

Gonorrhea wasn't the only sexually transmitted disease to come a cropper with silver — it was also used to treat syphilis at the turn of the 20th century.

Years ago, people would place real silver dollars in their milk to delay it spoiling.

Thousands of years ago, ancient Romans and Greeks discovered that liquids stayed fresher for longer when they were in silver containers.

Often we describe our royalty as having "blue blood". This comes from the fact that they didn't get ill as often as us commoners. Health historians attribute this to them eating and drinking from silver cutlery and goblets!

Silver in medicine

> ### Silver the bug killer
>
> Silver is the most effective pathogen killer known. It can remedy and prevent colds, flu and infections.
>
> It will kill the spirochete bacteria associated with Lyme disease.
>
> It will kill warts and verrucas within a few weeks, when continually applied topically to the problem area.
>
> When put into your ear it will destroy any pathogens and so cures earache.

Silver is so powerful, it can even neutralise sodium fluoride poisoning. Over the years, as antibiotics became more popular, silver went out of favour. Now, because of the way antibiotics are failing and causing ill-health, silver is being championed once again.

The results of using silver include more energy, less stress, and faster healing.

A silver compound is used in most of the major burn centres in the USA because it fights infection so readily. Even some elastoplasts contain silver!

How does it work?

Silver disables the invading organism's internal functions within six minutes of coming into contact with it. It does this by attacking their metabolic enzyme, also known as their chemical lung. Viruses are left unable to reproduce as their internal protoplast collapses and they can no longer reproduce. Once the invading organism is destroyed, the lymph and other elimination systems clear it out of the body. Now, you can see how all the detox helpers even help each other! Taking silver to kill invaders, and then skin brushing (as outlined in the next section) will really cleanse your system.

Pharmaceutical antibiotics destroy beneficial enzymes in our bodies, but silver doesn't.

In addition, normal doses of silver don't kill the good bacteria in our guts, which is also something that traditional antibiotics are very guilty of.

Can everyone use it?

Yes, unless you have an allergy to silver! It is totally non-toxic, non-addictive and has no known side-effects. Therefore it is suitable for people of all ages, anyone on prescribed medication and even pregnant women. It has no smell or sting, so you can even use it in your eyes and on your pets. When you taste it, it might produce a strange flavour — this is just the silver going to work destroying the pathogens in your mouth!

How do I use it?

Ionic silver comes in bottles, sometimes with a dropper. The common way to take it is orally. You drop the prescribed amount under your tongue, wait a minute and then swallow it. The average dose is about a teaspoon a day, but it varies from brand to brand due to potency differences. As it sits under your tongue, the tiny particles start to be transported around your body.

You can also take it vaginally or anally if you have infections or troubles in those regions. Used in the eyes or on skin, you should apply it every few hours, but when taken orally you only need to take it once a day or every other day for it to work perfectly.

You will feel the benefits in a few hours, or a few days, depending on what the silver is having to fight, and how healthy your body is. You can take more under qualified supervision for quick results.

Skin brushing

If you haven't yet tried skin brushing, you're in for a treat! You can stimulate and cleanse your lymphatic system by using a soft dry vegetable bristle brush. You can buy the brush from health food shops and cosmetics stores. It has a long handle which should be detachable for ease of use.

Some people also use the loofah to skin brush, as it is the traditional Chinese method, but I feel it's very harsh and not as effective as bristles.

Why skin brushing is great for you

We need to take action against the toxic stagnant fluid in our lymph nodes. One of the easiest ways is to stimulate the nodes with skin brushing.

The skin is the largest organ in the body and a quarter of your daily elimination comes through your skin. Therefore it makes sense to assist it if we live any life other than a totally natural one.

Body products such as deodorants, soaps and lotions as well as synthetic clothing can all play a part in causing more toxins to enter your body via your skin. Skin brushing can coax them out.

When you skin brush, you help your lymph system clean itself and you also keep your skin pores open. This encourages your body to discharge its toxins and metabolic waste.

If you skin brush for just three days in a row, you will start to notice your skin texture become smoother, your colour might change and lose any grey tinge, and your body will tone up so cellulite is less visible.

How it works

Many toxins are supposed to go to the colon to get ready for passing out of the body. Skin brushing causes the lymph to drain itself more readily of toxins and dump them in the colon. Then they are discarded.

Once the lymph is cleaner, it can get on with its proper job of keeping the blood and other vital tissues clean.

How to skin brush

This is such a simple technique for something so valuable. Just brush your skin once a day when you get up in the morning as you're waiting for your bath to run or your shower to warm up. When detoxing, you might feel the benefit of doing it twice a day.

> Taking only about two to five minutes a day, experts say that it's the equivalent of a twenty minute exercise programme!

You can buy dry body brushes from many supermarkets, wholefood stores and beauty shops. Look for a natural vegetable bristle, which gives a little but isn't too soft.

Go into a warm room, make sure your body is dry, and remove all clothes.

You can use circular motions or stroke in one direction, towards the heart. Do it in this order:

Soles of feet, ankles, calves, thighs, tummy, buttocks, hands, arms, back and chest.

When working on your tummy, make sure that you brush from the left of your body to the right in a circular motion. Imagine that you're following the direction of your colon.

You can brush your face with a smaller and much softer brush, or you can omit it. Don't brush across your nipples, as they might get a bit sore!

Once you've brushed yourself all over, you can do it once or twice more, or you can go and enjoy your bath. If you can bear it, have a cool rinse after your bath or shower, as this will help your blood circulation.

After a few days you will automatically be less tentative on yourself, as your skin becomes used to the brush.

As most household dust comes from the skin we shed, you can imagine how your skin brush may end up! It will last for years, and will stay beautiful if you wash it in a mild shampoo every few weeks and let it dry naturally.

Benefits of skin brushing
- Skin becomes tighter
- Dead, clogged skin is removed

- Cellulite is reduced
- Digestion improves
- Cells are renewed at a faster rate
- Your lymph is cleaned
- Your immune system is strengthened
- Your whole body is stimulated and so will work better

Side-effects

A few days after you first start brushing, you may pass some mucous when you go to the toilet. Don't worry about it, it's just some toxic lymph fluid which has drained into your colon due to your skin brushing efforts!

Further information

Book

Reveal Your Glow
Brush Your Body Beautiful
Donna Rae
ISBN: 0966328639

Donna has been a natural beauty consultant for over fifteen years. In this book, she teaches you how to glow using her four-step bodybrushing system.

The Tibetan Rejuvenation Rites

In the 1920s, a Colonel Bradford from the UK heard about some monks who seemed to defy the tests of time because of some exercises they practised.

He went in search of the hidden Tibetan monastery and did indeed discover ageless monks. They taught him the rites and the Colonel started turning back the clock.

A month after finding the Tibetan Monks, the Colonel stumbled across a mirror: "I stared in amazement, so changed was my appearance. It seemed that I had dropped 15 years from my age. It was my first intimation that I was growing younger; but from then on I changed so rapidly that it was apparent to all who knew me. Soon the honourary title of The Ancient One was heard no more."

A while later, a friend of the Colonel heard a knock at his door. When he opened it, he greeted a man who he presumed to be the Colonel's son. Needless to say, he was more than taken aback when the visitor declared that he was in fact the Colonel.

What is it?

My experience with the rites has also been remarkable. I can only describe the effects as feeling like you are going back in time. Though it has a grand title, the rites are not much more than simple play-like exercises, and almost anyone can do them.

You will notice a difference after a few days, though after a month you'll start to feel the mental and physical rejuvenation for which these rites are so famous. As you continue into the tenth week, you'll notice fantastic changes on all levels of your being.

There's no reason to delay practising your rites. Do it as you begin your detox, or even before. Imagine yourself rejuvenated in just a month — simply by doing five minutes of easy exercises a day!

What to do

Start your rites by doing five repetitions of each exercise. Each day, add another repetition until you are doing a total of 21 repetitions per exercise. Do these in the morning when you've just got out of bed and you'll really feel set up for the day. If you want to do them in the evening as well, feel free.

As with any exercise, you must check with your doctor before starting if you have any doubt as to your body's current capabilities.

Exercise one

Extend your arms out to the sides, and make sure your palms are facing downwards. Relax your shoulders. Bring your arms up in line with your shoulders. Slowly start to spin around in a clockwise direction. One spin is one repetition. Keep looking straight ahead, not up or down, as this might make you dizzy. When you've spun round five times, stop and take three deep breaths. Put your hands together and raise your arms overhead as you inhale. Exhale as you lower your arms out to the side and down.

Exercise two

Lie flat on your back on the floor with your arms down by the side of your body, placing your palms down. Breathe in through your nose and raise your head off the floor. At the same time lift your legs off the ground, keeping them straight. As you exhale, lower your head and legs back down, remembering not to bend your knees. This is one repetition. Relax for a second and then repeat four more times. When you've finished, put your hands over your tummy and take three deep breaths.

Exercise three

Kneel with your knees under your hips. Tuck your toes under. Put your hands on your bottom or thighs. Exhale as you lower your chin towards your chest. Inhale and arch your back. As you go back, drop your head right back. This is one repetition. Repeat four more times. When you've finished, put your hands on your tummy and take three deep breaths.

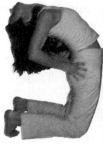

Exercise four

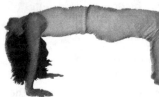

Sit on the floor with your legs out in front of you. Place your feet hip-width apart. Put your palms face down on the floor and point your fingers forward. As you exhale, tuck your chin into your chest. Slowly inhale as you raise your body off the ground. Drop your head back. When in this position, hold your breath and tighten all the muscles in your body. As you exhale, slowly lower your body down back into the sitting position. This is one repetition. Rest for a second and then repeat four more times. When you've finished, lie flat on the floor and take three deep breaths.

Exercise five

Come down on to all fours, so that your knees, feet and hands are on the floor. Make sure your hands are shoulder-width apart, and your knees and feet are hip-width apart. Tuck your toes under. Inhale and pull yourself up into an upside-down V shape, like the downward dog in yoga. Tuck your chin into your chest. Exhale and lower your body down and forward, bending your arms. Then straighten your arms and bring the top half of your body up, like the cobra in yoga. Tilt your head back and look up. Keep your shoulders back, not hunched, pushing your chest forward. This is one repetition. Repeat these movements four more times and then lie flat to relax for three breaths.

Exercise six

There is a sixth exercise, which is used to channel sexual energy. You don't have to practise it with the other exercises. It's good to practise this whenever you have an excess of sexual energy or wish to be celibate. Don't attempt it if you have no sex drive, as it won't have any effect. Practise the first five rites until your sexual urge returns, then you can turn your attention to this rite.

If you want to practise the sixth rite, be aware of its power: Tibetans say that it will turn you into a superbeing!

Close your eyes. Stand and exhale as you bend from the waist, placing your hands on your knees. Make sure all air is expelled from your lungs. Without taking in a new breath, return to an upright position. Put your hands on your hips with fingers at the front. Press your hands as hard as you can while sucking in the abdomen. Your shoulders and your chest will come up. Keep holding in the abdomen. Squeeze your pelvic floor muscle upwards. While holding this position, focus your closed eyes on the point between your eyebrows. This causes lower chakra energy to rise up to your higher centres. When you need to take a breath, do it through your nose, and exhale through your mouth as you relax your arms back down to your sides. This is one repetition. Breathe normally through your nose for a while before repeating.

How it works

The theory goes that these exercises work on your chakras, causing them to spin at the correct speed and in the correct direction. Once the chakras are spinning correctly, you achieve vibrant health. The feeling is like the exhilaration you remember as a child, and that makes sense, because most children have open and correctly spinning chakras.

Further information

Books

The Five Tibetans
Five Dynamic Exercises for Health, Energy, and Personal Power
Christopher S. Kilham
ISBN: 0892814500

As well as describing the Tibetan rites, the author discusses kundalini, chakras and breathing.

Ancient Secret of the Fountain of Youth
Book 1
Peter Kelder
ISBN: 038549162X

This book describes Kelder's experiences with Colonel Bradford, as well as a practical guide to the rites.

Vipassana

This is emotional detox, big time! When you sit for hours in one position, turning your attention to the space beyond your nose, for 10-21 days without uttering a single word or writing anything down, you face and overcome your biggest demons. This is not for the faint-hearted, yet if pursued correctly, it can transform you in less than a month.

Vipassana means insight, or to see things as they really are. It's an ancient Indian meditation technique, which was rediscovered by Gotama Buddha over 2500 years ago. By meditating vipassana-style, you aim to eradicate all mental impurities and gain the highest happiness of full liberation. Advocates say that having completed a vipassana course, they achieve healing at a profound spiritual, mental and physical level. Further, they promise that love, peace and compassion will engulf you.

The successful after-effects of vipassana means that the courses are becoming more widespread and accessible. They are even being taught in prisons. To go on a vipassana course, you just need to agree to the rules, and book yourself on. There is no accommodation or food charge. The centres rely solely on donations from previous attendants who have benefited and want to give back.

What they say

My good friend Shoshana outlines how vipassana has influenced her: "In the late half of my twenties I moved to India and dedicated myself to the study and practice of Yoga asana and meditation. I found India to be a fascinating lab for observing the mind-body interaction. I "sat" (meditated) through several vipassana retreats as taught by Goenka in which one spends 14 hours a day for 12 days of silent meditation, observing sensations on the body with an alert yet equanimous mind. I was pleasantly surprised to find that this resulted in the release of innumerable pent-up "Sankharas" or imprints, on a very deep level, causing among other progressive and psychic changes, an emotional cleanse and a physical detox on a cellular level.

"Having since been part of a 100% raw food eco-village in Spain as well as co-guiding and participating in 8-day juice/water or shivambu fasts, I can still say that vipassana meditation was the most powerful physical and mental detox I have experienced."

The courses

Once you are in the centre, expect to agree to a code of discipline. You will not talk or communicate with anyone for the length of the course. As you learn and practise the method, you will gain enough experience to continue at other times, as well as benefit on your particular course.

To calm your mind and allow for self-observation while on the course, you are required to not kill, steal, have any sexual activity, speak falsely and take no drugs. Very simple vegetarian food is served at the centres. You will concentrate on the flow of the breath, and this in time helps develop mastery over your mind.

After four days, as your mind is calmer and more focussed, you can observe body sensations, and understand their nature without reaction or judgement.

> The meditation of loving kindness or goodwill towards all is also learned.

Vipassana is a mental training, and helps to cultivate a healthy mind. Though your mind won't be totally purified in the ten day course, it will happen over time through continued practice. However, you will learn everything necessary to carry vipassana on in your everyday life. The more you practise, the closer you come to total liberation.

Though meditation is something you can practise alone, I would recommend that you first practise vipassana under the guidance and care of a trained teacher.

Further information

Book

The Art of Living
Vipassana Meditation As Taught by SN Goenka
William Hart
ISBN: 0060637242

This book shows how vipassana can be used to problem solve, develop unused potential, and lead a peaceful, productive life.

Web sites

www.vipassana.com — Many vipassana resources, including an online meditation course, so now there's no excuse!

www.dhamma.org — Find your nearest vipassana centre here.

Yoga

I didn't put yoga in the exercise section as it is so much more than exercise. It's a total mind, body and spirit unifier, it's a way to bliss, as is meditation, and certain forms of yoga aren't even physical.

Types of yoga

Our interpretation of yoga is frequently the one which uses asanas (postures or poses) to clean out the body and cultivate stillness. However, as yoga becomes more well-known to us westerners, we realise that there are many non-physical types of yoga:

Abhva yoga — Yoga of self-annihilation through meditation. The aim is to withdraw the senses to achieve a state of non-existence.

Ahara yoga — This states that our mind, body and spirit are made up of what we eat. This yoga is very relevant to this book!

Bhakti yoga — This is also known as devotional yoga, and uses the love of God to influence and change your life's direction through prayer, meditation and mantras.

Buddhi yoga — Uses the development of intuition and intellectual thinking to achieve enlightenment.

Karma yoga — The devotee takes the path of selfless action of serving others to achieve healing and spiritual powers.

Maha yoga — The practitioner seeks out-of-body experiences through awakening kundalini energy and shaktipat energy.

And I could go on! There are many many types of yoga that most of us in the western world wouldn't recognise as such. However, there are also many forms of yoga which use the physical body and asanas. Here are some of the popular ones:

Astanga yoga — Made famous by Madonna and Geri Halliwell, this is my preferred practice. It's a flowing, dynamic type of yoga which uses a very controlled method of breathing.

Bikram yoga — This is hot yoga, designed to expel more toxins and stretch muscles further. The room you practise in has a temperature of about 40 degrees celsius.

Hatha yoga — This is the yoga that most people recognise. Its aim is simple: for you to learn how to control the body to enable it to absorb the universal life force energy known as prana.

Iyengar yoga — This is a systematic, disciplined approach to align the mind, body and spirit.

Kundalini yoga — Movement, breathing, sound, meditation and chanting are used to awaken kundalini energy. This energy is spiritual and healing, and needs to be guided through the chakras, purifying as it goes, before it is fully released.

There are so many more forms of yoga, so I can't mention them all here. It's well worth you reading more about them all, as there is a type of yoga to suit everyone.

Why yoga?

Despite the many types of yoga, there really is one common aim: To create unity. This is done by cleansing and purifying the mind, body and spirit simultaneously. It's a great way to achieve equilibrium, so if you feel unbalanced in any way at all, yoga will be of great relief to you.

As well as detoxing you on a physical level, by promoting your lymph fluid to move, yoga detoxes your emotions. The great thing about yoga is that it works on everything simultaneously.

Further information

With the millions of resources available for yoga, this is the hardest section I've had to write! I eventually decided to list my personal favourites, but please explore further into the wonderful world of yoga, as it really is the practice for everyone. I do recommend that you find a yoga teacher, as well as using these aids, as postural adjustments can make all the difference to your practice.

Books

Power Yoga
Connect to the Core with Astanga Yoga
Liz Lark
ISBN: 1858689368

This book has been my constant companion from the moment I bought it. If you're learning Astanga yoga and would like a good reference book, this is the one. The design is fab, and the pictures push you on when you think all is not possible.

Yoga Mind, Body, Spirit
A return to wholeness
Donna Farhi
ISBN: 0-7171-3155-6

This book has over 200 pictures, and details of over 75 asanas. It's a wonderful reference book, describing the history and philosophy of yoga.

Magazine

Yoga Magazine — This is a relatively new and beautiful UK magazine which is being distributed worldwide. It looks at yoga from all aspects, from Abhava through Tantra and to Zen. For more information, please visit **www.yogamagazine.co.uk**.

Videos/DVDs

Raw Yoga
Kim Sol with David Wolfe

Raw Yoga is the leading edge in yoga practice and nutrition available today. Led by Kim Sol, accomplished Astanga yoga instructor and raw foodist, Raw Yoga offers solid, guided instruction for practising yoga students.

Dynamic Yoga
Godfrey Devereaux

A challenging video, not for beginners. If you want to build both strength and flexibility and become more relaxed, this is the video for you. It's a straight-talking video, which aims to push you to your yoga limit.

Learn Yoga
Beginners Class 1
Quantum Leap Group

If you've never practised yoga before, this is a wonderful introduction. The video has very good instructions and is easy to follow. There are then sequel videos to purchase once you are confident and well-practised at this one.

Web site

www.yoga.com — this is an American web site, which encompasses an online store and teacher's directory. However, there are articles and discussion forums which are useful to everyone in the world.

Things to do

- Find a local yoga class, and join up. Start at the level you're comfortable with, and remember there is no competition. Always practise to the level which suits you.

- Put pictures of celebs with fantastic yoga-toned bodies in your journal or scrap book for inspiration. Gwyneth Paltrow, Madonna and Christy Turlington will get you motivated!

- Fall in love with a beautiful yoga mat! The best I've found is the eco-friendly jute and rubber mat. it comes in some beautiful colours, and is also biodegradable. When you have beautiful yoga accessories, you often have more inspiration to practise.

All about food

Let's explore why you eat food, what effect it has on you, and which types of food are good, bad, ugly or beautiful.

What's the best way to eat food?

It might not surprise you by now to hear me say that the best way to eat food is to eat it as you would find it in nature. Natural animals might spend a while eating from the fruits of one or a few trees, but they would never mix twenty ingredients up to make one meal. When you eat like a natural animal, you may feel better than when eating any other way. When you eat the fruits from just one tree, this is known as mono eating. This is a great way to cleanse your whole body, and free up much-needed energy.

This doesn't mean get hungry, eat a packet of biscuits, and then lie on the sofa all day because you're too stuffed to move! If you look closely enough, biscuits are made up of more than one type of food — there's usually flour, sugar, salt, water, fat and flavourings and additives of all kinds. So that doesn't count, right!

Great duos and trios

To ensure you get enough variety and greens, try eating two or three types of food at a time.

Great twos:

- Celery, avocado
- Cucumber, macadamias
- Mango, watercress
- Figs, lettuce

Great threes:

- Celery, cabbage, walnuts
- Avocado, courgette, tomato
- Almonds, peppers, kale
- Galia, watermelon, cantaloupe

You will be surprised at how you can create really tasty and filling dishes by becoming simple!

So what does count? One type of food is something like a bunch of grapes, a head of celery, a plate of figs, a bag of baby spinach (oh, yes!), or just a bowl of apples. Mono eating like this is very popular amongst all primates, of which we are one type.

After you've eaten like this, you notice something happening, just as we discussed in the colonics section. Your gut moves! It's called peristaltic action: your gut literally starts to spasm and passes out the food that it's finished processing. This rarely happens with food that's combined, cooked, or processed. When this happens, your gut can finally start pushing out waste, rather than having to rely on you stuffing in more food in order to create enough pressure to force the other end open! A few meals of eating like this and you will start to feel lighter and cleaner immediately.

There can be a lot of waste in your back passage, which is called impacted faeces. It even sounds horrible, doesn't it? You're so lucky because when you've detoxed, your poo will smell pleasant. You'll also be able to go without straining — and it will look totally different! The more your meals are made of one or two foods, the quicker this will happen. What a great detox prize! Many people have even cured haemorrhoids by eating this way.

If you would like to cleanse deeply, and fasting isn't an option due to time or medical concerns, mono or duo eating is a great option. Remember that when eating like this, you're putting in a very different type of meal than is normal for you. Drink live water when you are thirsty. If you are hungry after a meal, wait an hour (drinking water as you need it) and then eat another type of food. If you don't wait, the food might not be gone from your stomach, and will be partially digested, causing fermentation and gas. Mono and duo eating is a beautiful way to eat, and I do it if I ever snack, and for at least one meal a day. But if you don't want to have all your meals like this, what's your next best choice? It's...

Food combining

Combining food has been made into an admirably complicated sport. Nutritionists say that your body can only release one type of digestive enzyme at a time, so if you mix two conflicting foods (such as a carbohydrate and a protein), one of them won't get digested, or they both might only get partly digested — giving you tummy ache, wind, and not nice poo.

When you eat naturally, most food combining concerns are eradicated. As I don't eat fish and chips, I don't have to worry and think "I'll have to have fish and vegetables instead"! While some will say that beans are flawed by nature because they contain protein and carbohydrates which can't be digested simultaneously (and they produce gas to prove the point!), I would say that it's then very obvious that beans aren't made for human consumption, so why eat them? Just because humans can eat something, it doesn't always mean we should. My diet is lovely and simple, I follow the laws of nature, and I'm only ever enthused by it. This is because I love simplicity. The simpler things are in life, the more you are opened up to reality, beauty and joy. Your diet shouldn't have to be complicated, and full of do's and don'ts — it's a natural act, just like sleeping and running. Eating techniques such as food combining only exist because people often eat food that their bodies weren't designed for. Rather than getting back to reality they'll search for every single possible way of staying with their addictive food, while trying to feel a bit better in the process. It's very interesting and entertaining, once your eyes have been opened, to see how people deal with the stuff they call food.

On a detox diet using my recipes, I would recommend that you don't worry about food combining. If something doesn't agree with you, don't eat it for a while. Usually, once you're cleaned out and functioning correctly, you may find that intolerances or allergies no longer exist. You can assist this by doing a three month course of MSM powder at one dessertspoon a day.

The easy way to combine food when eating my recipes is to realise your own limitations. Most people agree that as fruit digests in about fifteen minutes and nuts take considerably longer, you wouldn't want to combine them on a daily basis. Eat melons alone or with other melons. Eat fruit before other food, and wait an hour or more. Eat fats with plenty of greens. This could mean you'd have something like a fruit smoothie, followed two hours later by a large green avocado and olive salad.

Juice

We know the importance of eating green food for health, cleansing and rebuilding yet it's not nice or practical to chew through two pounds of vegetables a day! Also, we're advised to eat at least five portions of fruit and vegetables a day, but most people struggle with this.

Juice offers you an easy to drink power-packed meal that's really easy to digest. The nutrients are easily assimilated because they've been removed from the tough cells. If you ate the food simply by chewing, you wouldn't have access to all of these nutrients because they'd stay locked up in the cells. Juices help you massively increase your antioxidant intake, they detox you and they rehydrate you.

Juice has most of the fibre removed. We need fibre in our diets, and if you eat from this book most of the time, you'll have plenty, so it's not an issue.

Fresh juice is the most optimal choice. Nutrient levels are lower in bottled and heat treated juices. Organic and wild juices are better for you than juices laced with agrochemicals.

The most well-known juice health promoter was Dr Norman Walker. He invented a juicer, wrote many books on juice and health, and lived to 99 years young. I've noticed that people who drink a lot of juice look ageless. Dr Walker said this: "I can truthfully say that I am never conscious of my age. Since I reached maturity, I have never been aware of being any older, and I can say, without equivocation or mental reservation, that I feel more alive, alert, and full of enthusiasm today than I did when I was 30 years old. I still feel my best years are ahead of me. I never think of birthdays, nor do I celebrate them. Today I can truthfully say that I am enjoying vibrant health, I don't mind telling people how old I am: I AM AGELESS!"

Types of juice

I love drinking about 2-3 pints of green juice a day. My favourite ingredients are kale, beetroot (a great blood cleanser), cucumber, peppers, parsley, coriander and a touch of lemon. You could invent a different juice every day, and you can adjust it to suit your taste and nutritional requirements.

The best juices for health are green juices. Juicing offers the perfect opportunity for you to get lots of good quality minerals into your body. In the beginning, when changing your diet, this will prove invaluable. A good green juice can kill all cravings, as well as prevent you bingeing. When starting out with green juice, adding a small amount of sweetness such as apple or carrot makes the perfect balance. As you get used to green juices, the need for sweetness in your juice goes away.

Fruit juices are lovely to drink, and offer some of the tastiest meals on the menu. When I lived in Spain, I got big crates of fruit, and spent afternoons hand-stoning hundreds of cherries and then making pints of juice. That was the closest taste to heaven imaginable! However, drinking that much sugar all in one go isn't something you want to do too often. It can affect you adversely, so take it easy when enjoying the taste of fruit juices.

Which juicer to buy

There are some great juicers available. Some juice fruit better than greens, others juice greens better than fruits — then there are the juicers which juice both equally well. My advice with juicers is this: Buy or borrow a centrifugal juicer and see how often you use it. If you don't use it almost every day, stay where you are. If you use it constantly, then see about upgrading to a masticating juicer. They are much more expensive, but last for years, are extremely heavy duty, get more juice out of the food than the others, and do other party tricks such as making pâté, banana ice cream, and creamed coconut.

 I use a Green Power Kempo as it has the best juicer technology I've ever seen. Juice can stay fresh for much longer when juiced with the Kempo.

How to drink juice

Because digestion starts with the smell of the food (smell something you love and notice the dribbling!), and then with the saliva in the mouth, you must drink your juice in the same way you eat your food. Smell the juice, think about how it will feel in your body, and take small sips. Chew those sips, or at least swish them around in your mouth. This will ensure sufficient saliva gets mixed up with the juice, as it would with food, ready for the next phase of digestion in the stomach.

Food for thought

Here's where you learn some home truths. We're going to deal with the baddies that might be affecting your life. Remember, when I write about the baddies, I'm not saying "all things in moderation" as that's a very dangerous statement. Ultimately you'll need to decide if you want these baddies out of your life, literally, for good.

Dairy

Milk is heavily promoted as the best source of dietary calcium. This is all false propaganda, delivered by powerful milk marketing companies throughout the western world. Milk is actually a very poor calcium source for a couple of reasons.

- Most milk is cooked (pasteurised), rendering the calcium unrecognisable by the body. It is largely treated as a toxin.

- The correct calcium/phosphorous ratio for bone building isn't right. The ideal ratio is 2 to 1 or higher. The ratio in cows' milk is only 1.3 to 1. Too much phosphorus leads to progressive bone loss because it blocks the assimilation of calcium.

And of course, there is more

Ovarian cancer rates can be compared to worldwide dairy eating patterns. This is due to galactose, a simple sugar which is broken down from the milk sugar lactose. One gynaecologist says that women with this cancer often have trouble breaking down galactose. Yoghurt, cheese and other fermented dairy products are the richest sources of galactose and should be avoided.

Pesticides become more concentrated in the milk of farm animals and humans. Do you really want those toxins travelling into you or your baby?

When you drink milk, your immunity could be lowered or start to malfunction, as cows' milk proteins damage human immune functioning. Removing dairy from the diet has been shown to shrink enlarged tonsils and adenoids. Doctors experimenting with patients on dairy-free diets often report a marked reduction in colds, flus, sinusitis, and ear infections.

It's well known that dairy is a mucous producer, and causes great strain on the respiratory, digestive and immune systems. With around 50% of children in the USA having allergies to cows' milk, it's obvious that it is not a substance made for humans. The only milk made for humans is human breast milk.

Benefits of wiping off your white moustache for good

If you decide to give up milk, you may also find asthma, sinus infections, diarrhoea, constipation and fatigue making a quick exit, too.

Cows' milk is known to cause or aggravate these conditions in humans.

If you are diabetic, or think you have a high chance of developing diabetes, it's doubly worth considering giving up all dairy products. Studies have shown that the milk protein bovine serum albumin (BSA) triggers an auto-immune reaction which impairs the pancreas' ability to produce insulin.

If all this is true, why do "they" say that milk is good for you?

Because money talks louder than truth. Again, use your instincts.

What perversion of thought brought us to shove a baby calf to one side and spend the rest of our lives unweaned on food designed for another species?

Do you really feel it's natural to push a baby calf out of the way, and stick your head under its mother's belly? Do you really think it's natural for humans to be the only animal in the world who can't or won't wean themselves, ever? Maybe this is the breast or mother obsession manifesting? Maybe if adults had more of their own mother's breast as a baby, they wouldn't feel the continual need to steal the food of another baby.

Cows' milk is designed by nature for baby cows. Human milk is designed for baby humans. Once you are weaned and start eating grown up food, you have absolutely no need to resort to the baby food of another animal. It's just not logical, is it?

But what do you drink instead?

I only ever drink water, fresh juice, smoothies, herbal teas or coconut water but some people like the feeling of downing a pinta. If you want to give up milk but feel like you need a substitute, even if it's just for a while, then make the tasty and satisfying almond or another nut milk, as outlined in *The recipes*.

Meat and fish

Anything that comes from a dead animal fits into this category, so it could be fried octopus, a rump steak, snail's bottoms or sheep's eyeballs. Whatever part of a dead animal you're eating, don't you think it's only fair to eat it if you catch it and kill it yourself? Aside from the destruction of the planet because of mankind's unnatural addiction to meat, the distasteful and cruel raising and killing practices of animals for meat, and the ensuing politics, ask yourself one question: "Could I kill an animal to eat it?" If the answer is "no" or even "I don't like to think about that", then you're not alone. Most humans in the world are vegetarians. The massive non-meat eating populations of Asia see to that. On average, vegetarians suffer less from diseases than meat eaters. A vegetarian diet is also lighter on the karmic load, whether you believe in it or not. I don't advocate the common vegetarian diet, as I don't believe it contains enough nutrients to keep the body healthy, but it's one of the single most important steps most people can take on their path to en-light-enment.

The dark side of meat

Meat, especially cooked meat, is full of pathogens, negative karma and damaging chemicals. The foodborne pathogens are carried and shed from the manure of apparently healthy animals. According to Eric Schlosser in the fantastic **Fast Food Nation**, this can only mean one thing:

> "...a simple explanation for why eating a hamburger can now make you seriously ill: there is shit in the meat."

These pathogens are not harmless. They are bacteria such as E. coli 0157:H7 which carry and release the Shiga toxin. This toxin can liquefy the organs of the (human) victim. Most of the hundreds who have died from this toxin are children, but thousands of people of all ages have been hospitalised due to this bug — many of whom now suffer permanent disabilities.

Natural meat

Personally, if I ate meat, I would give up for the sake of my health! The processed, packaged, non-organic stuff available for sale to most people today will not assist you in your quest to become the best you can be. The only natural way to eat meat is to put yourself in a situation where you can catch it yourself.

Primates catch and eat small mammals, insects and other bugs. Some primates eat very few of these bugs, preferring the plant-based diet. As we have access to high-protein plant foods, it isn't even necessary for us to eat bugs if we don't want to!

The protein myth

One of the most common questions people ask me is "Where do you get your protein from?" Protein is constantly recycled in the body. I eat a high-green diet, so get lots of high quality assimilable amino acids. Hemp seeds, goji berries and maca are all high in protein. Even good quality organic fruit contains enough amino acids for us to make protein. Cooked meat, on the other hand, contains a protein that your body can't use. It has to waste energy converting it into amino-acids before it can use it. Consider this: A baby grows faster in its first six months than any other time, and so has higher protein requirements than when it is older. At this time its natural diet is mother's milk which contains less than 2% protein. Any well-balanced raw plant diet easily matches that.

The iron myth

While we're on the myths tip, I'll cover iron. Again, it's a total myth that meat-eaters have more iron than vegetarians. However, what is true is that new vegetarians need time for their bodies to adjust to the different type of iron. Once this has happened, anaemia is rarely an issue, especially when there's a good intake of organic greens. I know a few raw-plant-eating mothers who had blood tests during their pregnancies. Without fail, each mother had higher than normal levels of iron. None of these women had eaten meat for over 10 years.

You can test your iron levels by looking at the inside of your eyelid. If it's bright red, then you aren't anaemic. If it's pale pink then you probably are.

Because this is a detox book, and not an anti-meat book, I am not suggesting you give up anything immediately. What I will suggest is that after embarking on a detox plan, you hold off from eating meat for about three months, while reading some of the recommended books. If you decide to go back to eating meat after that, please make sure you do it very infrequently, you only eat organic meat, and you eat it with a big salad to buffer the harmful acidic affects that it can cause.

Grains

Grains stored for longer than 90 days often start to ferment. This is the perfect environment for mycotoxins to develop. Studies have linked oesophageal cancer and stored grains.

A nation's addiction

Think back to the times when smoking was considered fashionable, good for your lungs and an all-round health treat. If anyone was to say at that time "smoking is addictive and damages your health" you can imagine that they'd be laughed at. So everyone continued to smoke, and slowly the truth became known. This is how it is with grains. Though the damage is less obvious, it is there.

Grains are addictive because of the peptides called opioids. These make our body produce exorphins. Exorphins cause addiction, cause the appetite to increase, and they cause food cravings.

Because we didn't evolve to eat a grain-based diet, we are faced with a major food being unnatural to us, just as with dairy. Think about how many times you eat grain products. Is it in your morning cereal, toast or mid-morning snack bar? Is it in your lunch-time sandwiches, your healthy pitta bread, or your mid-afternoon biscuits? Is it in your evening pasta, pie, or sausages? Is it in the crackers you have with cheese just before you go to bed? Grain is everywhere! Even when we don't know it, we're more than likely eating it, as it's used as a cheap filler in many products.

What we do know is that as soon as we stop eating grain products, even for just a few hours, we start to feel withdrawal symptoms caused by the exorphins. This is why most people think about food as soon as they wake up, and eat a grain-based breakfast.

If you crave one particular type of food, eat more frequently than normal, are constantly hungry unless absolutely stuffed, feel anxious, are tired or feel overweight, then you may well be addicted to something in your diet.

Breaking the habit

When you break the addictive cycle of grain products you notice many positive results, so it is worth persevering. Replacing wheat pasta with corn pasta, wheat bread with rye bread, and cereals with non-wheat muesli all help without making you feel like you're missing out.

It's healthiest to come off wheat products gradually. Stopping overnight will cause cravings and can lead to bingeing and other food disorders.

Treat yourself to the **Freedom from junkfoods** CD from InnerTalk, and know that you have the power within you to change this destructive and controlling habit.

Salt and pepper

Fake salt

If you still want to use salt and pepper, use small quantities, mixed with dried herbs, or follow this **Fake salt** recipe:

1 head of celery
Juice of 2 lemons

Chop the celery into small pieces, and soak it in the lemon juice. Dehydrate the celery until totally dry, then grind in a mill.

Table salt is very toxic to your body, as it's cooked, bleached and processed in countless ways. If you want to use salt, then use unbleached sea salt, known as Celtic or Atlantic sea salt. This salt is grey in colour and slightly moist. It has many different minerals in it, and is actually health-giving in small doses. Pink Himalayan salt is another great choice and is really high in minerals.

Black pepper is used so much in our cuisine to reflavour the food after cooking the flavour out! It's long been accepted that it's carcinogenic, and so many people avoid it for that reason.

When detoxing for life, gradually cut down your pepper intake, and only use the salts I mention. Use lots of lovely fresh herbs for flavour, too. You will soon get used to less amounts of salt and pepper on your food, even if you smother it now because your tastebuds will start to come alive again.

Further information

Books

Fast Food Nation
What the All-American Meal Is Doing to the World
Eric Schlosser
ISBN: 0141006870

This is one of my favourite fact books! Find out about the gruesome working conditions, the cruel livestock conditions and the corruption in the farming industry. Your jaw will drop more than once when reading this book!

Dietitian's Guide to Vegetarian Diets
Issues and Applications
Mark Messina, Virginia Messina
ISBN: 0834206358

This is one of those technical books that some people lap up. It's mainly for dieticians and those counselling vegetarian clients, but gives great facts and figures to all of us.

Mad Cowboy
Plain Truth from the Cattle Rancher Who Won't Eat Meat
Howard Lyman
ISBN: 0684854465

Lyman is the man famous for telling America the truth behind their burger on Oprah. Oprah publicly declared that she'd never eat a burger again, and a court case ensued. With angels by their sides, Oprah and Lyman came out on top and the cruel, murderous and torturous meat industry is still reeling from the impact. This book is down-to-earth, good-humoured and well researched — just for you.

CDs

Freedom from junkfoods
Freedom from sugar
InnerTalk

These CDs will help change your mind about eating destructive foods.

Web site

www.notmilk.com — This is a well-known hard-hitting web site, which will give you all the information on milk that I didn't have space for.

Things to do

Get creative with a new fruit or vegetable every week!

Wild and organic food

You weren't designed to eat food sprayed with random chemicals, food engineered beyond recognition, or food that can't survive without human intervention. It's no wonder then, that if you eat this food, you won't be as strong and healthy as you could be. As more and more people are switching to organic food, prices are dropping and availability is increasing. The early adopters of organic food are to be thanked for this, and so are you, if you are now doing the same. My uncle often says to me "But if you have an organic field, and it's surrounded by non-organic fields, the organic field will also be affected by the sprays, so it's not worth buying it." Thankfully, those who have been buying organic for years didn't think like that, so the chances of that one organic field being next to another organic field are a lot higher now. Please don't be defeatist when it comes to making health choices. Too many people are critically ill just after middle age because they didn't seek out the optimal choices for themselves earlier on.

> ## Prevention is not only better than cure, it's an awful lot easier.

Introducing wild food into your diet

Nobody ate non-organic food a few generations ago, because it didn't exist. However, as crop strains become weaker through selective breeding and genetic modification, it's necessary to put a load of sprays on, otherwise the plant dies. Ask yourself: "Do I want to eat a plant that isn't strong enough to live without human intervention?" This kind of weak, low-life-force food will not keep you strong and healthy, it will ultimately make you weak and low in life-force, too. Why do you think weeds seem to grow anywhere? It's because they are perfectly adapted to the climate they grow in, and are naturally resistant to many of the diseases which kill lesser plants.

> ## Give me a weed to eat any day!

I'm not joking here: eating wild food, or what we would sometimes call weeds, can make you stronger than any other food. Try it by going on a nature walk with a good wild food book. Pick leaves, flowers, berries, fruits and nuts which appeal to you, and using the book as a guide, taste them, and feel the potent effect they have on you. If it's strength and power along with a deep connection to the earth that you're looking for, you'll find it in wild food.

All non-captive animals eat wild food.

Think of the majestic lion in your nature video, perfectly toned, and able to do its job without calling in sick. Think of the active monkeys, playing and loving all day long without shouting at each other "I don't feel like it today". These animals can do what they're supposed to do in life because they are eating the best food that nature can provide them. We can make that choice, too!

Lion's teeth

I am so passionate about wild food that I'll source it whenever I'm outside. After a while you just know what's edible, even though you might be in a strange area or country. If you don't know what to look for, go into your garden and check out the dandelions.

Dandelion fan club

Dandelions are a good source of calcium, potassium, vitamin A and vitamin C.

They have twice as much vitamin A in a one-cup serving than most vitamin pills. They also have more calcium than most other vegetables.

They are high in iron, phosphorous and the B vitamins and other trace minerals.

Most importantly to me, they are high in life force, because they're naturally strong. I let all dandelions live in my garden!

Their botanical name is Taraxacum Officinale, which means the official remedy for disorders, and they truly are medicinal. The leaves have a bitter-sweet taste, the roots are full of juice and life, and the flowers taste like angels made them. This plant will provide you with outstanding nutrition most times of the year.

In the same way that we grow lettuces, the French grow dandelions, and it's from them that we derived the name. Dent de Lion means "lion's tooth", and this refers to the tooth-like jagged points on the leaves. Although you can eat them any time of year, dandelion greens are sweetest and most tender if you pick ones that are not in mown grass. The best time to gather is long before the last frost of spring.

Eating just a few dandelion greens with your meal will assist in the whole digestive process, help you to assimilate more nutrients, and reduce gas and indigestion.

Go wild

Once you're used to eating something recognisable such as dandelion, take a look at what else you can see. Nettles (containing calcium, magnesium, zinc, iron, cobalt, copper, potassium, and B complex vitamins), chickweed (reported to be a lymph stimulant, containing calcium, iron, copper, magnesium, zinc, and vitamin A), burdock, lambsquarters (like spinach, but wild and free!), purslane (with EPA, vitamins C, E and beta carotene), shepherd's purse and many others are all there for the picking.

Ponder on this. countless money is spent on garden weedkiller. Then once we all have nice lawns, with no weeds poking through, we drive off to the hypermarket to waste even more money on buying lettuce! There's nothing wrong with good quality organic shop-bought lettuce, but it doesn't come close to the great nutritional value of wild, freshly picked leaves. Spare a thought for the conservation of the world and eat free wild food whenever you can. It's so nutritious, you'll feel better than ever!

When eating a low toxin diet, it's easy to see where you should be getting most of your minerals! These powerful leaves, stalks, shoots, roots and flowers can all be eaten direct from the source, or put into salads. It's best to eat them immediately, so you benefit from all the nutrients available. Strong leaves such as these are also your best source of amino acids, which are converted into protein. It's in a form that your body can instantly recognise and either use straight away or store until it's needed.

> A weed is just a flower that's in a place you don't want it, but they're all loved in nature's garden.

In nature you would eat wild food all the time, there's nothing strange about it. A low-toxin diet resembles nature as closely as possible. Go and eat some safe wild food today.

Fruit

Nutritionist Shane Heaton analysed studies which suggested that levels of vitamins, minerals and other nutrients are affected by different farming methods. As we are fruit-eaters, we need to be eating high-quality fruit. Over the past 50 years, mineral levels in fruit and vegetables have declined. While more research is needed in this area, it's one more reason to eat organic food because it's less messed-with than non-organic food.

> The average non-organic UK apple has about 20 to 30 artificial toxins on the skin.

Artificial chemicals on food

The public have been warned to peel their fruit and vegetables to reduce the risk of chemical exposure, but at what expense? If you peel something that is designed to be eaten whole, you will surely become deficient. The good bacteria on the outside of your apple or carrot is necessary for healthy colon function, and is a source of vitamin B12. Peeling your fruit and vegetables obviously isn't the answer to agrochemicals in food.

Organic food

Contaminated breast milk
A study of 1,400 women in the USA on widespread pesticide contamination of human breast milk found that contamination levels were twice as high among the meat- and dairy-eating women as among vegetarians.

Because it's unlikely that you'll be eating massive amounts of wild food (though I'd love you to prove me wrong!), making up the rest of your diet with as much organic food as possible is vital.

Eating polluted food won't give you vibrant energy!

I have seen, smelt, tasted and felt the difference in organic food. Most of it (not all, as there are always exceptions to every rule) is stronger, tastier, juicier, sweeter, and generally a lot more like it should be! I remember clearly my first organic mushroom. I licked my lips and said "Mmm, that tastes just like mushrooms in the olden days". Like I remember the olden days! I meant that they had the flavour people reminisce about with home food preparation. That first organic mushroom made me realise that it didn't matter if my weekly shopping bill was a little bit more, I'd finally found food that tasted like it should. My venture into organic food was half a health quest and half a taste quest. I loved food, and so anything that gave me better flavours naturally was worth having. I noticed that I stopped using so much flavourings and sauces on my food, because the organic food was so tasty.

Little stepping stones like this create a pavement to greater overall health choices.

Buying your produce

In the UK and the USA, organic delivery services are cropping up all the time. Most supermarkets now have a wide selection of organic produce. The Internet has a great choice of organic delivery, where you can order to your specifications online. This all results in much less hassle, petrol and wasted time for you. The USA has large organic farmer's markets, where the produce is sold direct by the farmer. This is now becoming popular in the UK, and means that you get the produce fresher and there's no middle man to pay. Some only happen once a month, so know that the more they are frequented, the more frequent they'll become! If you don't buy organic because of the price, think back to the early adopters who were sometimes paying up to five times as much for the organic option. The difference isn't so great these days, and sometimes it's cheaper, especially if you look at the bargain shelves in the supermarkets.

Start thinking longer term. The fewer toxins you'll take in today, the less you'll spend on healthcare, pills, potions and therapies tomorrow. When you think about the costs of non-organic farming and you widen your vision, there really is no comparison. The BSE crisis of the early 2000s cost UK taxpayers around £4 billion.

Organic food and the health link

Those who work with non-organic foods have much higher instances of cancer, respiratory problems and other major diseases than those in organic farms. Those working in developing countries have it even tougher, so please buy organic cotton as well as food wherever possible.

When I lived in Andalucia, southern Spain, I was aware just by looking at the rows upon rows of trees that it was the top produce grower for the whole of Europe. The weather there is subtropical in parts, and exotic mangoes, papayas, cherimoyas and other delights are easy to grow. In addition, other more everyday foods such as lettuce, celery and tomatoes are also grown commercially there. Over in the so-called "Tropical Zone" there are mountains covered in plastic, so farmers can double their crop quantities.

However, this extra work brought extra problems. Few locals would work in the vast non-organic plastic tunnels. Illegal immigrants were usually the only people to work in these very dangerous conditions. The locals knew the dangers of breathing in these toxic fumes, yet the immigrants were so desperate they had no choice. It makes sense that if these plastic tunnels are poisonous to the humans working there, the produce will be poisonous to the people eating the produce. Doesn't it? The only difference is the amount of poison, and that's why it's important to detox your body, to allow any stored chemicals to come out, thus giving you a stronger body to fight future infections, a clearer mind to make excellent life decisions, and a more content spirit to guide you to your higher purpose.

The more organic food you buy now, the more choice there'll be for you and your children tomorrow. Vote for healthy food with your wallet.

Some people insist that organic food is no more nutritious than pesticide-ridden food, and studies frequently come out sitting on either side of the fence. The studies I'm inclined to believe say that fresh organic produce contains an average of 50% more vitamins, minerals, enzymes and other micro-nutrients than non-organic food.

However, even if you just think it's no more nutritious in terms of vitamins, minerals and all the thousands of other chemicals that scientists are yet to recognise and label, consider the stuff that's sprayed onto them. "*icides" conjures up horrible images of criminal acts, violence and blood. Think about it: homicide, suicide, pesticide, herbicide! Why do we happily pay someone to give us food covered in *icides? These things don't belong in our body, our atmosphere, our land or our water. Don't let your body, environment, animals or children become victims to the *icides.

Non-vegetable food

Although I don't recommend or condone it for a million reasons, it's a fact that some people eat animals and their products. If you're one of those people, be aware that intensively-reared dairy cows and farm animals are fed a dangerous cocktail of antibiotics, hormones, anti-parasite drugs and many other medicines on a daily basis, whether they have an illness or not. These drugs are passed directly onto the consumers of their dairy produce or meat. This has to be a contributing factor to meat-related diseases such as coronaries and high blood pressure.

Try to eat more recipes from this book, have as much organic food as possible, and give intensively reared animal consumption a wide berth. Organic animals are stronger and at the time of writing, there has never been a case of BSE in organic cattle in the UK.

The environment you live in

People often talk about "the environment" as if it's a separate issue to our lives. Choosing to take care of the environment or not is seen more as a lifestyle choice rather than a necessity.

The facts, though, are cold and hard. If we don't "look after the environment" today, there won't be a tomorrow for humans.

Your children,
or their children,
will suffer the effects you caused.

We are using resources at an alarming rate, with little or no regard for the consequences. The diverse wildlife that makes up our ecosystem is supported by organic farming yet it's killed by conventional farming.

In the last 30 years, this is what has happened in the UK:

- Intensive farming has caused major soil erosion.
- There are about 70% fewer wild birds in some parts of the country.
- Hedgerows are destroyed.
- Many butterflies, frogs, snakes and wild mammals are near extinction.

> By simply choosing organic food,
> you are starting to do "your bit"
> for the environment.

Genetic modification

When you choose certified organic food, it is guaranteed not to be genetically modified, so you will naturally get a stronger and more tried-and-tested strain of food. Don't allow yourself to be a human guinea pig in this commercial venture. GM-reliant farmers are now unable to self-seed and have to constantly line the pockets of giant uncaring and unethical companies. My best advice to you is to stay well away from this monstrosity.

> In the UK, about 99% of non-organic
> farm animals are now fed
> GM soya products.
> That's another reason for taking
> a fresh look at the meat on your plate.

The low-down on non-organic food

This is such a horror story. Take a look at just two of the chemicals sprayed onto your food:

Lindane — also known as gamma-HCH, a dangerous pesticide which was still used until the early 2000s in Europe. It is a known endocrine disrupter and has been linked to breast cancer. Traces have been found in 8% of non-organic UK milk samples.

DDT — was banned years ago due to its effect on the nervous system and its link with cancer and the reproductive systems. Traces of DDT are still found in non-organic butter.

Pesticides, herbicides and other agrochemicals shouldn't be in our food — they are poison.

Middle ground

Because organic foods are not yet as accessible as non-organic, there will be times when you might buy non-organic. Here is a list of the best foods to eat as non-organic: Avocado, banana, broccoli, cauliflower, onion including spring onion, plum, sweet potato, watermelon.

And here are some to avoid when not organic if at all possible: apple, apricot, cherry, cucumber, grape, green bean, peach, pepper, spinach and strawberry.

Being realistic, there will be times that you eat food which is high in pesticides, even when you do your very best to avoid them. Bearing this in mind, it makes it worthwhile to always undertake at least one or two detoxes a year where you only eat organic food.

Interestingly, the Green Power/Kempo juicer claims to strip out around 70% of agrochemicals from the food it juices. If you are going to get into juicing, it's worth you looking at this model for that feature alone.

Fertilisers and the mineral connection

Non-organic food isn't just about *icides, it's about fertilisers. Here lies a big problem:

Nitrogen, phosphorous and potassium is collectively called NPK. It was discovered in the mid 1800s by Baron Justus von Leibig and used as a fertiliser to replenish over-farmed soils. At the time, he wasn't aware that using NPK prevented plant uptake of trace minerals.

For NPK to reach the roots underground, it's converted into the salt version of the chemical. As salt is water soluble, rain causes NPK to reach the plant roots. Without trace minerals, the growing plant has no immunity and so is often sick and weak. This makes it susceptible to insect attacks.

Remember that you are made of this material, too.
You can only be as whole as the
ingredients you're made of.

Animals who ate the sick and weak plants also became sick and weak. When the Baron realised the destructive nature of NPK it had already become popular with farmers, and although he tried to reverse its damage, he was unable to do so.

How plants and minerals get together

Green-leafed plants can only absorb minerals once they have been pre-digested by a particular fungus. Just as the green leaf converts sunshine into carbohydrates, the fungus converts ground minerals into digestible molecules.

When NPK salt reaches the plant's roots, it also surrounds and kills the friendly fungus. When the fungus tries to grow back to once again live symbiotically with the plant it gets hit again by another dose of NPK.

At first, the plant looks healthy. It's having its physical needs met by the addition of NPK, but it is weak. In this weak state, it broadcasts infra-red waves known to us as heat. Air-breathing fungus spores and insects are attracted to it, and they begin to feed on it, slowly destroying it. This is just nature's way of keeping weaklings out of the survival loop.

Because the plant is being attacked, the farmer sprays his field with insecticides and fungicides, and we already know why we don't want them in our lives.

Strong wild plants such as weeds are rarely
attacked to death like farmed plants.

The only way to avoid becoming mineral deficient, overloaded with agrochemicals, and ill from these effects is to go as organic and wild as possible — today.

If you believe you have a mineral deficiency, then supplement for a while with ionic minerals. These are fully absorbable by the body, you can't overdose on them, and they don't get trapped in your cells. I've used these minerals and recommended them to many people. They are the best isolated minerals currently available in the world.

Think your baby is safe?

We all know that breast is best when feeding your baby. Nutrients aside, feel-good hormones found in breast milk but not in formula milk make for a more contented child. However, toxins are powerful and will get into breast milk if they're floating around the body looking for a way out.

Luckily, women can minimise the amounts of pesticides in their breast milk very easily. The breast milk of vegetarians (and vegans even more so) shows lower levels of the pesticides DDT, chlordane, heptachlor, and dieldrin, and industrial compounds or by-products, such as polychlorinated biphenyls (PCBs) and polychlorinated dibenzodiozins. Virginia Messina and Mark Messina explain this all in the **Dietitian's Guide to Vegetarian Diets**.

This information confirms many other studies:

- Over twenty years ago the breast milk of many vegans was analysed. The levels of 17 chemicals were markedly lower than in non-vegans.

- A few studies have linked frequent consumption of meat, dairy, and fish to breast milk contamination.

- In the 1970s a study revealed that pesticide levels were far lower in the breast milk of vegetarian women.

The above results should make everyone think twice about eating animal products.

> I've always said that if I wasn't a vegan for ethical reasons, I'd certainly be one for health reasons!

Because plant foods don't store pesticides in the same way as animals do, they are much safer to eat, even if they have been sprayed. This means that weight for weight, non-organic fruit will have much lower amounts of pesticides than animal flesh or milk.

So if you're breast feeding or even planning a baby, take great care to ensure most if not all of your diet is organic and plant-based. This way you won't be passing on such high levels of toxins to your precious little one. And even if you're already breast feeding, please don't switch to formula, as you have more superior nutrients and feel-good hormones that bottled milk can't match.

Further information

Books

The Organic Baby Book
Tanyia Maxted-Frost
ISBN 187009879X

www.theorganicbabybook.co.uk — Read more about the dangers of commercial food, and the benefits of organic food. This book has an excellent web site too.

Super Nutrition Gardening
How to Grow Your Own Powercharged Foods
William S Peavy
ISBN: 0895295326

Peavy discusses links between the health and condition of the soil and the nutritional value of its food. Gardening and nutrition enthusiasts alike will benefit from this book.

Great Garden Companions
A Companion-Planting System for a Beautiful, Chemical-Free Vegetable Garden
Sally Jean Cunningham
ISBN: 0875968473

Instead of using chemicals, many organic gardeners use companion planting. This book offers you a workable way of growing pest- and pesticide-free.

Web site

www.organicfood.co.uk

Billed as the UK's premier organic food magazine web site, there is a whole host of free information here, and message boards for you to interact with.

Things to do

- Discover the beauty of wild food by foraging one day. Make a green juice with the edible goodies you find and add apple juice to taste.

- Start increasing your organic food intake right away. This is especially important if you're planning on having a baby or are currently breast feeding.

- If you are mineral deficient, or would like a nutritional-building-block boost, have a course of ionic minerals.

Cooking your food

People cook food for a variety of reasons. If they eat meat, they usually prefer the taste of cooked meat. Raw and undercooked meat is riddled with live parasites which can be dangerous or even lethal for a weakened human. Most nutritionists will tell you to cook your meat before you eat it.

Other food is cooked because it's inedible or not flavoursome when in its natural state. Cooked potatoes, beans and grains are invariably preferred over raw ones. However, as I have this lifetime obsession with "what is natural", I know that cooking your food for the reasons above just isn't right. If you can't eat it in its natural state, then surely, unless you are starving hungry, you shouldn't eat it at all, should you? Cooking to improve the taste, and to make the food more palatable is harder to argue against. It's an art, and art is an intrinsic part of our being. But again, I wonder. Cooking potatoes and grains turns starches into sugars, or complex carbohydrates, as nutritionists would say. As we're naturally frugivorous, it's those sugars that we want.

We crave sugar because it's our number one energy source in nature.

Cooking our food for nutritional reasons means we have no faith in nature. Did nature make a mistake by only offering 3025 micrograms of lycopene in 100 grams of raw tomato, when its cooked counterpart has twice that? Or could it be that we really only need 3025 micrograms of lycopene in 100 grams of raw tomato? And do we need another substance which is destroyed in the cooking process to utilise the lycopene or other tomato nutrients in our bodies? Scientists don't have all the answers, otherwise they'd never be discovering new information every day. Putting your faith in the hands of a scientist is not going to win you health, happiness and liberty. Trusting nature and rediscovering your intuition will.

Chemical changes in food

Cooking causes major chemical changes to the food and cooked food contains new and unrecognisable chemicals. Your body doesn't recognise them and treats them as toxins. It creates an immune response, and produces many white blood cells to go and disarm the invaders. Ultimately, your immunity really suffers because it's made so many attacks on the "food" you've eaten, and so becomes depleted.

A good example of this is the simple potato, which is used in some detox programmes. When it is baked, it contains over 400 more chemicals than when it is raw. As we're undergoing a detox, we want to remove ourselves as far from all known sources of toxins as possible, so we spend this time eating a diet which has not been cooked.

In my recipe book, **Detox Delights**, I've created over 100 delicious and sometimes sinful-looking recipes which will make you love food that loves your body. In this book, there are another 100+ recipes. This all goes to show that you don't lose out on variety or enjoyment when eating healthily.

If this looks a bit too different for you to try, please trust me for a while! The detox plans are carefully worked out so that you gain maximum energy with minimal cravings.

The hot news from Sweden

A recent finding at Stockholm University's Department of Environmental Chemistry revealed that high levels of acrylamide exist in foods such as bread, rice and potatoes. The US Environmental Protection Agency classifies acrylamide as a medium hazard probable human carcinogen. It has already been proven that it causes cancer and nervous system damage in non-human animals.

This is all down to a carbohydrate found in cereals and potatoes which transforms into acrylamide when cooked or heated.

This amazing find caused "crisis meetings" around the globe. Can you imagine: the food you eat every day, once, twice or three or more times, could give you cancer? Don't wait for the scientists to prove something that natural law tells us, as you could be risking your life. Cut out or cut down on cooked food — especially bread, pasta, cereals and potatoes.

Your body has an immune response when you eat cooked food

When you ingest cooked food, your body acts as if it has been poisoned. White blood cells are produced and rush to your defence. This immune response is known as leukosytosis. If you eat raw food, or at least 50% raw food by weight in each meal, this doesn't happen.

All forms of cooking change the structure of the cells within the food, such as the baked potato's 400 chemicals mentioned above. Your body has to try and do something with these new and unrecognisable chemicals. When your body has to deal with this chemical assault on a daily basis, over weeks, months and years, it doesn't have the time or energy to do normal housecleaning and repair. It also has to find safe places to put the chemicals that it doesn't have time to remove. This long term storage of toxins accounts for many of the diseases prevalent in our society.

Even hotter: the lowdown on microwaves

Lots of research has shown that microwaved food suffers severe molecular damage. The molecules are literally torn apart and deformed. As well as becoming susceptible to viruses, fungi and other micro-organisms, these cells can't repair themselves properly. When in the process of repair they would normally produce water and carbon dioxide, but they are so deformed that they produce hydrogen peroxide and carbon monoxide. And then you eat it.

As with conventionally cooked foods, your body doesn't recognise these molecules and so, when eating microwaved foods, you produce even more leukocytes. This means that your body senses a bigger danger. Tests have show that foods cooked in a microwave cause a more drastic case of leukosytosis than foods cooked any other way. Ask yourself if you can afford to put such a strain on your immune system.

Cooked food causes untold and unnecessary stress on your body, but of all the commonly used cooking methods, microwaved food is the worst. In addition to leukocytosis and its associated risk of lower immunity, there is the risk of lower haemoglobin levels and HDL (good) cholesterol. Tests have concluded that anaemia, contagious diseases and heart disease are very real threats when eating lots of microwaved foods.

If all that science stuff does nothing for you, think about this. When blood is used for transfusions, it is sometimes warmed first. Once, a nurse warmed the blood in a microwave instead of the normal way. The patient was killed, and of course a law suit followed. If microwaving doesn't do anything other than simply heat food, then this couldn't have happened.

Further information

Books

The Sunfood Diet Success System
36 Lessons in Health Transformation
David Wolfe
ISBN: 0965353362

When you start to change your life, a book full of motivation and inspiration such as this can make all the difference. The words are electrically charged and full of a special magic. Amongst the magic, you also get sound nutritional and transitional advice.

The UnCook Book
Raw Food Adventures to a New Health High
Elizabeth & Dr Elton Baker
ISBN: 1887314202

Although this book is out of print, you can still buy it on the Internet, and it's well worth it. Elizabeth describes how she and her husband healed themselves of cancers and other diseases by detoxing on raw food, fasting, and drinking watermelon juices.

Web sites

www.rawfoodsupport.com, **www.rawfood.com** and **www.welikeitraw.com** are all dedicated to educating the world on the science, facts and fun of eating food in its natural state.

Things to do

- Read as many books on natural living as you can, and observe how other animals succeed in their lives.

- If you want to stop eating cooked food, do it gradually and make some like-minded friends by joining web groups or going to raw pot lucks. A pot luck is an American term: everyone turns up to a meeting with a dish and you all share the food around to get ideas about what's possible.

- If you don't want to stop eating cooked foods, then make the decision to cut out microwaved foods and to have at least 50% raw food in each meal to stop yourself suffering from leukocytosis and a suppressed immune system.

The food you will be eating

Here's a list of the food you'll be tucking into during your detox plan. Of course, it's not comprehensive, as there are many local-grown variations. However, it does give you an idea of the variety that you can come to expect to eat on a regular basis both during and after your detox. Once you've been on a detox plan, use this list when going shopping or planting your garden as it might give you ideas that you wouldn't otherwise have thought of.

Fruit

Ripe fruit, picked straight from the tree, gives you the best feeling in the world. However, if you live in a temperate climate, your experience with tropical fruit might have left a sour taste in your mouth. Fruit is frequently sprayed, picked before it's ripe and then exported thousands of miles for us to "enjoy" — quite often, we just don't.

Whenever possible, eat local organic or wild fruit, for the sake of the planet and you. When eating a high fruit diet in the UK you may have to eat imported fruits as well as enjoying local berries, apples, pears, plums, and even peaches. Wherever you love, enjoy your local fruit the most. We all make environmental sacrifices in this modern world, so eat the food you love with a thankful heart.

> **About durians**
>
> Durians are a white-chocolate-onion-tarty-creamy-custard-heaven food. They are the favourite food of the orang-utan. It's reported that a tiger will kill a human who is carrying a durian, leaving the dead human and walking off with the prize fruit in its mouth!

> **About avocados**
>
> The creaminess of avocado makes it great for salads, dressings, dips, ice creams and puddings. If I eat it on its own, I peel the skin right off and bite into it. Then I rub the remains into my hands just like a moisturiser.

Fruit for energy

Fruits have an abundance of energy to give us. This is why we have a naturally sweet tooth, so we choose fruits over other foods. When we rid ourselves of calorie-packed yet detrimental and nutrient deficient foods such as pasta, bread, rice and potatoes, we turn to fruit to supply us with our energy needs.

A high fruit diet frees your body up to use its energy on repair as it doesn't have digest heavy food. You also get more nutrients, as they haven't been destroyed or denatured by cooking. This all adds up to a glorious and fruit-filled life.

Some fruits you will come to know and love

Apple, apricot, avocado, banana, blueberry, cherimoya, cherry, courgette, cucumber, durian, fig, goji berry, grape, Incan berry, kiwi, lucuma, mango, melon, papaya, persimmon, tomato, okra, olive, orange, peach, pear, pepper, pineapple, raspberry, strawberry, ... and many many more.

Seek wild fruits like rosehips, brambles and yew berries (minus the poisonous pip). These are available free, and provide you with the nutrients you need for that season.

What to do with fruits

You can make the best meals in the world with fruits. Try a smoothie made with just orange juice, banana and mango — just three ingredients make for a great taste sensation. Or how about a savoury fruit salad with tomato, avocado, okra, pepper and cucumber? Experiment with all the fruits that are available to you and appreciate the abundance of nature.

A high fruit diet must be buffered with lots of greens for you to get all your nutrients. Try making fruit smoothies and add a couple of handfuls of dark green leaves

Dried fruit

This is a great addition to the store cupboard and snack bag. These fruits are very concentrated, so don't make a whole meal out of them. Look for dried apricots which are dark brown instead of bright orange, as these have no sulphur on them. Look for raisins, sultanas and currants that haven't got vegetable oil on them, and check out banana chips that haven't been sweetened with honey.

Further information

Books

Detox delights
Shazzie

My first book contains over 100 recipes which make massive use of all kinds of fruits to make your mouth water.

A Produce Reference Guide to Fruits and Vegetables from Around the World
Nature's Harvest
Donald Heaton
ISBN: 1560228652

There's a ton of information here, from all the different available fruits and vegetables to nutritional guides. It's a great reference book to have on hand.

Web site

www.thefruitpages.com — this is one of the sweetest web sites. There is so much information here, and it's beautifully and simply presented.

Greens

Greens are frequently referred to as "nature's medicine" because for so many thousands of years, people relied upon them when they were sick. In fact, it's not only humans who practise this — have you ever seen a dog eating grass to make himself vomit when he has a stomach bug? This is the natural world using greens as medicine. We know that greens are very potent and life-enhancing, and we should all eat some greens each day for optimal health.

A high green diet causes your body to become stronger, more alkaline, more flexible, less toxic and more oxygenated, to have a higher immunity and to feel more alert. It's also reported that greens emulsify cholesterol and fat in the body. Even if you just eat an organic green leafy salad before each meal, you will make massive improvements in your health.

Phytochemicals (plant chemicals) are found in all plant food, including greens. Scientists know relatively little about them, but they do recognise they are essential for us to fight off disease and stay healthy. Amino acids, chlorophyll, enzymes, fibre, essential fatty acids, vitamins, minerals and antioxidants all make an appearance in greens, and they are all recognised as being detox-friendly elements.

Because greens are low in calories when comparing volume, they are the perfect ingredients to pad out your detox meals.

> Tuck into as many greens as you want,
> any time of the day.

Chlorophyll

> ### Green reports
>
> Studies suggest that foods containing chlorophyll can halt tooth decay. If you have a tooth issue, chew on some dark green leaves for a while, as if it is chewing gum. Repeat this every day and note if the discomfort goes away.

This is the green colour in vegetables. It's the blood of the plant, and has been associated with the ability to block carcinogens, reduce cancers and act as an antioxidant. Some people find the use of wheatgrass juice extremely beneficial during detox. However, if you are on a standard diet, start off with very small amounts, as it is extremely potent, and can set off a string of cleansing reactions to the unsuspecting drinker.

Some of my favourite greens

This list is by no way extensive — there's a whole world of edible greens out there. Look around you when you're outside in nature, most of it is green! I think this is a great clue as to how much of it we should eat. Check out your local markets and seed centres to see what you can buy or grow for yourself.

About batavia
Also known as escarole, this is a really well structured lettuce. This lettuce stays fresh when all others around it wilt and wither, so if you can only do your shopping once a week, stock up on the longer-lasting batavia. The leaves are large and strong, making them perfect for roll-ups. Put your favourite filling in them, roll up the ends and tuck in.

Batavia, butterhead lettuce, celery, chard, Chinese leaf, cress, dandelions, endive, frise, iceberg, lamb's lettuce, lollo rosso, mizuna, oakleaf lettuce, radicchio, red mustard, sunflower greens, rocket, romaine lettuce.

What to do with greens

Greens provide you with endless salad possibilities, as well as soups, dips and smoothies. Many people use greens instead of bread, making elaborate or simple roll-ups. The recipes in this book all make the most of greens, but do remember that your experiments will always be the best, because they come straight from your heart.

Sprouts

Sprouts used for eating fall into three categories. There are easy to digest seed sprouts, such as alfalfa, sunflower, radish, mustard cress, clover, broccoli and onion. Then there are pulse sprouts such as lentil, mung bean, chick pea, aduki and pea. Finally, there are the grain sprouts, such as wheat, rye, buckwheat and quinoa. Some of these sprouts could quite easily fit into two of the categories, but this is a rough outline of what you might encounter. I find seed sprouts very enjoyable, the pulses very hard to digest, and grain sprouts mucous forming if I have too many.

If you want to experiment with growing sprouts, then make a note of which ones "agree with you" and which ones don't. There are many books and web sites around which explain exactly how to grow them.

Benefits of sprouts

Sprouts offer you optimal nutrition very inexpensively. When you buy the seeds in bulk and grow the sprouts regularly you will find that your budget can breathe again.

Because you harvest the sprouts as you want to eat them, they are bursting with life, electricity, antioxidants, protein (amino acids) and other nutrients. They are indeed an excellent detox and rejuvenation food.

The guys at The Hippocrates Health Institute in Florida, USA have taught many people to heal themselves using various techniques and lots of wheatgrass and sprouts! They believe that it's your birthright to experience good health and free will. In the UK, Jill Swyers uses the same techniques to work with people who need healing, detoxing, rejuvenating or energising.

Green superfood

Green superfood is a generic term for many foods that are nutrient-packed. The superfood I refer to is called Nature's Living Superfood in the UK, or Nature's First Food or Vitamineral Green in the USA. I've been using this product since 2000, and it has greatly contributed to my health. I also use the life-force-packed Pure Synergy superfood. These superfoods are 100% raw and vegan, so can be used by everyone. It doesn't have inexpensive fillers, and all the ingredients are organic or wildcrafted. If you don't have regular access to wild greens, then I thoroughly recommend that you use this superfood daily to ensure you get all those little nutrients which are lost in modern food.

Other greens

> **Green heart**
>
> Green is the colour of the heart chakra, which governs your feelings, emotional connections to others, to the universe and to life.
>
> Start to heal any emotional pain by meditating on green and eating green food throughout your day.

Chorella, spirulina, algae and other aquatic green foods are also classed as greens. These are single-celled organisms which have been used by many as health-promoting and detoxifying foods.

These green foods are fantastic sources of vitamins, minerals, protein and other nutrients, making them some of the most beneficial foods you can eat.

My favourite is AFA algae in the form of E3Live and Crystal Manna, which comes just from one lake in Oregon, USA. E3Live is frozen and shipped all over the world. When you defrost it, you can see these gorgeous fractals forming. Crystal Manna is freeze dried and is so tasty on salads. When detoxing, AFA algae cleanses and boosts you.

People have used these greens to heal themselves of cancers. Mouth and cervical cancers (which have the same mucous membranes) are reported to be particularly vulnerable to the healing powers of these greens.

If you have appetite issues when detoxing, spirulina could help you. Alongside cacao and AFA algae it contains the amino acid phenylalanine, which is reported to be an appetite suppressant.

Further information

The Raw Gourmet
Nomi Shannon
ISBN: 0920470483

This recipe book is based upon the healing principles outlined by the Hippocrates Health Institute. All of the recipes are uncooked, and Nomi makes the most of greens more than any other book I've seen. With this book in your collection, you'll never be confused by chard or baffled by butterhead again!

Living Foods for Radiant Health
The Natural Way to Boost Immunity and Detoxify Your System
Elaine Bruce
ISBN: 0007121172

This is a practical guide and recipe collection showing the simplicity of eating live foods. Amongst the recipes, you'll find broths, ferments, juices, blends, grain breads, and sprouting information. www.livingfoods.co.uk.

Retreats

Hippocrates Health Institute
1443 Palmdale Court
West Palm Beach, FL 33411
USA
+1 (561) 471 8876
Reservations: +1 (800) 842 2125
Fax: +1 (561) 471 9464
info@hippocratesinst.com
reservations@hippocratesinst.com
www.hippocratesinst.com

If you are seriously ill, then I would highly recommend you go here to mend yourself. This is where I would go if I needed to. The director Brian Clement is at the cutting edge of living foods nutrition and healing, so you can be sure you're in the most capable of hands. Even if you are not ill, but feel like you need a little help getting started in this new way of life, then why not do it in the Florida sunshine?

Tree of Life Foundation
Rejuvenation Center and Health Practice
PO Box 1080, Patagonia, AZ, 85624
+1 (520) 394 2520
Fax: +1 (415) 598 2409
healing@treeoflife.nu
www.treeoflife.nu

The Tree of Life is directed by Gabriel Cousens MD, author of Conscious Eating, Spiritual Nutrition and the Rainbow Diet.

The Tree of Life Rejuvenation Center is an innovative eco-retreat center committed to the integration of all healing life forces for complete body, mind and spiritual renewal. They offer the art of physical rejuvenation, combined with psychological and spiritual development. I've visited this place and have felt the powerful energy of the place. This is one retreat that is run on 100% pure love. The food is so good, too!

Things to do

- Bring more green into your diet. Pick out a new green food every week when out shopping and invent a recipe with it. You may end up being the next Nomi Shannon!

- Make an indoor sprouting garden and harvest your greens as you want to eat them!

- Make a green juice if you ever feel tired, and add some E3Live to it for a power kick.

Nuts and seeds

Nuts and seeds give us a wonderfully healthy source of plant fat, which is essential to our well-being. Nuts can be quite tough to digest, but you can enhance their digestibility by soaking and blending them before eating them. Seeds appear to be easier to digest, and are so versatile, you need never eat them the same way twice!

A few nuts and seeds

About gingko biloba nuts

As well as having very nutritious leaves, the gingko (or ginkgo) gives a fruit and a nut. The fruit looks like a persimmon, yet really smells, so people in our culture don't use it to get to the nut. However, in China and Japan, the nuts are gathered from the wild trees and sold. Though the hulls also smell, the edible nuts inside don't. gingko is a very interesting plant to many, and is reported to help brain development. If you pass by a tree, pick a few leaves to chew on. They're quite strong, but very edible. You're unlikely to find a female tree in public places because of the smell of the fruit!

Almond, brazil, cashew, chestnut, coconut, filbert, ginkgo biloba, hazel, hemp, macadamia, pecan, pili, pine nut, pistachio, pumpkin, sesame, sunflower, walnut.

A word about the apricot seed

The apricot is related to the almond, and they contain similar seeds. The apricot seed is a bit smaller, and is found inside the hard stone in the centre of the fruit. It's a controversial little seed because it contains B17, which destroys cancer cells. The hulled nuts have been banned in the USA and in Australia, reportedly because they contain a small amount of cyanide. If you taste the nut, you'll notice it's like marzipan or Bakewell tarts. People who want to take advantage of its alleged health properties add 5-35 a day to smoothies or they eat them straight.

Spice seeds

We often forget that most spices are seeds. As spices were used in the past to disguise rotting food, they are regarded by some as unnecessary today. However, I feel that there are tiny elements in many plants that we sometimes need. When detoxing you won't be using spices very heavily, but they can make a big difference to the taste of this new food food, which may be welcomed when you first start making changes for life.

Spice is the variety of life.

Remember nutmeg, cardamom, cumin and coriander when flavouring your new food.

What to do with nuts and seeds

Try not to have a packet of nuts on your desk and eat them all day long. This will play havoc with your digestion and won't be the most nutritious option for you. Enjoy creating some of the delicious pâtés, dips, drinks, and main meals from *The recipes*.

Almonds are a great nut to use when cleansing your body, because they are the least acidic of all nuts.

Make a trail mix of nuts, dried fruits and seeds. The variety is endless.

It's best if you soak seeds and nuts in water for at least two hours before eating or using in recipes, as the enzyme inhibitors are then destroyed. Soaking overnight is usually the easiest option.

Butters (not the dairy variety!) are a great way to eat nuts. Try raw nut and seed butters spread on flax crackers, in smoothies, topping soups, as a salad dressing ingredient or sandwiched between a banana! My favourite is almond butter — if figs are in season try flax crackers spread with almond butter and a big blob of fig on top, it's better than any peanut butter and jelly sandwich!

Further information

Book

Raw
The Uncook Book
Juliano
ISBN: 0060392622

I love Juliano's book for its style and cheekiness. The recipes are fabulous, too! He will stun you into creating food which is great for you! Making the most of nuts and seeds for every occasion, this is the best recipe book around that features much nut use.

Things to do

- Go to a wholefood store and check out all the different nuts and seeds. Ask the staff what to do with them if you're not sure!

- When it's walnut season, climb a walnut tree and take the wet walnuts. They are succulent, juicy, full of flavour and very satisfying. They taste totally different to dry walnuts.

Other plant foods

There are some types of foods which don't fit into the above categories. Some of these, though they're eaten by many people, aren't suited to a detox diet.

Legumes

These can be sprouted and eaten, but because of the protein and starch in them, they do not digest well. For that reason, I stay away from them most of the time. If you want to try them, sprout mung beans, chick peas or aduki beans. Do not sprout red kidney beans as they are highly toxic and can cause death.

Peanuts

We all know and have probably loved the peanut in our childhood years, and we also know that it's not a nut, it's a legume. It can harbour a powerful toxic mould called aflatoxin, so if you do eat them, be careful that they do not have mould on them.

Of the 12,000 kinds of legumes, peanuts are one of the most easy to digest.

Peanuts contain about 30% protein and 50% oil. If you have the right climate you can easily plant peanuts, and you will be given a prolific crop in return. Peanuts are also called groundnuts or monkey nuts.

Carob

Carob is another legume, and I use it dried, powdered and mixed in with sweet things to substitute and complement chocolate. I have also enjoyed eating the pods from the tree. If you get them at just the right time, they are like a toffee-chocolate bar — quite amazing! The attractive trees grow to about 15 metres, are native to the Mediterranean areas and probably the Middle East but they have now spread further afield. Carob came to Spain via the Moors, who planted them alongside citrus and olives. The pod is also known as the locust bean. The pods are a rich in sugars and contain about 8% protein.

Herbs and spices

Herbs and greens are both in the same group, really, but for eating purposes, I've put the herbs here, as we use them mainly for flavourings, and not for bulk. As well as the spice seeds mentioned earlier the following are all used to spice up your life: basil, bayleaf, cinnamon, cloves, cumin, dill, garlic, lemon grass, mace, paprika, onions, rosemary, sage and thyme. There are countless more herbs and spices, and they differ from country to country. Have a look at your regional flavours and add them to the recipes in this book for an authentic local-flavoured dish.

Special superfoods

These don't belong in one food class, so I'm mentioning them all here as they're often eaten together and are very special indeed. There are thousands of foods that can be classed as superfoods, but there are only a handful that really stand out from the crowd. Raw cacao (real raw chocolate), maca, goji berries and AFA algae are my favourite superfoods. I've already mentioned AFA algae, so here's a brief description of the others.

Cacao

In 1753 Carl von Linnaeus, the 18th-century Swedish scientist, thought that cacao was so important that he named the genus and species of this tree himself. He named this tree: Theobroma cacao, which literally means "cacao, the food of the gods."

In its raw state, the bean offers many properties and nutrients to those in the know. Experimental provings of chocolate by homeopaths indicate its stimulating effect when cooked yet when the same decoction was made with raw, unroasted beans no effects were noticeable. David Wolfe and myself wrote the world's first book on raw chocolate, called **Naked Chocolate**, which has had a profound effect on the health food revolution.

Maca

Maca is a root from Peru. It looks like a little turnip or radish. It's been used since before the ancient Incan times. These days, many millions of people throughout the world are starting to hear about its properties. It's helping people with male impotence, menopause, osteoporosis, chronic fatigue syndrome, depression, menstrual difficulties, and much more. It's also a really nutritious food to add to smoothies and desserts.

Goji berries

Goji berries took media by storm in 2006. Billed as "the weight loss fruit", they have been given extensive coverage in the media worldwide. Goji berries are an extremely nutrient-dense fruit. They contain 18 amino acids (six times higher than bee pollen) including all 8 essential amino acids.

The Goji berry is a deep-red, dried fruit about the same size as a raisin. It's very sweet and tastes something like a cross between a cranberry and a cherry. I love adding them to smoothies, trail-mix, cereals, teas and cakes. I also just eat them by the handful!

Your detox plans

You can make up your own detox plans, but if this is your first detox, then following one of the plans in this section will make it easier for you. When you're a seasoned detoxer, you can just choose recipes from this book or its companion **Detox Delights** and know that you're doing great things for your body. Remember to make the most of the *Detox helpers* too — that's the luxurious part of detoxing!

It's time to remember: if you're putting fewer toxins in your body than are coming out, you are detoxing. Keep working on this principle all the time and you'll soon be a beautiful butterfly.

Read through the detox information that precedes the plans. This will help you choose the best one plan for you at this time. You'll also find out what to expect when detoxing.

For the best results, follow these plans as closely as possible. However, if for social or other reasons, you can't do that, then do what you can — you'll benefit much more than by doing nothing! If you suddenly find yourself eating something that isn't in the plan, don't worry — you're just having a learning experience! Calmly say to yourself "OK, now I'm ready to continue the detox, and I learned so much from my little detour". Don't reprimand yourself and don't think you've fallen off the wagon so you can't carry on — neither of those things are constructive or necessary. Pick yourself up, brush yourself down, and carry on. No harm done.

How to detox

When using this book and these plans, you are in total control of how far and how quickly you detox your body.

If you want to start slowly, simply add variety to your existing diet by using a few of the recipes each week or by drinking a smoothie a day. If you want to detox as much as possible, use one of the detox plans or eat only the recipes in this book.

On a long detox plan, note which recipes decelerate or accelerate the detox process and use this to control your progress. To detox for life, take a look at the suggestions, and very slowly but surely alter your lifestyle habits to make you a lighter, cleaner and purer being.

Taking your time

Although some people recommend that you plunge headlong into a totally new diet for the rest of your life, I don't. If you do this, you are more likely to:

- Suffer from uncontrollable cravings

- Miss your old life too much

- Have detox symptoms which are too great for you to continue your everyday life

If you've never detoxed before, do it gently. There is no rush unless you're seriously ill. To ease into detoxing, try cutting down on coffee, cooked chocolate, tea, fizzy drinks, wheat products, and anything with cooked fat in it. Just by doing these things first, you'll feel some detox benefits and reactions. If you have a very toxic diet, I recommend that you cut down on the above foods for a couple of weeks before you even start on one of these plans.

Before starting the plans

If you have never detoxed, follow the above advice, then eat at least one recipe from this book a day for a couple of weeks before starting any of the plans.

The week before you start your plan, don't eat any grain or dairy products. That means you are going to say "no" to pasta, bread, wheat-based cereals, yoghurt, butter, milk, cheese and cream. It also means you will check for ingredients containing wheat or dairy products on all your meals.

Lighten your duties while detoxing, making space for leisure and pleasure.

If this is your first detox, start with the three day plan. After finishing the plan, keep eating at least one or two recipes a day from this book or its sister book, **Detox Delights**. Wait about four weeks before starting the seven day plan or the *Detox for life* plan. You're much more likely to succeed and attain great results this way than by plummeting head first into a bucket of "cold turkey".

Dealing with detox effects

If your detox effects are too strong for the situation you are in, there are ways of relieving the symptoms. Just by eating heavier food for a while, such as the flax crackers and walnut burgers listed in the recipe chapter, you will come back into a workable comfort zone. When you feel ready to continue, slowly go back to your full-on detox.

Whatever you do, don't take any drugs to make cleansing symptoms go away. This will just put more strain on your body as it fights to deal with another bombardment of toxins. Though the experience may be new to you, sit with any feelings of discomfort, and celebrate the fact that toxins are being released from your body. Know that when it passes you will be at a new level of health and happiness.

If you can, take as much time out as possible to sit with and observe all emotions and feelings. If you are keeping a journal, write your emotions and feelings down, and refer to them if you experience another set of detox symptoms. You might be surprised at how different and less strong each subsequent set of symptoms are.

Think back to Betty, cleaning her beloved hats out from her room. She felt pangs of loss at the same time as feeling lighter, and more spacious. Like Betty, your symptoms are releases. Go with them, don't fight them, trust that your body knows what's best. Know that after the healing signals have gone, you will have a better life for yourself.

Detoxing with herbs

Just like all animals, some people use herbs to detox. Some herbs, for example, stimulate the liver into releasing stored toxins. You can look at this in two ways:

- This adds extra strain to organs which are already under pressure.
- This gets the toxins out quicker so your body can revel in being clean.

> ### Detox on the wild side
>
> Wild animals use herbs medicinally to detox, to remove parasites, to gain strength after giving birth and as medicines when ill. Herbs are valuable to us when used in conjunction with our instinct and ancient knowledge.

I personally prefer to use the more natural methods of correct nutrition and conditions, though I agree that some organs can be so dysfunctional that they could do with a gentle prod to get them started.

If you wish to use a herbal detox product, then read up on it thoroughly, to ensure it will leave you in a safe and balanced place rather than an enervated and bankrupt one. I have used the Ejuva cleanse before, which is a four-week course of herb-popping. I lost a piece of gristle in my wrist on week three, and gained very clear skin. However, herbs are not necessary to detox, so if you don't want to spend a lot of money on becoming healthy, you don't have to.

A while ago, I was talking with a taxi driver about this book. He stated: "Oh, I nearly bought a bottle of that detox stuff from the chemists, but put it back on the shelf when I saw the price." As I mentioned to him, you do not buy a detox — detox doesn't come in bottles. You can buy products which stimulate your body to clean out at a faster pace, or to support certain organs, but you do not need to do this. Your body is cleaning itself all the time, all you need to do to benefit from this is to stop taking in so much rubbish.

Once you've detoxed a certain amount, a good herbal cleanse might be a turning point for you and your health. However, don't rush into this, because for now, just lightening your load will cause you to detox gently while you get on with your everyday life.

If you agree to compromise your health, then every part of your life will suffer.

Further information

Web site

www.detox.org — A wonderful resource of information, offering experts' opinions, books and hints and tips.

Making your detox work

You won't stick to a detox programme that doesn't satisfy you. There is no point in eating food that isn't gorgeous, satiating and good for you. Every recipe and meal plan in this book has been created to taste fantastic, without compromising your health.

The plans are made to fit to your lifestyle. Your lifestyle may change through a long transition period, but forcing it to happen on a detox plan isn't necessary. Ensure you succeed on your quest for a beautiful mind, body and spirit by listening, learning, and implementing new behaviour patterns slowly and continuously.

Helping yourself

As we've seen in the *Detox helpers* chapter, there are many pleasurable ways to help you detox.

By detoxing, you are taking responsibility for your future, for your life. Even if you have a hectic lifestyle, and can't fit any more self-help into your personal equation, you can do this. Detoxing this way is simple, requires less effort than eating "normally" and it will give you more energy to pursue the things in life which are important to you.

Taking up yoga, walking and deep breathing will not only make you feel great — these activities assist in the detoxification process. You can also try dry skin brushing, self-massage, wearing natural fibres, having your windows open, preparing your food with love, and meditation. All of these tools will ensure that your transformation is a delightful and stress-free time for you. You don't need to go through every detox helper, just pick and choose a few which appeal to you, and note how you feel afterwards.

With your new outlook, increased energy levels and lack of aches and pains, you will feel ready to take on new challenges in your life.

Let go of all that does not serve you.

As your mind, body and spirit will be stronger, fully embracing your future will be easy. You'll automatically analyse everything in your life and change those things that don't make you feel 100% wonderful 100% of the time.

The best time for you to detox

As you'll be eating fresh products, and nothing pre-frozen or from cans or packets, find a time when there's an abundance of food in the shops, markets and gardens. These days, in many western countries, it's easy any time of the year, as the shops are always full of good, fresh food.

Most people choose to detox in January, either as a New Year's resolution or to knock some Christmas stuffing out of them. My chiropractor says that they do it to detox their emotions after being stressed out with relatives, which probably holds much truth!

If you choose to detox when the weather is cold, take advantage of some of the warming foods, and meals such as soups which you can heat to a warm temperature without ruining the goodness in them. Add saunas, steam rooms, exercise and invigorating massages to your programme and you won't even notice the weather.

How it works

Detox with this book in two consecutive ways: Purge the bad stuff out of your body, and (maybe for the first time in your life) put health-enhancing goodies into it. Instead of caffeine, alcohol, nicotine, refined sugar and distorted food chemicals dominating your diet, delicious fresh fruits and vegetables steal the show. There's no wonder you might sometimes feel dizzy!

> Enjoy the masses of intact vitamins, minerals, enzymes and phyto-nutrients skating around your body giving you more love and attention than a bag of chips could ever do!

These nutrients ensure that as your body systematically rebuilds, it's doing it with the best possible materials. When you detox for long enough, you literally become a different person.

Puffy bread people

If the saying "You are what you eat" is true, would you like to be made out of soggy rice, greasy meat, and puffy bread, or super juicy wild greens, extra strong nuts and ultra sweet fruit?

You can start to notice the results within a day, especially when you take action on this little gem of information:

Magic midnight

From around midnight to 8am, your body is in super cleaning mode. This is because your body has rested, hasn't eaten for a while (hopefully) and is able to take advantage of the quiet time it has to itself. For this reason eat your evening meal quite early on, to allow maximum detox to happen overnight.

Morning glory

> If you aren't hungry in the mornings, don't eat.
> Let your body tell you when it does
> and doesn't want food.

From 8am to about midday, your body is still cleansing quite heavily. By eating only fruit (or nothing if you aren't hungry), you'll allow your body to continue doing what it needs to.

Is breakfast the most important meal of the day?

As I just mentioned something which may upset some nutritionists, I'll expand a little bit here.

> Eating breakfast when you are not hungry is not only
> counter-intuitive, it's bad for your health.

If you eat when you're not hungry, you're just adding to a load that your body would rather not deal with. It's far more sensible to take food to work with you and eat it when you do want it, than to stuff it down when your body is clearly asking you not to.

Throughout this book, I've written some pretty challenging statements, and it's fine if you don't believe me. However, I urge you to just give them a try, and then draw your own conclusions. Whatever you decide to do, follow your instinct and not the advice of a profession which changes its guidelines as often as it changes its white coats.

Midday munching

After midday, your digestion is at its strongest. This is when it's best for most people to eat their biggest meal of the day. Here's a good experiment for you to try: for a few days, make lunch your main meal. Then do the same with your dinner as your main meal. Note down the differences you feel, such as morning grogginess versus alertness.

Evening energy

If you find that eating your main meal at lunch time works best for you, then eat a light evening meal before 7pm. If hunger strikes, make a green juice or eat some sweet fruit.

Dealing with a cold or flu

When you feel like you're getting a cold or the flu, rest completely and don't eat until the symptoms have passed. If complete rest isn't possible because of necessities such as work or children (and you really can't find someone to take your place for a short while), then eat small portions of just one type of fruit (melon is a good one) or make fresh green juice until the symptoms have passed. This method allows your body to continue functioning, as well as release toxins.

Green juices and sweet fruits are both super ways of keeping hunger at bay. If you eat a heavy meal late at night, your body won't be able to finish digesting it, and so your nightly detox will also be hindered. When you respect the evening meal guideline, it will benefit you more than you can imagine.

Turning detox theory into practice

Having read this far, you now know that holistic detoxing makes sense. Now you know why you'd want to do it, let's get started! Before we do, here's a quick refresher course.

By detoxing, you can reduce or remove common (but unnatural) ailments like these:

- aches and pains
- bloating
- constipation
- dark circles around the eyes
- flaking nails
- furry tongue
- menstrual pains (including PMS)
- skin eruptions
- vague, annoying, indescribable symptoms

These are all symptoms of a toxic body, desperate to clean itself. Eating fresh whole ripe raw plant foods for a period of time will allow the body to divert its energy to repair and cleaning. These foods also supply great building materials for your next phase in life.

Even if you don't suffer from the above, detoxing will benefit you by giving you younger-looking skin, stronger nails, shinier hair, improved circulation, better digestion and elimination, better weight control and more energy.

Getting started

Although I encourage you to make gradual life-long changes towards better food choices, you can kick-start this new lifestyle by setting a particular amount of time to eat fresh, organic energy-giving food. This can also uplift your tired mind, body and spirit. If you have been overworking at the game called life, the lightness of this food rests your digestive system, and you'll be cleansed and enhanced.

Because you might not be able to put your life on hold, I've devised several detox plans: choose the one that fits in with the time and lifestyle you have. Finding free time is often easier than we think. It's amazing how much time is wasted due to lack of energy, cooking elaborate meals, watching soaps (is the life of a soap character one that you really want to have?) and working to keep up an expensive lifestyle. When detoxing, take a good long hard look at your life, and make changes to anything that stops you being a superbeing.

When you detox, take note of your feelings. How much cleaner does your mind feel? Do you feel like you want to change anything else in your life? Detox isn't just physical, so make other shifts as and when you feel the need to.

Please remember, if you have serious health problems or are pregnant, seek the care of a natural health practitioner before embarking on any detox plan.

Staying strong

Because our eating habits are mixed up with our social habits, there will be times when you feel like you can't escape that big toxic world. This is when you need to stay positive, and know that your new lifestyle will serve you so much more than your old one. You aren't losing anything, you're gaining a whole new reality.

How much to eat

When making recipes or snacking, remember that this isn't a calorie restriction diet. There is no weighing or measuring! Eat until full but not bursting and stick to the recommended foods — you will soon notice a big difference in yourself. All the recipes mentioned are listed at the back of the book. Feel free to substitute anything unavailable with something similar.

You'll also notice that you have a snack bag. You'll make this up in the morning and carry it round with you all day. It will help you when you are hungry and there are only burgers all around!

Your detox shopping list

There is a specific shopping list for each detox plan. I don't give amounts, as you can eat as much as you like on the plans (unless otherwise stated for a very few specific foods). Feel free to vary ingredients according to the seasons and what's available.

Make sure that as much of your food as possible is organic. If you don't remember why, read the section on *Organic and wild food* in *All about food* again.

If you are on a standard western diet, all of the recipes in this book will contribute to your detoxification simply because they're less toxic, so your body can clean itself more efficiently. After your detox, continue shopping for ingredients mentioned in the plans and recipes.

A few notes for women

La luna

When you are pre-menstrual, you will need to take in more calories. Some medics say the calorific intake goes up by about 500 a day for the week before your period. It's a time to eat more dense food, and to feel in tune with what your body is asking for. I have found the following to be invaluable to myself and others.

A week before your period

Eat lots of watermelon, melon, mangoes, bananas and avocados. Keep nuts and dried fruit to hand in your snack bag so you don't reach for a more unhealthy choice. You might feel happier eating five small meals a day at this time.

Make the most of the hormone-regulating and nutrient-dense dried root called maca. You can blend it into any smoothie, though I just lick the powder! Enjoy some raw chocolate.

Make an appointment with a massage therapist, reflexologist, or other therapist. If you can't do this, get a friend or partner to pamper you in total silence for at least an hour.

Soothe your soul with the power of touch.

Remember that stress is toxic. Keep your blood sugar and hormone levels stable by snacking on lots of fresh fruit throughout the day and insist on an abundance of snuggles.

The day before your period

When you eat very lightly, any next-day bloating and cramping will be a lot lighter. As your body diverts energy away from digestion, towards menstruation, you can sometimes be left with various tummy troubles. A diet consisting of only juices, smoothies and soup the day before your period will help enormously.

Creeping cravings

As menstruation is a time of detox, remember that cravings will appear. Be extra kind and loving to yourself at this time, so you don't feel like you're missing out on anything.

Take more time out, and allow yourself to be alone, just with your feelings, to observe which emotions come up. You will notice this change over time, as feelings such as "It's the end of the world" get replaced by feelings such as "I'm so peaceful today". Note all of this down in your journal, so that you can really see your progress. This will encourage you to continue.

Before you have totally detoxed, if your period bothers you in any way, remember how lucky you are to be a woman. We can actually track, month by month how our bodies are clearing up, as the period gets lighter and less painful. If you don't believe this, write it down in your journal, or make a chart to track your own progress.

Period pains

To rid yourself of any pain, try doing some yoga postures which have been specifically recommended for menstruation. Also, check out the Senza drug-free magnetic device. Look for other ways to relieve period pains without resorting to toxic tablets.

> Detoxing your world means that you could
> say goodbye to your period pains.

I was sure I could never cure my extremely painful periods. Yet when I detoxed I noticed a difference after six months. From that moment on, I have never taken another painkiller. Now, I rarely feel any pain at all. Time for celebration, indeed.

Let's go!

Now you're all set to detox! Choose one of the following plans, make use of all the hints and tips, and enjoy the process. You're about to turn into a butterfly!

Hormone balancing maca root

Your peaceful three day detox plan

If you haven't detoxed before, I recommend you start with this plan, as it will give you an insight into how you might feel when on the longer plans. It will also rest your body sufficiently to see some changes, such as higher energy levels, less bloating and fewer aches and pains without putting you into full-blown detox mode!

If you work normal weekdays, it's easier to start this detox on a Friday and finish on Monday morning. When starting this detox, don't plan any heavy duties — it's about creating time for you to nourish yourself with what you need so you can give back more when you're ready.

If you have young children, try to get someone to look after them for at least some time during the day so you can rest and partake in the detox helpers.

Sleep is an important part of detox, so for these three days allow yourself to sleep and rest as much as you want.

Writing in your journal while on this detox plan is a great way to remember the emotions and feelings that you'll encounter. Don't watch television! If there's a television on in the house, go into another room, and read, meditate or write in your journal. Be peaceful.

Two days before the detox

If you eat meat, poultry, fish, soya products or dairy products (milk, cheese, eggs etc), give them up for the two days before this detox. If that leaves you stumped for what to eat, take a look at some of the recipes in this book. You can add rice, boiled vegetables, potatoes or bread to them if you need to.

Book an appointment for a lymph drainage massage on day two. If you can't get a lymph drainage massage, book a different type and state that you want it for detoxification. If you can't book any massage or find a friend to massage you, then you will give yourself a massage.

Book a yoga class or teacher for day two. If you can't do this, then buy or borrow a yoga video to suit your level.

Buy a notebook to use as a journal to record your feelings and changes.

Buy or pick a bunch of flowers, and set them by a well-lit window, with a chair.

One day before the detox

Now cut out all wheat and potato products. This means that for today, and for the detox days, you won't be eating bread, potatoes, pasta, meat, fish, soya meat, soya milk, milk, cheese, butter, eggs, cakes, cookies, crackers, sweets, chips or crisps!

If it's sounding scary already, remember that you are about to embark on a high-energy boost for your total self. You'll be guided all the way, so there's nothing to be scared about.

Give me sunshine

Contrary to popular belief, the sun is good for you. All animals go to where it is warm, raise their body temperature or sunbathe when ill. This helps to detox the body.

The ultraviolet light in sunlight is lethal to most pathogens, and so can help you remove toxins that are being released from your cells. Love some sun today!

Things to do in your free time

As you won't be watching television, you may have more free time than you are used to. This detox is a peaceful time, so make the most of resting, relaxing and just being. Creative activities such as painting, sewing, or light gardening are also great, but don't overdo it.

Most people aren't used to doing "nothing" and find it hard to switch into this way of being. However, when you persevere, you'll rediscover your serenity, you'll feel peaceful, you'll begin to appreciate your surroundings and you'll feel connected to all that's around you.

If you get "bored", go for a walk and take in your surroundings with new eyes, phone a friend you haven't chatted to for ages, or write a wish list of the top ten things you want to accomplish in the next year — that should keep you occupied!

Shopping list

Buy these ingredients fresh, ripe and organic the day before your detox starts. It might seem that there are lots of ingredients at first glance, but some of them are so small, you won't fill up too many trolleys! If any of the foods are out of season or unavailable to you, replace them with a similar substitute.

Eight litres of mineral or pure water. It's better to have too much than not enough, and I recommend that you don't shop over the three days of the detox.

A selection of dried fruits such as currants, dates, figs, gojis, mango, papaya and pineapple.

Acai powder	Alfalfa sprouts	Almonds
Apples	Apricots, dried	Avocados
Bananas	Beetroot, raw	dark Berries
Broccoli	Cabbage, red	Carrot
Celery	Cinnamon powder	Coconut, brown
Coriander, fresh	Courgette	Dates
Dulse powder	Figs, dried or fresh	GarlicHerbs,
Italian, fresh	Lemon	Lime
Macadamias	Mangoes	Melons
Mint, fresh	Oat groats, raw	Onion
Oranges	Paprika	Pear Pecans
Peppers, yellow and red	Pumpkin (or other squash)	Pumpkin seeds
Pineapple	Romaine lettuce	Spirulina powder
Spring onions	Strawberries	Sunflower seeds
Superfood, green	Tahini, raw	Tomatoes, fresh
Tomatoes, sundried	Vanilla pods	

Snack bag

Carry a snack bag with you at all times as it will help you with hunger, cravings, and emotions. Renew it each day. If there's anything you don't use, have it with your breakfast or lunch the next day to avoid wastage.

- Chop up a quarter of a cantaloupe or honeydew melon, or a whole cucumber or six stalks of celery into bite-sized pieces. Put in a plastic container.

- Mix two handfuls of raw almonds with two handfuls of currants, dates, gojis or any other dried fruit that you like (check out dried mango and papaya, for example!). Wrap these in foil or put in another plastic container.

- Buy a half-litre water bottle, and add your fruity water to it (see below).

- Add two ripe bananas, apples, oranges and any other easy-to-eat fruit.

The night before your detox

Make fruity water by adding a squeeze of lemon or orange to a two-litre bottle of water. Put this beside your bed for the next morning.

Make your **Muesli** and **Almond milk**, keeping them separate until the morning.

Day one

Wake up when you want. Don't set an alarm clock unless you have to go to work. Before getting out of bed, drink about half a litre of the water you prepared last night. If it isn't comfortable to drink that much, just drink the amount you can. If you're at work today, do some simple stretching exercises in bed for five minutes (act like a cat) and then prepare for work. If you're not at work today, do the Tibetan Rejuvenation Rites before breakfast.

Snack bag

Throughout the day, if you ever feel hungry, reach for your **Snack bag**. If you're hungry just before a meal is due, have some water and try waiting until you eat the meal. Read the information on hunger in this book.

Throughout the day, drink plenty of your special fruity water. You will become more thirsty throughout the detox, so don't be alarmed by your rise in water intake.

Breakfast

Muesli with **Almond milk**. Chop bananas, apples, mango, pineapple or any other fresh fruit into the muesli. Have as much as you want. Sit quietly beside your window with the flowers.

Before lunch

If you have time, go for a twenty minute walk or jog. Whether you walk or jog depends on your fitness level, so if you don't already run, walk today. If you don't have time, walk for five minutes, and then in the evening do yoga for fifteen minutes before you go to bed. If the weather is too bad to go outside, walk up and down the stairs for ten minutes. Remember that this exercise gets your lymph moving, which greatly helps the detoxification process.

Lunch

Make simple **Romaine roll-ups**, as many as you want.

Before dinner

Sit quietly for five or ten minutes, where no-one can disturb you (outside if possible or by your window). Take slow, deep breaths, and as you breathe out, release the events of the day. For the last minute, close your eyes and repeat the word "relax" over and over each time you breathe out. Let yourself know that the next two days is "my time". Slowly start to move, first by rolling your shoulders, and then move your neck, and then the rest of your body. Know that this evening will relax you like never before.

Dinner

Two ripe **mangoes**. Eat these, and then wait thirty minutes before your soup.

Sweet beet soup with **macadamia cream**.

Evening

Prepare fruity water (put this beside your bed) for the following day.

Detox helper

Epsom salts

Epsom salts are made from magnesium sulphate. They originate from Epsom, a village in the UK. In the 17th Century, people would come from miles around to drink the healing waters of the village well, as it was high in these salts. These days most people soak in the salts, instead of drinking them. This can ease aches and pains as well as help expel toxins.

Before bed time, run a warm bath, add 2-4lb (1-2kg) of Epsom salts, and stir until dissolved. Brush your skin before getting in, soak for about 5-10 minutes, and clean your skin with a sponge or soft mitt and natural soap or a freshly mashed papaya.

Once you're out of the bath and dried, go straight to bed, and cover yourself up even if you aren't cold — after the Epsom salt bath you need to keep warm. Switch off the lights, close your eyes and repeat "relax" on each out breath.

Day two

Today is a no-work, no-obligation day. Remember that television isn't on your list of things to do, so if you think you might get bored make sure you have some new books or peaceful projects such as gardening or painting to do.

Snack bag

Throughout the day, if you ever feel hungry, reach for your **Snack bag**. If you're hungry just before a meal is due, have some water and try waiting until you eat the meal. Read the information on hunger in this book.

Throughout the day, drink plenty of your special fruity water. You will become more thirsty throughout the detox, so don't be alarmed by your rise in water intake.

Wake up when you want — don't set an alarm today. Before getting out of bed, drink about half a litre of the water you prepared last night. If it's not comfortable to drink that much, just drink as much as you can.

Take your time getting up. Make sure your feet don't touch a cold floor (have slippers or socks ready if that's likely). Keep very warm today at all times. Wear extra clothes, and have a blanket ready for resting time. Remember that feeling cold is a cleansing signal, so if you do feel cold, just smile to yourself and know that it's working already!

Detox helper

Do five each of the Tibetan Rejuvenation Rites, then sit cross-legged (or in lotus if you can do it without forcing or straining) with a straight back for five minutes and keep your mind as calm as possible. Use a meditation technique if you like. Today's mantra will be "still", so you can say that over and over to keep your mind from getting in the way. If you can't sit cross-legged for five minutes, lie down, with your palms upwards and your feet falling outwards, and relax. If you have a bad back, put yourself into any comfortable straight-backed position.

After the five minutes are up, make a note in your journal of this "still" feeling you have, and tell yourself you can recreate that feeling whenever you want throughout the day just by repeating your mantra. Draw a sketch of your feelings. This could look like anything, and it doesn't matter how well you can draw, as no-one else will see it. This is your personal record of transformation.

Breakfast

> ### Superfoods
>
> **Big green** smoothie has green superfood in it. This is a powdered blend of organic plant foods which are high in life force. There are many green superfoods around, and you can find some in your local wholefood store. The two I use are **Nature's Living Superfood** and **Pure Synergy**.

You're going to take your time with breakfast today. Make a **Big green** smoothie. If you can't finish it all, put it in ice cube trays in the freezer to have as a snack another time.

When your smoothie is ready, take a lovely glass and a blanket if necessary and sit outside or at your window. Remember to keep warm.

Take your time drinking the smoothie. Take small sips and chew it, so it starts to digest in the mouth. Concentrate on the flavour, texture and feeling you get when drinking. If any other thoughts come into your mind, gently sweep them away by repeating "still" and concentrate on your food. Focus your eyes on the green outside (or your flowers if there is no green outside) at all times.

After finishing your smoothie, sit and look at your greenery or flowers for a further ten minutes. Allow calm to fill you. Think of the "still" mantra of today and incorporate it here if you feel like it.

In your journal, make a note of how you feel after the ten minutes are up. Compare your feelings now to your feelings a week ago. There will be some positive feelings and also some negative feelings, as you start to detox emotions.

Detox helper

Go for a ten minute walk, jog, or rebound, and then prepare for your massage.

If you booked an appointment for a lymph drainage massage, enjoy! Let the therapist know that you don't wish to talk on this occasion. Use your "still" mantra throughout or another meditation technique. After your massage, remain still for ten minutes if you can, before getting dressed.

If you are giving yourself a massage make sure the room is warm. Adding candles, relaxing music and incense will help detox your mind and spirit. Use a cold pressed oil with a couple of drops of your favourite essential oil if you like.

Drink some water and relax for at least half an hour after your massage, before doing anything else. Make a note of how you feel in your journal. Ask your back how it feels. Ask the same of other body parts — you might be surprised at the answers you receive.

Idea
If you're hungry just before a meal is due, have some water and try waiting until you eat the meal. Read the information on hunger in this book.

Lunch

Lunches will always be bigger than dinners on a detox as we want to take full advantage of the detoxing that occurs at night.

Make **Chakra salad** with **High vibe** dressing. If it's warm enough, eat outside. If not, eat it inside by your window with soothing music and a quiet mind. Remember and use today's mantra: "still".

Detox helper

Yoga. It's great if you can go to a class. Otherwise use a borrowed, hired or bought video or DVD. Always stay at the level you're happy with. There is no physical punishment associated with this detox: this is the peaceful detox. Relax after yoga for at least ten minutes before moving on to anything else.

Dinner

One **papaya**. Eat this and then wait thirty minutes before the next course of **Fig stew**.

Evening

Prepare fruity water (put this beside your bed) for the following day.

Before bed time, run a hot bath and add therapeutic clay or mud to it. The amounts will vary according to the type you use, so refer to the manufacturer's instructions. Brush your skin before getting in, soak for twenty minutes and clean your skin as you did yesterday.

Go straight to bed, and keep very warm. If you're not tired, write in your journal how you feel, and then relax with today's mantra: "still".

Day three

Today is also a no-work no-obligation day. Remember that television isn't on your list of things to do, so if you think you might get bored, make sure you have some new books or peaceful projects such as gardening or painting to do.

Wake up when you want — don't set an alarm today. Before getting out of bed, drink about half a litre of the water you prepared last night. If it's not comfortable to drink that much, just drink the amount you can.

> **Snack bag**
>
> Throughout the day, if you ever feel hungry, reach for your **Snack bag**. If you're hungry just before a meal is due, have some water and try waiting until you eat the meal. Read the information on hunger in this book.
>
> Throughout the day, drink plenty of your special fruity water. You will become more thirsty throughout the detox, so don't be alarmed by your rise in water intake.

Take your time getting up. Make sure your feet don't touch a cold floor (have slippers or socks ready if that's likely). Keep very warm today at all times. Wear extra clothes, and have a blanket at the ready for when you're resting. If you feel like using a hot-water bottle all day, then do!

Detox helper

Do eight each of the Tibetan Rejuvenation Rites and then sit cross-legged (or in lotus if you can do it without forcing or straining) with a straight back for ten minutes and keep the mind as calm as possible. Use a meditation technique if you like, or today's mantra: "renew". If you can't sit cross-legged for ten minutes, lie down, with your palms upwards and your feet falling outwards, and relax. If you have a bad back, get into any comfortable straight-backed position.

After the ten minutes are up, make a note in your journal of this "renew" feeling you have, and tell yourself you will feel that for the rest of the day. Draw a sketch of your feelings. This could look like anything, and it doesn't matter how well you can draw as no-one else will see it. This is your personal record.

Breakfast

You're going to take your time with breakfast today. Make a **Coconut drink**. If you can't finish it all, put it in ice cube trays in the freezer to have as a snack another time.

When your drink is ready, take a lovely glass and a blanket (if necessary) and sit outside or at your window. Remember to keep warm.

Take your time with the drink. Take small sips and chew it, so it starts to digest in the mouth. Concentrate on the flavours, texture and feeling you get when drinking. If any other thoughts come into your mind, gently sweep them away, by repeating "renew" and concentrate on your food. Focus your eyes on the green outside or your flowers at all times.

After finishing your drink, sit and look at your green or flowers for a further twenty minutes, allowing calm to fill you. Use today's mantra if you like. Green is a very healing colour, relating to the heart and working on your immunity. If you have a known immunity problem, you could keep a turquoise stone on you, which may also help. Concentrating on green and opening up your heart will steer you towards generosity, harmony, a long life, compassion and love. This should be our primary goal in life.

In your journal, make a note of how you feel after the twenty minutes are up. Use a green pencil or pen and draw on a whole page whatever is in your head (or heart).

Detox helper

If you can get to a swimming pool, swim for 20-30 minutes, and then have a Jacuzzi and sauna. Take care in the sauna — if you feel faint, get out, sit down and drink water until you feel well again. Even if you are a seasoned sauna goer, you may be more susceptible to dizziness because you are detoxing quite profoundly now.

Lunch

Sunflower pâté with **Cucumber salad**. If it's warm enough, eat outside. If not, eat it inside by your window with soothing music and a quiet mind. Note how slowly you chew, and how much more you appreciate the food when there is no television or hurried conversation. Write this in your journal, as it will help you keep this feeling again once your detox is over.

Detox helper

At least two hours after lunch, stretch! Do this on the floor or bed. Pretend you're a cat, and stretch out your body in all directions that feel good without challenging your body for thirty minutes. If you get adventurous and want to do forward rolls on the bed, then do them! Allow your inner child out to play.

Dinner

Eat half a cantaloupe melon, and wait thirty minutes before your main meal of **Cream of pepper** soup.

Evening

Prepare fruity water for the following day.

Before bed time run a warm bath. Brush your skin before getting in, soak, and clean your skin with a flannel and natural olive soap or a freshly mashed papaya.

Go to bed before you are tired. If you can't sleep, read a book or write your feelings down in your journal. Then relax and repeat today's mantra "renew" in your head.

After your detox

The day after

When you wake up, immediately write down or draw any feelings or dreams that are in your mind. Have your morning fruity water. Continue eating recipes just from this book for the next five days. If you feel hungry, add more nuts to your snack bag. Sleep as much as you need if possible, and continue moving your lymph by exercising.

One week later

Continue with the morning fruity water and Tibetan Rejuvenation Rites. Make sure that at least 75% of your diet consists of fresh raw fruit and vegetables and recipes from this book and **Detox Delights**. If you are going to re-introduce cooking into your diet, then remember to steer clear of cooked animal fats, fried foods and foods containing refined sugar and/or flour.

One life later

Keep experimenting with the *Detox helpers* until you've tried all those which appeal to you. In your journal, note the ones that make you feel good. Use them regularly, and enjoy discovering other ones — there are hundreds out there.

Try to eat a minimum of 75% raw fresh fruit and vegetables and recipes from the books I recommend whenever possible. This can take the form of two fresh raw meals a day and a cooked meal at night, or lots of fruit and salad before every small cooked meal or two green juices and some superfoods each day. It's your choice — and now that you're aware of the effect food has on your body, you'll always want to make the most appropriate one.

Keep noting in your journal the changes you feel while eating the detox way. Very soon, you will have made and assimilated many significant lifestyle choices, and it will feel so natural that you hardly notice.

Your next detox

Now you know what to expect, you can make up a whole new detox based on the structure of this one. Substitute the food for other recipes in this book and use different detox helpers.

Your seven day chakra rejuvenation detox

This detox plan is for you if you have already completed the three-day detox, or if you eat a healthier-than-average diet. It isn't as detailed as the three-day detox, though you can take the procedures from that and incorporate them here. This detox puts great emphasis on cleansing your chakras through meditation and rejuvenation rites. Because it spans seven days, we can take advantage of juices to clean you out even further. If you are working while on this detox, make sure that the two juice days fall on a weekend or light-duty days.

About chakras

There are seven main or common chakras in your body, these are also known as energy centres. They follow the rainbow colours, starting at red and ending at violet.

Chakras influence your mental, emotional, spiritual and physical health. Various methods of meditation, yoga and exercise will open your chakras, and allow energy to flow effortlessly through you. When your chakras are all spinning correctly, your energy levels are consistently high, you feel well and you feel in harmony with everything around you.

Two days before the detox

If you eat meat, poultry, fish, soya products or dairy products (milk, cheese, butter, eggs etc), give them up at least two days before this detox. If that leaves you wondering what to eat, take a look at some of the recipes in this book, and add rice, boiled vegetables, potatoes or bread to them if you feel you need to.

Book an appointment for a lymph drainage massage on day two. If you can't get a lymph drainage massage, book a different type but stress that you want it for detoxification. If you can't book any massage, or find a friend to massage you, then you will give yourself a massage.

Book a yoga class or teacher for day three. If you can't do this, then get a yoga video or DVD to suit your level (either buy one or borrow one from a friend or library).

Buy a notebook to use as a journal to record your feelings and changes.

Buy a sheet of paper for each colour of the rainbow: red, orange, yellow, green, blue, indigo and violet. Wrapping paper is good, as it's big. You will be meditating with these papers, so find somewhere on a wall to stick them; you'll be using one each detox day. You'll be meditating in the morning to set you up for the day, so if you are working you'll need to wake up an hour earlier to squeeze this in. If you're not working, meditate two hours after breakfast. If you are working, meditate and then eat breakfast.

Eat all meals in front of your coloured paper, in silence or while listening to soothing music. Wherever possible, relax for ten or twenty minutes after you've eaten.

One day before the detox

Now cut out all wheat and potato products. This means that for today, and for the detox days, you won't be having bread, potatoes, pasta, meat, fish, soya meat, soya milk, milk, cheese, eggs, cakes, cookies, crackers, sweets, chips or crisps!

If it's sounding scary already, remember that you are about to embark on a high-energy boost for your total self. You'll be guided all the way, so there's nothing to be scared about. Imagine being the best you ever!

Things to do in your free time

As you won't be watching television, you may have more free time than you are used to. This detox is a transformative time, so make the most of resting, exploring and discovering, outwardly and inwardly. Rekindle your love for hobbies you used to have, or try your hand at new creative activities which stretch your mind but don't tire you out.

If all this sounds like too much, don't worry — you'll get all the help you need this coming week, and you will be left transformed and raring to live a life which you could only dream about.

If you get "bored" at any time, ask yourself what it is you're wanting. If it turns out that you're craving the anaesthetic effect of television, write in your journal, read, go for a walk or meditate while looking at your colour of the day.

Unless you have to go to work, don't set your alarm. Sleep with the curtains and window open, so you can make the most of the fresh air. This will help you when you are detoxing: breathing in stale air for eight hours won't!

Shopping list

Buy these ingredients fresh, ripe and organic as much as possible the day before your detox starts. It might seem that there are lots of ingredients at first glance, but some of them are so small, you won't fill up too many trolleys! If any of the foods are out of season or unavailable to you, replace them with a similar substitute.

Twenty litres of water. It's better to have too much than not enough. As most of the food you will be eating is fresh, you will probably have to shop mid-detox. Make the most of online shopping and let the supermarket or organic farm come to you!

A selection of dried fruits such as currants, dates, figs, mango, papaya and pineapple.

Acorn squash, or other type of squash		Almonds
Apples	Apricots, dried	Atlantic sea salad
Avocados	Bananas	Basil, fresh
Blueberries	Butternut squash	Cabbage, red
Carob/cacao powder, raw	Cardamom pods	Carrots
Cashew nuts, raw	Celery seed	Chilli, hot, red
Chives, fresh	Coconut meat, brown	Coriander, fresh
Coriander, powder	Courgette	Cucumber
Cumin, powder	Dill, dried	Dulse or other sea vegetable
E3Live or other edible algae		Galangal, fresh or dried
Garlic	Ginger, fresh	Grapefruits, pink
Hemp oil	Kale, or savoy cabbage	Kumquats
Lemon grass, fresh	Lemons	Lime
Little gem lettuce	Macadamias	Mango
Marrow	Mint, fresh	Mushrooms, button
Mushrooms, portabello	Olive oil, cold pressed	Okra, fresh
Onion, red	Onion, white	Oranges
Oregano, dried	Papaya	Paprika, powder
Parsley, fresh, flat leaf	Peanuts, raw	Pears
Pecans	Pepper, yellow, orange, red	Poppy seeds
Pumpkin, or other squash	Rocket	Romaine lettuce
Sea lettuce, dried	Sea salt	Sesame oil, cold pressed
Spring onions	Strawberries	Sunflower seeds, hulled
Superfood (optional)	Tahini, raw	Tomatoes
Tomatoes, sundried	Turmeric, powder	

Snack bag

Your snack fruit will change daily to reflect the colour of the chakra which you are detoxing. In addition, for the first three days only, make this up:

- Mix two handfuls of raw almonds with two handfuls of currants, dates or any other dried fruit that you like (check out dried mango and papaya, for example!). Wrap these in foil or put in a plastic container.

- Buy a half-litre water bottle, and add your fruity water to it.

The night before your detox

Add a squeeze of lemon or orange to a two-litre bottle of water. Put this beside your bed for the next morning.

Day one

You might want to weigh yourself this morning. If so, make a note of your weight in your journal, then forget about it until after the detox!

Red snack
Throughout the day, if you ever feel hungry, reach for your **Snack bag** or as much of one red fruit of your choice such as strawberries or apples.

Do five each of the Tibetan Rejuvenation Rites before breakfast. If you are working, do your meditation and then eat breakfast.

Breakfast

Chocolate orange smoothie

Meditation

Pin your red paper up on a wall, so it's right in front of your eyes when you sit on the floor. Red is the colour of your base chakra. Many wise people say that you don't clean out the attic before cleaning out the basement, so this is where we will start today.

Red is the colour of energy, rejuvenation, strength, power, love, passion, courage, vitality, and self-confidence, and some of these are the words you'll be concentrating on during this meditation. Either memorise "energy, rejuvenate, power, love, confidence" or write them in large letters on the red paper.

You will be sitting for an hour, so make sure you are comfortable. Keeping your back straight, find a good position, maybe with a cushion or two. Once you are comfortable, look at your red paper, and imagine all your energy is flowing to your base chakra, located at the base of your spine. Concentrate on the first word. In your mind, repeat "Energy" over and over again, as it becomes your mantra. After about ten minutes, move to the next word, and continue like this for each word. For the last ten minutes, concentrate on your base chakra, allowing the warmth created here to go anywhere in your body which needs healing with love.

Meditating for an hour might seem like a long time, but you will get lost in time. Making sure you repeat the words will help keep you on track if you're not used to meditating.

Once you have finished meditating, continue with your day, knowing you can always use the power of your base chakra to help you.

Lunch

Squash and kumquat soup served with **Basilled tomatoes**.

Detox helper

Choose from the detox helper section. A reflexology session or some time on your rebounder would be great, as it stimulates your organs to start kicking out toxins.

Do this either two hours after lunch, or after you have finished work.

Dinner

As much of your red fruit as you like. Wait twenty minutes before eating your meal below.

Champiñónes au natural and **The gratest salad in the world**.

Evening

Take an Epsom salts bath, as outlined in the three day detox.

Day two

We are going to get a bit lighter on food today, but there is still your snack bag to eat from. Remember to replenish this every day, and always have your fruity water to hand.

> ## Orange snack
>
> Throughout the day, if you ever feel hungry, reach for your **Snack bag** or as much of one orange fruit of your choice such as oranges or peaches.

Do six each of the Tibetan Rejuvenation Rites before breakfast. If you are working, do your meditation and then eat breakfast.

Breakfast

Seaside smoothie

Meditation

Pin your orange paper up on a wall, so it's right in front of your eyes when you sit on the floor. Orange is the colour of your sacral chakra and is related to emotions, sexuality, and your reproductive, respiratory and intestinal systems. It's the colour of food, happiness, confidence, success, pleasure, goals and action, and resourcefulness. You'll concentrate on some of these words during this meditation. Either memorise "happy, success, pleasure, active, resourceful" or write them in large letters on the orange paper.

You will be sitting for an hour, so make sure you are comfortable. Keeping your back straight, find a good position, maybe with a cushion or two. Once you are comfortable, picture your base chakra for a minute and feel the energy move up to the sacral chakra. From there, look at your orange paper, and imagine all your energy is flowing to your sacral chakra, located in your lower abdomen. Concentrate on the first word. In your mind, repeat "Happy" over and over, as it becomes your mantra. After about ten minutes, move to the next word, and continue for each word. For the last ten minutes, concentrate on your sacral chakra, allowing the warmth created here to go anywhere in your body which needs healing with happiness.

Meditating for an hour might seem like a long time, but you will get lost in time. Making sure you repeat the words will help keep you on track if you're not used to meditating.

Once you have finished meditating, continue with your day, knowing you can always use the resourcefulness of your sacral chakra to help you.

Lunch

Golden gazpacho soup

Detox helper

Choose from the detox helper section. A full body massage would work well here. You need to be treated today, as the first few days of detoxing are always the hardest, so ask a willing friend to give you an unconditional massage if you can't get to a therapist.

Do this either two hours after lunch, or after you have finished work.

Dinner

As much of your orange fruit as you like. Wait twenty minutes before eating your meal below.

Thai salad with **Seeded noodles**

Evening

Take a mud bath, as outlined in the three-day detox.

Day three

Apart from the snacks you will be on liquids today. Some foods are juiced, and some are blended, so it's taking more pressure off your digestive system to allow your energy to divert into the areas which need detoxing. Remember to drink your fruity water, too!

Yellow snack

Throughout the day, if you ever feel hungry, reach for your **Snack bag** or as much of one yellow fruit of your choice such as bananas or melon.

Do seven each of the Tibetan Rejuvenation Rites before breakfast. If you are working, do your meditation and then eat breakfast.

Breakfast
The candy floss tart juice

Meditation

Pin your yellow paper up on a wall, so it's right in front of your eyes when you sit on the floor. Yellow is the colour of your solar plexus chakra and is related to your colon, stomach, liver, nervous system and eyes.

Yellow is the colour of personality or ego, clarity, awareness, curiosity, wisdom, intelligence, learning and self-esteem. You'll be concentrating on some of these words during this meditation. Either memorise "clear, aware, curious, wise, intelligent" or write them in large letters on the yellow paper.

You will be sitting for an hour, so make sure you are comfortable. Keeping your back straight, find a good position, maybe with a cushion or two. Once you are comfortable, picture your base chakra for a minute and feel the energy move up to the sacral chakra, stay there for a further minute, and then feel the energy move up to your solar plexus chakra. From there, look at your yellow paper, and imagine all your energy is flowing to your solar plexus chakra, located beneath your chest. Concentrate on the first word. In your mind, repeat "Clear" over and over, as it becomes your mantra. After about ten minutes, move to the next word, and continue like this for each word. For the last ten minutes, concentrate on your solar plexus chakra, allowing the warmth created here to go anywhere in your body which needs healing with wisdom.

Meditating for an hour might seem like an age, but you will get lost in time. Making sure you repeat the words will help keep you on track, especially if you're not used to meditating.

Once you have finished meditating, continue with your day, knowing you can always use the clarity of your solar plexus chakra to help you.

Lunch
Spicy pear juice

Detox helper

Choose from the detox helper section. Yoga would be the best choice for you today, as it helps stimulate and internally massage your organs. If you can't get to a class, either buy or hire a video and do it in the comfort and privacy of your own home.

Do this either two hours after lunch, or after you have finished work.

Dinner

As much of your yellow fruit as you like. Wait twenty minutes before eating your meal below.

Cardamom cooler (keep the papaya peel)

Evening

Walk up and down the stairs, jog on the spot or rebound for ten minutes to get your lymph moving. Use your body brush, and then run a hot bath.

Grate a handful of fresh ginger, and add this to the bath, inside a muslin bag or an old stocking. Soak for about twenty minutes, before cleansing your whole body and face with the inside of the papaya peel. Once you're out of the bath, dry yourself as soon as you can and go to bed, keeping very warm.

Green snack

Throughout the day, if you ever feel hungry, make a green juice out of cucumber, apple or celery for the base, and add some wild leaves from your garden or good organic greens such as watercress, spinach or kale.

Day four

Now, just for two days, you're going to drop your snack bags, and only have juices. This will enable your body to spend even more time on cleaning itself instead of digesting. If you feel hungry, go to your meditation paper, and repeat one of your mantras for the day. Drink as much water as you need today, your body will make good use of the liquid. Try to do today and tomorrow on days when you aren't working, and make the most of relaxing.

Do eight each of the Tibetan Rejuvenation Rites before breakfast.

Breakfast

Cucumber and apple juice

Meditation

Pin your green paper up on a wall, so it's right in front of your eyes when you sit down on the floor. Green is the colour of your heart chakra and is associated with your heart, blood circulatory system and the whole chest area.

Green is the colour of universal love, breath, harmony, renewal, peace, protection, healing, abundance and kindness. You'll be concentrating on some of these words during this meditation. Either memorise "harmony, peace, protection, abundance, kindness" or write them in large letters on the green paper.

You will be sitting for an hour, so make sure you are comfortable. Keeping your back straight, find a good position, maybe with a cushion or two. Once you are comfortable, picture your base chakra for a minute and feel the energy move up to the sacral chakra. Stay there for a further minute, and then feel the energy move up to your solar plexus chakra. After a minute on that chakra, look at your green paper, and imagine all your energy is flowing to your heart chakra, located in the centre of your chest. Concentrate on the first word. In your mind, repeat "Harmony" over and over, as it becomes your mantra. After about ten minutes, move to the next word, and continue like this until all your words have been used up. For the last ten minutes, concentrate on your heart chakra, allowing the warmth created here to go anywhere in your body which needs protecting and kindness.

Extra help

Because you're deep into detox now, you can utilise the power of the heart chakra by hugging. Ask someone you love to hug you, unconditionally for at least ten minutes. During the hug, picture green, and feel your heart chakra open.

Meditating for an hour might seem like a long time, but you will get lost in time. Making sure you repeat the words will help keep you on track if you're not used to meditating.

Once you have finished meditating, continue with your day, knowing you can always use the universal love of your heart chakra to help you.

Lunch

Rocket Fuel juice

Detox helper

Choose from the detox helper section. A conscious breathing session would be great today as you are working on your chest area in your meditation.

Do this either two hours after lunch, or after you have finished work.

Dinner

Runny romaine juice (keep the mango peel)

Evening

Walk up and down the stairs, jog on the spot or rebound for ten minutes to get your lymph moving. Use your body brush and then run a warm bath.

Soak in the bath for about twenty minutes, before cleansing your whole body and face with the inside of the mango peel. Once you're out of the bath, dry yourself as soon as you can, and go to bed, keeping very warm.

Day five

You are doing so well! A whole day just on juices will make today very easy as you should now be feeling some of the benefits to lightening your life. Remember to conserve your energy as much as possible so your body can continue cleaning at full force. Today is another juice-only day, so keep the snack bag at bay just for another 24 hours!

Blue snack
Throughout the day, if you ever feel hungry, make a juice out of cucumber, apple or celery with blueberries.

Do nine each of the Tibetan Rejuvenation Rites before breakfast.

Breakfast

Supercharged celery juice

Meditation

Pin your blue paper up on a wall, so it's right in front of your eyes when you sit down on the floor. Blue is the colour of your throat chakra and controls the throat, neck, arms and hands.

Blue is the colour of communication, expression, creativity, manifestation, fulfilment, relaxation and balance. You'll be concentrating on some of these words during this meditation. Either memorise "express, manifest, fulfil, relax, balance" or write them in large letters on the blue paper.

You will be sitting for an hour, so make sure you are comfortable. Keeping your back straight, find a good position, maybe with a cushion or two. Once you are comfortable, picture your base chakra for a minute and feel the energy move up to the sacral chakra. Repeat this with your solar plexus chakra and heart chakra. Look at your blue paper, and imagine all your energy is flowing to your throat chakra, located in the base of your throat. Concentrate on the first word. Repeat in your mind "Express" over and over, as it becomes your mantra. After about ten minutes, move to the next word, and continue like this until all your words have been used up. For the last ten minutes, concentrate on your throat chakra, allowing the warmth created here to go anywhere in your body which needs to be balanced and relaxed.

Meditating for an hour might seem like a long time, but you will get lost in time. Making sure you repeat the words will help keep you on track if you're not used to meditating.

Once you have finished meditating, continue with your day, knowing you can always use the expression of your throat chakra to help you.

Lunch

Fractal fortnight juice

Extra help

Because you're deep into detox now, you can utilise the power of the throat chakra by writing in your journal. Really get to grips with expressing your feelings using the written word. Otherwise, you can be vocal and use a tape recorder to communicate with your deepest self.

Detox helper

Choose from the *Detox helpers* chapter. How about an energetic session on a rebounder, or going for a light run? With your new-found energy you should enjoy this exhilarating time, but remember not to overdo it as you are in big-time detox mode.

Do this either two hours after lunch, or after you have finished work.

Dinner

Strawberry patch juice

Evening

Walk up and down the stairs, jog on the spot, run up and down your stairs or rebound for ten minutes to get your lymph moving.

Detox helper — body scrub

You're about to make a luxury scrub which will make you glow all over. Make sure your bathroom is warm before starting this.

1 cup of cold pressed sesame oil

1½ cups of sea salt

1 lime

1 teaspoon of grated ginger

Juice the lime and mix all ingredients together.

In your bathroom, stand on an old towel and work the scrub into your body starting from your feet and working upwards. Don't use this on your face. If you have someone to help you, then rope them in! Gently massage the scrub into your skin, concentrating on elbows, knees, thighs and buttocks

After about ten minutes of massaging, turn the shower onto warm and wash all the scrub off with a pure soap. Now, if you can — turn the shower onto cold for 30 seconds. Turn all the way round so all of your body is covered in cold water and then turn the water onto warm for a minute. Repeat this five times, and finish with a lovely warm shower for as long as you want. Once you're out of the shower, dry yourself as soon as you can and go to bed, keeping very warm.

Day six

As you approach the finish line, you will notice many changes in your mind, body, and spirit. Journal these changes, and think about what you'd like to continue once the detox is over. Today we reintroduce solid foods, but we're keeping it gentle. The snack bag is different today, so have a look at what you are going to eat.

Snack bag
Your snack bag today can contain as much fresh fruit as you wish for, and soaked almonds.

Indigo snack
Throughout the day, if you ever feel hungry, eat as many plums or blackberries as you would like.

Do ten each of the Tibetan Rejuvenation Rites before breakfast. If you are working, do your meditation and then eat breakfast.

Breakfast

Melonlemon drink

Meditation

Pin your indigo paper up on a wall, so it's right in front of your eyes when you sit on the floor. Indigo is the colour of your brow chakra, also known as the third eye chakra. It's associated with the forehead, temples, lower brain, central nervous system, nose, eyes, ears, lymph system and pituitary gland.

Indigo is the colour of the unconscious self, intuition, imagination, creativity, psychic powers, mysticism and understanding. You'll be concentrating on some of these words during this meditation. Either memorise "intuition, imagine, create, psychic, understand" or write them in large letters on the indigo paper.

You will be sitting for an hour, so make sure you are comfortable. Keeping your back straight, find a good position, maybe with a cushion or two. Once you are comfortable, picture your base chakra for a minute and feel the energy move up to the sacral chakra. Repeat this with your solar plexus chakra, heart chakra and throat chakra. Look at your indigo paper, and imagine all your energy is flowing to your brow chakra, which is located in the centre of your forehead. Concentrate on the first word. In your mind, repeat "Intuition" over and over again, as it becomes your mantra. After about ten minutes, move to the next word, and continue like this for each word. For the last ten minutes, concentrate on your brow chakra, allowing the warmth created here to go anywhere in your body which needs psychic healing.

Meditating for an hour might seem like a long time, but you will get lost in time. Making sure you repeat the words will help keep you on track if you're not used to meditating.

Once you have finished meditating, continue with your day, knowing you can always use the psychic abilities of your brow chakra to help you.

Lunch

Yellow pepper and almond soup

Detox helper

Choose something from the detox helper section. More meditation exercises would work well today, as you have done a lot of spiritual clearing over the past few days. If you can't face any more meditation, then going for a quiet walk in nature for at least an hour is also a great detox helper.

Do this either two hours after lunch, or after you have finished work.

Dinner

I can't believe it's not Waldorf salad

Evening

Walk up and down the stairs, jog on the spot or rebound for ten minutes to get your lymph moving.

Detox helper — face treat

This face treat is great for all skin types. If your skin is dry, add extra avocado.

½ avocado, peeled and stoned

¼ papaya, peeled and de-seeded

Using a hand blender, blend both ingredients together and smooth over the face. If you have some cucumber to hand, mash some of that up and place it on your eyes. Relax for 10-15 minutes, then wash off the face treat.

Have another Epsom salts bath as outlined in the three-day detox, then go straight to bed.

Day seven

It's your final detox day today! Well done for getting this far. By now you should have lost a lot of bloating, and you should have more energy than you have had for years. You should also look younger in the face. If you weighed yourself at the beginning, wait until tomorrow morning before you weigh yourself again.

Do eleven each of the Tibetan Rejuvenation Rites before breakfast. If you are working, do your meditation and then eat breakfast.

Snack bag
Your snack bag today can contain as much fresh fruit as you wish for, and soaked almonds.

Breakfast

Cucumber number juice

Meditation

Pin your violet paper up on a wall, so it's right in front of your eyes when you sit on the floor. It's the colour of your crown chakra, also known as the cosmic consciousness centre. It's associated with the top of the head, the brain, and the nervous system.

Violet snack
Throughout the day, if you ever feel hungry, eat as many fresh figs, plums, brambles (blackberries) or purple grapes as you would like.

Violet is the colour of the spiritual self, purity, weight control, inspiration, artistic talent, ideals, spirituality, beauty and self-assurance. You'll be concentrating on some of these words during this meditation. Either memorise "pure, control, inspire, talent, beautiful" or write them in large letters on the violet paper.

You will be sitting for an hour, so make sure you are comfortable. Keeping your back straight, find a good position, maybe with a cushion or two. Once you are comfortable, picture your base chakra for a minute and feel the energy move up to the sacral chakra. Repeat this with your solar plexus chakra, heart chakra, throat chakra and brow chakra. Look at your violet paper, and imagine all your energy is flowing to your crown chakra, which is located at the top of the head. Concentrate on the first word. In your mind, repeat "Pure" over and over again, as it becomes your mantra. After about ten minutes, move to the next word, and continue like this for each word. For the last ten minutes, concentrate on your crown chakra, allowing the warmth created here to go anywhere in your body which needs purifying.

Meditating for an hour might seem like a long time, but you will get lost in time. Making sure you repeat the words will help keep you on track if you're not used to meditating.

Once you have finished meditating, continue with your day, knowing you can always use the spiritual abilities of your crown chakra to help you.

Lunch

Japanese okra with **Carrot nests**

Detox helper

Choose something from the detox helper section. A swim and a sauna will work well today. Go easy in the sauna, and swim in many positions so your whole body moves.

Either do this two hours after lunch, or after you have finished work.

Dinner

Crudités with **Creamy herb dip**. For the crudités, use sticks of your choice of raw baby sweetcorn, baby carrots, courgette, cucumber, peppers and celery with cauliflower florets, broccoli florets, tomato halves.

Evening

Walk up and down the stairs, jog on the spot or rebound for ten minutes to get your lymph moving.

Detox helper — mud wrap

If you can get someone to help you with this, it will be easier. You'll need:

Therapeutic clay or mud, enough for your body

Water to mix with the mud if necessary

3 bin liners

1 sleeping bag

Old towels

Old socks

Where to get mud and clay
Herbalists and specialist online stores sell all kinds of mud. Check out green clay, Fuller's earth and kaolin.
If you're lucky enough to get good clay from your garden, then use that, diluted with water.

Put your old towels on the floor before starting. Put your sleeping bag on the floor, opened up. Cut the bottoms off two of the bin liners and tape all three liners together so you have created one long bag.

If you have to mix water to the mud, do that now. It's more comfortable to mix warm water with it. Cover your whole body in mud. Depending on the type you use, you can often put it on your face, but check for sensitivity first. Jump into the bin liners, pop yourself into the sleeping bag, zip it up and then wriggle right in. Make sure all your body is covered, and you are very warm.

After twenty minutes, get out of the bags and put your old socks on to go to your shower room, shower off the mud and go straight to bed to keep warm.

After your detox

The day after

When you wake up, immediately write down or sketch any feelings or dreams that are in your mind. Have your morning fruity water. Continue eating recipes just from this book for the next seven days. Continue doing your Tibetan Rejuvenation Rites, adding one extra each day. If you feel hungry, remember what you did to counter the hunger before and do the same now. Sleep as much as you need if possible, and continue moving your lymph by exercising.

The week after

Continue with the morning fruity water. Continue with your Tibetan Rejuvenation Rites, adding one extra each day until you reach twenty one. Make sure that at least 75% of your diet consists of fresh raw fruit and vegetables, utilising recipes from this book and **Detox Delights**. If you are going to re-introduce cooking into your diet, then remember to steer clear of cooked animal fats, fried foods and foods with refined sugar and flour in them.

215

For life

Keep experimenting with the detox helpers, until you've tried them all. In your journal, note the ones you like, the ones that make you feel good. Use them regularly.

Try to eat a minimum of 75% raw fresh fruit and vegetables and recipes from the books I recommend whenever possible. This can take the form of two fresh raw meals a day and a cooked meal at night, or lots of fruit and salad before every small cooked meal. It's your choice — but now you're aware of the effect food has on your body, you'll want to make the right one.

Keep noting in your journal the changes you feel when eating the detox way. Very soon, you will have made and assimilated many significant lifestyle choices, and it will feel so natural, that you hardly notice.

Your next detox

Now you know what to expect, you can make up a whole new detox based on the structure of this one. Substitute the food for other recipes in this book, and use different detox helpers.

If you feel like you want to go further, try out *Your juice detox* or the *Detox for life* plan!

Fasting and juice cleansing

Fasting is an ancient time-honoured process where you can deep cleanse and heal your body, by lying still and only drinking water. Some people fast for weeks, and some fast for one day a week. Some people fast for healing, some fast for a deeper spiritual connection and clarity. Whatever your reasons for fasting, please be careful. It is a beautiful process, and one which I regularly enjoy, but it is not something you should do without further research or support.

If you have never fasted before, then a juice cleanse might be a better option. If you are heavily toxic and want to fast your way to health, then please seek the supervision of a fasting counsellor.

If you are in relatively good health, then you can probably do a three day fast in your own home, though it is best to have someone with you.

There is some controversy surrounding fasting, and so juice cleansing is becoming increasingly popular. Whereas fasting totally relies on the body for detoxing and rejuvenation, juice cleansing offers certain nutrients as support to the body, while it can cleanse at a better rate than normal. I believe both methods are very valid and valuable.

Personally, I find juice cleansing difficult, because if I taste food I want to eat it until I feel full, but with fasting, I don't taste anything and so my desire for food isn't there at all. It's all a case of preference, so you could try both and then decide which suits you the best.

Emotional cleansing

When you detox, past emotions and events do come up, as your cells release their memories of these events. Meditating while deep cleansing is a great way to allow this to happen. Remember that you don't want to sweep your emotions under the carpet, as they will just store up and manifest in a worse way later. If your emotional cleansing becomes too much, please seek the help of a counsellor who will be able to work you through the arising issues.

Contraindications

If you are diabetic, pregnant or have a serious illness, please do not do either of these deep cleanses without the supervision of a trained practitioner.

Hunger and fasting

I've never been hungry when I've fasted, though many people say they are hungry for the first three days, and then it disappears. Obviously, you don't want to be in discomfort, but if you do feel hungry, or are hankering after something, try to understand why. It's often the case that you're not actually hungry, you're just used to putting stuff in your mouth on a regular basis.

Breaking a fast

It's important to break your fast correctly. If you haven't eaten for several days, make sure you have some fresh organic fruit and greens delivered to your house a day before you want to break your fast.

I like to break a fast with just a few spoonfuls of melon, though my last fast was broken with two apples. Some people break fasts on alkaline fruits such as papaya, while others like oranges. Some people even break fasts on freshly squeezed green juices. These are all valid ways to break your fast. If you have a variety of fruits and greens in the house, then smell them to let your body choose what it wants.

However you break your fast, make sure that the next three food days only consist of fruit and green leafy vegetables, with no fat. Make simple juices such as celery and apple or pear and rocket, to slowly let your body get back to normal. Make use of mono meals, or green and fruit meals, and eat little meals throughout the day.

Juice cleansing

Experts claim that fresh juices assist the body to deep cleanse and rejuvenate. Because fruit and juices are alkalising, they neutralise acids in the body. In addition, juices are easy to digest, and your metabolic activity doesn't slow down as in true fasting, so further cleansing is promoted.

I think that a juice cleanse is a good way to start your deep inner cleansing, as it isn't so harsh and dramatic as a water fast. However, nothing can compare to the feelings you get when you water fast, so do give the water fast a go, once you are sufficiently detoxed. I'd suggest you wait until six months after you have started detoxing before you water fast, but juice cleansing can safely be done much sooner.

Whichever method you choose or prefer, deeply buried pollutants and chemicals will be cleared out through your elimination channels. Make the most of removing them after you have finished fasting with the help of exercise, sauna and massage.

Further information

Books

Fasting and Eating for Health
A Medical Doctor's Program for Conquering Disease
Joel Fuhrman
ISBN: 031218719X

Once your eyes are opened to fasting, you will wonder how you lived without it! This book details medical facts and references for a life of health.

The Juice Lady's Guide to Juicing for Health
Unleashing the Healing Power of Whole Fruits and Vegetables
Cherie Calbom
ISBN: 0895299992

Containing over 150 tasty juice recipes, this book will help you treat an A-Z of ailments. Again, backed by scientific data, The Juice Lady brings you a veritable vitamin feast.

Web sites

www.fasting.com — Claiming to be the world's most informative, comprehensive and educational scientific fasting web site, all your questions will be answered.

Fasting and detox centres

If you want to complete a supervised fast or detox, then contact this centre. It is run by experienced fasting supervisors:

Rest Of Your Life Retreat
Drs Gregory & Tosca Haag
PO Box 102
Barksdale
TX 78828
USA

Tel: +1 (830) 234 3488 | Fax: +1 (830) 234 3599
www.roylretreat.com | greg@roylretreat.com

In Texas, USA, this retreat provides a peaceful, restful, relaxing and rejuvenating place for you to fast and rejuvenate, or just take a break.

Things to do

- When juice cleansing, make sure all your food is organic or wild. Toxic *icides don't belong in your body at any time, and will hinder your progress if you have them when cleansing.

- When fasting, turn to meditation for guidance and healing. Don't do anything strenuous, and lie down outside (out of the direct sun) as much as possible. Make sure you have fresh air, warm baths and plenty of peace.

- As fasting can make you more creative, complete a short fast before new big projects, and keep an ideas book close at hand for you to write in.

- If you have detoxed for six months or more and suddenly have a heavy workload, then take on a juice cleanse to give you mental clarity, more time and more stable energy.

Your juice detox

This is a workable alternative to a fast. When on a juice detox, your body can cleanse more than normal and you can still undertake light duties. If you are working, start the detox on a work day and then take two days off (such as the weekend). If you can take more time off, you can extend this detox for five days just by repeating the same recipes or by using other juices from the recipe section of this book.

Before your detox

This is going to be a great time for you. You will feel lighter and have more energy, so try to conserve or channel it as much as possible. A week before, cut out all tea, coffee, alcohol and grain-based food. Two days before, eat only raw fruits, vegetables, nuts and seeds.

Water

Stock up on bottled water. Buy enough for two-three litres per day. You might drink less, but it's best to have enough so you don't have to go shopping. As with the other detox plans, squeeze some fresh fruit juice into the water a day before you drink it.

How to eat your juice

When your juice is freshly made, take slow sips and chew it, to get the digestive system working, then swallow. Finish the juice within fifteen minutes of making it and don't store any leftovers.

What a relief!

Buy an enema kit. When you sometimes really feel the need to go to the toilet, but can't, an enema kit comes in really useful. Use your bottled water in the enema and find the relief you need, whenever necessary.

Relax and keep warm

This is a time for you to relax, so clear all responsibilities before starting. This is "me time".

Throughout the detox keep well wrapped up if it's cold weather and wear socks at all times. However, even if it's cold, go outside for fresh air for at least an hour a day, even if that means sitting in your garden inside a sleeping bag!

Shopping list

| Apples | Blueberries | Cabbage, white |
| Carrots | Celery | Cinnamon, powder |

Chilli, medium	Cucumber	E3Live or Crystal Manna
Ginger	Grapefruits, pink	Kale or savoy cabbage
Lemons	Little gem lettuce	Mango
Melon, cantaloupe or piel de sapo		Mint, fresh
Okra	Orange	Peaches
Pears	Pepper, yellow and red	Rocket
Romaine lettuce	Spinach	Strawberries
Tomatoes	Wild leaves such as dandelion, dock, plantain	

If you can't find some of the items of food on the list due to seasonal fluctuations, you can easily replace one item with something similar. If you have access to edible wild leaves, by all means juice some of these with your recipes — be aware that they are very strong, and you should go easy on drinking them if you aren't used to it.

It's important that you buy organic food, as you will be eating peel — and you don't want to ingest poisonous chemicals, especially on a detox!

Day one

When you wake up, drink half a litre of lemon water or as much as is comfortable for you.

Drink plenty of fruity water throughout the day. Have five juices today, in any order, and at any time:

Wake up, ginger

Cucumber number

Apple and orange

Cabbage and carrot

The lady juiced her fingers

Day two

When you wake up, have half a litre of lemon water.

Drink plenty of lemon water throughout the day. Have five juices today, in any order, and at any time:

Spicy pear

Supercharged celery

Sweet grapefruit

Runny romaine

Sangria Maria

Day three

When you wake up, have half a litre of lemon water.

Drink plenty of fruity water throughout the day. Have five juices today, in any order, and at any time:

Strawberry patch

Cucumber and apple

Hot orange

Rocket fuel

Carrot top-up

After your detox

As you've done such an intense cleanse, it's very important to reintroduce solids slowly. For the first day, just have blended foods from the recipe section of this book such as soup, smoothies and other drinks. On the second day after your cleanse, add some whole fruits that are easy to digest and watery, such as melon, mango and papaya. Continue having juices, too, especially green ones. On days three to five, introduce some light salads and avocado if you like.

A week later

Slowly reintroduce other foods such as nuts and seeds into your diet, and stay at the point where at least 75% of your intake is fresh raw plant-based foods. For example, you could choose to eat fruit until noon, a juice every day, and have a big salad with every cooked meal. Remember how you felt during the cleanse by looking in your journal, and know that you can lighten your life any time you want by going back to the juice cleanse.

Your fast

Really, I should have left this page blank, because your instructions are to do nothing. OK, you do need to do a few things...

Important note

Do not fast if you are pregnant, if you are addicted to any drugs (remove them from your life first), if you are ill, or if you have a responsibility towards others, such as young children or work. Many fasting practitioners recommend that your first fast is supervised, and that all fasts over three or five days are supervised. Use your inner wisdom, and fast only to the point where you feel it is benefiting you and you are in control. It's worth being responsible when fasting because when you do it correctly, it detoxes your mind, body and spirit at a great rate.

If you haven't completed one of the previous detox plans and your current diet is a standard western one, I strongly recommend you complete a less intense detox plan before doing this. Otherwise, it could be like jumping off the top of a ladder, instead of gently climbing down it.

Before your fast

First of all — know that you will enjoy your fast. This isn't a time of deprivation, it's a time of new experiences, and new doors will open within you. A week before the fast, cut out all tea, coffee, alcohol and grain-based food. Two days before, eat only raw fruits and vegetables. One day before, eat only one or two types of food or juice (such as melons, or apple and cucumber juice).

Stock up on bottled water. Estimate two to three litres per day. It's best to over estimate as I promise that you will not want to wobble to the shop on day three!

Buy an enema kit. If you want to go to the toilet but can't, an enema kit easily and quickly solves the problem for you. Use your bottled water in the enema, as it's purer than tap water.

Buy a hot water bottle. When fasting, all your blood is diverted to clean out your organs, so your limbs can start to feel a bit cut off! Keep warm at all times, but do get out in the fresh air, or at least have your window open constantly.

Fasting days

If you are not supervised by a qualified practitioner, plan to fast for three to five days only. On the first day of your fast, stay in bed for as long as you can. Very few people can fast and go to work, so please don't try it. If you become "bored", then meditate. Play a chanting or meditation CD, and close your eyes. This is a time to journey inward and explore undiscovered caverns in your mind and imagination.

Sip room-temperature water when you are thirsty. Do not "dry fast" (fast without water).

If you feel hungry, return your mind to a meditative state, and know that it will pass.

Rest as much as possible. If you have ideas (this happens a lot when fasting), write them in your journal. Do not act upon them, as you will not have the stamina to see them through and you need to conserve your energy so your body can detox more thoroughly.

Remember to breathe deeply, and do so outside if possible. The extra oxygen will help your cells detoxify and rejuvenate.

If you have a garden, sit outside (weather permitting) and get at least an hour's exposure to the air a day. If it's cold, keep well wrapped up, as you will feel cold more when you fast.

If someone can give you a light massage each day, then accept graciously, but do not allow oils on your skin.

Breaking your fast

Breaking your fast correctly is necessary for best results. Experts' opinions vary, from eating a papaya to drinking green juice, but my experience tells me that a juice made from mild greens and non-sweet fruit is good. It gives your body some nourishment, but it's still very watery. Fresh young coconut water is also great.

Try juicing half a cucumber, two romaine leaves and one stalk of celery. If it's not sweet enough, juice two apples and mix them in. Sip it, chew it and swallow it very slowly — finish it within fifteen minutes.

An hour later, or when you feel like eating, have your first meal.

Take four to six lettuce leaves and two pieces of fruit. Eat them together, separately, or created however you want. You could blend them into a soup, or you could finely chop them and mix them up, or you could even juice them again. Eat this slowly and then rest for the day. If you want to eat more, make another juice.

For all this to work smoothly, you need to have food ready for you in the house, but not there when you start your fast as it won't be fresh enough by the time you finish. Either order the food for the day before you plan to break the fast and have it delivered, or ask a family member or a friend to do some shopping for you.

After breaking your fast

Your stomach will have shrunk and your insides will be cleaner, so go easy on what you put in. For the next five post-fast days, just eat lettuces, juices and fruit. Do not eat any fats or starches. That means: no avocados, olives, seeds, nuts, meat, bread, pasta, potatoes or rice.

For the next week slowly reintroduce other good, wholesome food to your life. Remember that from now on you will only accept the very best in your newly detoxed world.

Detox for life

This detox plan is different to any others that you might have seen or used. The aim here is for you to gradually alter things in your life to make you lighter, happier, healthier and more positive in all areas of your life. Do it consistently, changing something every week — and don't worry about missing some of the steps out or doing some things in a different order. Tailor it to your needs. So long as you keep moving with it, you will succeed in lightening your life.

When you begin your *Detox for life*, you'll see that you're not cutting anything out, you're just altering and adding things. When you add so much good stuff to your life, the bad stuff just melts away, without pain. This plan is devised so that you don't feel like you are on a plan, and because of that you can use the other detox plans simultaneously while detoxing for life.

I recommend that everyone follows this plan, because the benefits to you, the environment, and your family and friends are greater than I can explain. It's very useful to keep a journal when detoxing for life, as your memories of how you used to be will fade. If you ever find yourself doubting the effectiveness of your detox, reading about those dim and distant achy, painy, tired, depressed, overweight, emotions in black and white will be the biggest incentive for you to carry on.

Because there's no time scale for finishing this plan, there's no pressure with backsliding. If you do something contrary to the suggested guidelines, just make a note that you are changing it, now. If you take a month to feel comfortable with one change and a week to feel comfortable with another, it's not important. What is important is that you do it. It's that simple. Happy detoxing, for your life.

Stages to a detoxed life

Remember that this is a method of becoming less toxic and, therefore, healthier in all areas of your life — over time, gradually and easily. Use the detox plans when detoxing for life to accelerate cleansing, which will greatly assist this process.

Start at the top and work your way down, taking the time you need to feel comfortable with each change. You might want to do the first three changes all at once, or you might want to space them out over three months. It's up to you. Once you've made a change, view it as a change for life. Some things will evolve, such as drinking water — you won't need so much when you're hydrated and eating more watery food as you do in the beginning. very soon, you'll be in touch with your instinct, so will be able to determine what to tweak, and when.

I don't mention how to kick drug habits in this list, as it's not an area I specialise in. If you need help with that, then please consult an expert in that field. You can follow this list at the same time, and please tell your counsellor. Remember that the InnerTalk CDs and tapes can help you to easily change all addictive habits, including comfort eating and overeating. These CDs are there to help you, as they've helped thousands of others.

So without further ado, here's your list. Take your time, and enjoy it.

Go organic

This is your first change and you don't have to cut out anything that you eat or drink yet (that'll come later!) If you have any doubts about switching to an organic diet, re-read the organic section in this book and read other organic food and farming books. As well as it being much more interesting than docu-soaps, you get to fill your brain with positive information. Once you do that, the negative fear-based information falls away.

Make full use of supermarkets (they often offer online ordering and delivery so you can save time and petrol). Check out local farmers, organic delivery schemes, markets, wholefood shops, neighbours with gardens and wild places. Use your initiative, and make it a fun project. If you can't afford to change to 100% organic, or if you don't find the availability, at least make sure your greens are organic (especially in juice) as this is where your much-needed minerals come from.

Drink more water

Most people are so permanently dehydrated that many diseases can occur because of that alone. Refresh your mind by drinking some water and reading my section on water. Then prepare the following every day: in a 1.5 litre bottle of mineral water, squeeze some lemon or orange juice before going to bed at night. Put the bottle by your bed and drink a third of it upon waking. Drink the rest throughout the day. If you're out and about, transfer some into a half-litre "sports" bottle. If you are thirsty, drink more than the amount I've listed.

Tea, coffee and fizzy drinks are not health-giving and are toxic, so this could be the first thing you start to cut down on, as your water intake increases.

Get fruity in the mornings

Once you're happy eating organic food and drinking fruity water every morning, it's time to change your breakfast. If you eat everything naughty under the sun for breakfast, make the change gradually. For example, eat fruit for breakfast one day, and your old way the next day. Or eat fruit first every morning, and then if you're hungry half an hour later, eat half the portion of your old food. Gradually work up to eating fruit (or nothing if you're not hungry) at the beginning of every day.

Check out the smoothies and pudding sections in this book and **Detox Delights** for recipe ideas — you need never have the same breakfast twice! So from now on: make your first meal a fruit meal. This will prolong the amount of time your body has to detox. Remember that your body detoxes more when you're resting and not eating, so sleep is a great time for detoxing.

Eating very light easy-to-digest food in the morning gives your body a big helping hand, with "Detox" written across its knuckles.

Once you have detoxed yourself, you might want to swap your fruit breakfast for a green juice breakfast. Wait at least one month before you make this switch, and do it gradually if you need to, until you're used to the flavour.

Go green

Now it gets interesting! Maybe you've taken six months or six days to get to this point — it doesn't matter, so long as you feel comfortable with your pace. Check back in your journal at how you felt before you started, and record how you feel now. Now you're going to make a green juice, smoothie, soup or salad every day. In theory it might seem like a big change, but check out these examples:

- Juice two apples and eight handfuls of greens (for choice of greens see the greens section in the *All about food* chapter).

- Finely chop four handfuls of greens, make guacamole and mix together. Have this as a starter before your evening meal.

- Take the leaves off one head of romaine, spread sunflower pâté on a leaf, sprinkle on generous helpings of your favourite fresh herbs, roll up and eat like a sandwich. Do this until you're full.

- Blend two bananas with half an avocado, half a litre of water (or freshly squeezed orange juice), a pinch of lemon peel and one to four teaspoons of green superfood or one teaspoon of E3Live. If you think that's a lot, try half the quantity and work up.

- Blend your choice of greens with carrots and almond milk for a quick and satisfying soup.

- Mash an avocado with alfalfa sprouts, green superfood or E3Live and chopped garlic for a super charged guacamole, to use in sandwiches, burritos, with crudités or stuffed into tomatoes. Add spices and olives to really get your taste buds zinging.

- Take the stalks off a head of celery, make a pâté or dip from the recipes section and add lots of fresh herbs such as basil or coriander. Spread onto the celery.

As you can see, even this small list has endless possibilities and notice I didn't mention the word "salad" once! Salads are the best meals in the world, but not everyone's ready to think of them as enough of a replacement to their normal diet. If you love salads, your world of greens is as open as your mind. Remember to experiment, make full use of my recipes, and know you're giving yourself the best food choices in the world. Take your time with this one, let it come over weeks, and persevere. It's a big change for most people, and will produce great results. If you don't like dark greens (yet!) then start with light lettuces, and small amounts of green superfood or E3Live. When you become more alkaline and clean, you will grow to love the taste, and will naturally want more.

Read the sections on organic food, minerals and greens again, especially if you're in any doubt as to what greens will do for you.

Why detox your home?

Think back to when you had your first drink or cigarette — maybe you choked or were sick? This happens because your pure body recognises it as a toxin and wants it out. However, after a while of continuing to use these drugs, your body stops fighting, and ends up storing the toxins that it can't process.

On a more subtle level, you have also become used to the toxins in your home, so when you detox, you will notice they aren't so pleasant to live with anymore.

Detox your home

The next batch of changes aren't food-related, but they contribute greatly to your health and should be welcomed with open arms.

You need to detox your home simultaneously with your body because you are becoming more porous and will be more sensitive to the toxins that you once tolerated. This is perfectly normal and in fact desirable, as it indicates your body is starting to respond to poisons as it did when you were younger and cleaner. I'm sure you don't want to be this pure thing floating around your home with toxins lurking in every cupboard, so make your home fit to live in, not to die in.

When you have a spare few hours, go through all your cupboards. If you pick a day where the moon is waxing or full, you'll have consistent energy to complete the process. Buy non-toxic versions of household cleaning products. Remember that solutions our Grannies used are often much better for the environment than anything you can buy as a specific product.

From now on, every time you do anything, big or small, to your house, car or other place that you spend time in, consider which chemicals are used, and how you can substitute them for less harmful ones. For example:

- Next time you decorate, use low-toxin paints. I prefer the Ecos brand.

- If you need to do any restoration work, check out the environmentally friendly options, as well as eco-conscious workers.

- If laying new flooring, look at natural fibres, lino or wood.

- When you redesign a room, remember to add plenty of plants into the plan.

> **Remember**
>
> Have you been taking photos? Your whole body and face shape will change, so make sure you have some close up and full-length snaps to put in your journal. Even if you don't believe your words when you re-read your journal, you can't deny what your photos tell you.

Detox your wardrobe

Don't throw everything away — but from now on, keep a look out for pure clothing. It's next to your skin all day and sometimes all night long, so let it at least be natural (cotton, hemp, ramie, linen etc) and if possible let it be organic.

Your skin is a massive organ which plays a part in detoxification. Its functions are inhibited by clothing. When possible, keep your pants off (that's knickers to you Americans, not trousers, though you could keep those off too). This sometimes isn't practical, but try to do it sometimes. Remember that the concept of this book is that the more natural your lifestyle is, the less toxic you will be, and the healthier and happier you'll become. Clothes aren't natural, so do what you can to either minimise the wearing of them or minimise the stifling effects they can have on your body. Tights, shoes, bras, ties, shirts — argh! Have at least one day a week without them!

Make your house a living home

Now that your house isn't polluted with harmful chemicals, get as many houseplants in your home as possible. Houseplants absorb harmful chemicals, deliver oxygen to you, are often the healing colour green, and they look beautiful. Having living plants in your home changes the vibration of the place, and you will feel calmer with them around you. Consider putting an air purifier or ioniser in your bedroom and living room.

On to your body

Now you've made permanent changes to your diet and water intake, and your home is much less toxic, let's get the body pushing more rubbish out...

If you aren't already doing a regular type of exercise, now is the time to start. If I write "do twenty minutes a day" it's unlikely that you'll do it for more than three days, so I'm not even going to go there! Look for some exercise that you will grow to love, that is fun, challenging, possible, and fulfilling. Read the *Exercise* section in Detox helpers for more tips, and make the most of the InnerTalk CDs which specifically deal with activity.

Detox your mind

The best way to detox your mind is to fill it only with information that will serve you. This one is so easy, because all you have to do is just allow old information to be pushed out by new information. Now is the time to start reading more, going to health lectures/workshops, and opening your eyes to different perspectives. Your life is already spiralling upwards, and at this point you'll already be feeling that you want more. You may be thinking of a career change, or you might have a burning desire to rekindle your passion for that hobby you had long laid to rest.

As your new self emerges, many new doors of opportunity will open up to you. This is the law of attraction in action (watch The Secret DVD for more information on this). Get involved in any alternative healing, ancient practices or esoteric things which appeal to you. If it doesn't appeal to you, make a list of what does (such as sport or charity work), search for information on that subject, and take action!

Rest and relaxation

As you're eating a higher percentage of low-toxin food than you were, your body will be detoxing your old food quite readily. It will be glad of the opportunity, and taking full advantage of it. Assist it by resting in tranquil places, having massages, saunas, sleeping in the afternoon, going to bed early to read, meditating, hugging and practising yoga. As you enter a higher vibration, all or any of these things will greatly assist you. Watching the telly and web surfing aren't a part of rest and relaxation and should be kept to a minimum.

Go with your flow, and rejoice in the feeling that your stagnant stream is becoming unblocked.

Down in the mouth

As well as swapping toxic toothpaste for a better choice, get any mercury ("silver") fillings replaced as soon as you can. Take care choosing a good dentist and ask for a rubber dam and mask. For at least a week afterwards eat plenty of greens. Check out the special supplements available for people having mercury fillings removed. These are are usually made from coriander or seaweeds.

Back to food

It had to happen. Let's go one step beyond...

Eat something raw before or with each cooked meal from now on. For example:

- Have a green salad, then your meal.
- Have a big portion of juicy fruit, then your meal.
- Have a big salad with a third of your old meal.

By doing the above, you're taking advantage of all the goodness in living food, but not getting to a point where you are craving "forbidden" foods. This is quite a major step, so again, take time to get used to it.

> ### At the restaurant
>
> When out in restaurants, it's easy to order something uncooked first. Imagine a lovely plate of ripe tomatoes with fresh basil, some garlic and a little olive oil as the perfect starter. Delight at the thought of a fresh fruit salad as your sweet course. And don't forget the side order of green salad with your main course.
>
> **You can so do this!**
>
> Remember that most restaurants (worth going to!) will create you anything based on items on the menu, even if they aren't a suggested menu item.

Notice that you still haven't cut anything out of your diet! Write in your journal how you feel: Do you feel lighter? Do you have more energy? Have any aches and pains eased?

Have two raw meals a day

Once you're happy with the above step, take it a little bit further by ensuring two of your meals are totally raw each day. This will give you a massive energy boost, and will get you to the "high on life" stage that many detoxed people talk about. For recipe ideas, refer to this book and **Detox Delights**, plus all the raw recipe books to be found in bookstores or on the Internet. Experiment with what you like, as this way of eating is more diverse than the one you've left behind. This change isn't very drastic, yet it will change you! You're already having a raw breakfast, and something raw with every meal, so all you need to do is just alter half a meal a day. Easy!

Re-evaluate your drinking

If you still drink anything other than water, fresh coconut water, or juice that has been freshly squeezed in front of your eyes, you are still taking in toxins. These toxins contribute to feelings of tiredness, lethargy, illness and weight issues. Reduce and then let go of coffee, tea, fizzy drinks, alcohol and anything in cartons, bottles or cans.

Look back in your journal to see how much you were drinking, because you may have already cut down. if not, now's the time to cut down your tipple to a dose which suits the new you. If you only want to reduce your cups of tea or nightly glasses of wine (for now), that's fine. If you want to cut it out all together, that's also fine. This is your detox, and you're in full swing of taking responsibility for your well-being now.

Detox your wardrobe, part two

Go on — spoil yourself

You have worked hard to get to this point, and the results will be showing, and probably glowing.

If you can, have a colour consultation, to see which new clothes you are going to fill your spacious new wardrobe with. Otherwise, make an appointment with an in-store personal shopper (they are free), and let them choose designs and colours for you that they think work. You will be surprised how much space and money you save when everything in your wardrobe matches!

Now is the time to clear out all the clothes, shoes, bags, belts, ties and accessories that you haven't worn for a year. If you're not ready to give them up, just put them in boxes in the loft and have a look in six months to see if you really ever thought "Oh, I so wanted to wear that four months ago." Whatever you don't use, lose. Give generously to some of the good charity shops, and you'll feel light in your heart as well as in your home.

Take up something creative

Take up something to help you channel your new creative energy. Whether it's healthy food inventions, sewing, gardening, painting, writing or sculpture; when living this new life, you might find yourself in creative freefall — so many great ideas come to you. Either act upon them or write them in your journal for future use. Create a *future box* to put all new project ideas into!

We all enjoy such a deep sense of satisfaction from being creative. Completing our tasks isn't always important, so don't worry if you're short of time and think you can't finish what you started. Remember that it's the process and the journey, not the destination, which is important.

What's left on your plate?

Now you're eating lots of wholesome organic unprocessed raw food, there won't be much room for bad food in your tummy! But let's just check. If your one cooked meal a day consists of fried bacon, eggs, toast, tomato sauce and black pudding, it's obvious that you can still help yourself further. First of all; it will conflict with all the changes you've made. Secondly; the mixture of fresh and fried food will probably be playing up in your tummy. Depending on what you're eating in your one cooked meal, take your time in cutting out (or reducing to once or twice a month) the following foods:

- **Meat and fish** — replace with nuts, seeds, greens, avocado, sea vegetables and sprouts. If you want to keep eating fish, oily fish is your healthiest choice.

- **Dairy products and eggs** — replace with products from the *Your new dairy* section in *The recipes*, avocado and durian.

- **Grains** — replace pasta with **Courgetti** and squash noodles. Replace biscuits, breads and crackers with dehydrated cookies, breads and crackers or the healthier versions in wholefood stores. Look for sprouted rye breads and gluten-free crackers.

If you have these products occasionally, your new strong body will deal with it, especially if you work within the 75% uncooked guide. However, if you cut out all acid-forming, cooked or otherwise unhealthy foods for a while and then try to eat them, be prepared for some severe rejection reactions. Your body will soon tell you what it approves of, once it's been allowed to get real.

Did you start yet?

I hope some of the information I've given in previous chapters persuades you that detoxing your life is good for you, good for our planet and well worth trying. Start from the top of the list, work down, and do it at your own pace.

This isn't a race, yet you are allowed to make a rosette saying "I detoxed for life"! Award it to yourself when you've finished — when you glow, when you smile all the time and when you're walking on air. Hey, why don't you email me a photo of yourself before and after with your rosette and I'll publish you on my web site! You can let the world know of any particular hints and tips that worked for you, so others can succeed, too!

Success stories

Whenever you need some inspiration, turn to this chapter. The people who have generously given their stories here are about to uplift you and give bright hope to any dark corner which may exist in your life. These people have all detoxed their worlds, and are now soaring high, discovering new dimensions.

Their stories come to you in their own words, and make for great reading. Enjoy!

Arlyn Grant

Arlyn is in her 30s and lives in the USA. By detoxing her world, she overcame many illnesses, and gained control over others.

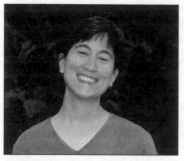

Arlyn after detoxing, free of illness.

In the spring of 2001 I became very ill after spending a week at a job away from home. I was so ill I couldn't get up off the couch. I didn't know if it was because of my severe allergies, my thyroid disease, or some other problem that I had developed. Around that same time, my gynaecologist had discovered a small fibroid tumour that had shown up on my uterus since the previous year. And I realised that I was looking at the warning signs that some serious health problems could be around the corner waiting for me.

So I took a good look at myself in the mirror. I was 35 years old with horrible acne, 50 extra pounds, out of shape (even though I had been working out twice a week with a trainer), allergies requiring three shots a week, a pill every night and prescription nasal spray twice a day, food allergies that could put me in the hospital, two different kinds of thyroid medicine, a fibroid tumour, irritable bowel syndrome, and high cholesterol.

Something had to change

I went to my acupuncturist who said that I needed to put a lot of lemon in my water and just rest. I thought he was a little crazy, but I put the fresh lemon in my water and literally felt my body grabbing for that lemon. After that first sip of lemon water, it became all about the lemon. All I could do was think about the lemon. And then I met a woman on an Internet thyroid group who was a raw foodist. While all the other thyroid sufferers were hassling her because of her food choices I remember thinking that everything she was saying made perfect sense. I contacted her through email and that is how I began my raw journey.

My SAD (Standard American Diet) was fairly healthy. I ate predominately steamed veggies and white rice and salads. Occasionally I would have meat. But I did eat a lot of cheese and ice cream.

My first jump into raw foods was at about 75%. I had fresh juice for breakfast and then salads for both lunch and dinner. And a couple of times a week, I would eat a SAD dinner. I did a lot of reading about juicing but the reality was that I didn't like it very much. In the meantime, my detox symptoms began in the form of extreme exhaustion. Fortunately, I was unemployed at the time so I could allow myself the time needed for rest. This exhaustion lasted for approximately three weeks before it started to abate bit by bit. I also had severe stomach pains which I finally realised were being caused by the raw peppers I was eating so I had to cut those out of my salads. And my irritable bowel syndrome went haywire when I put some raw broccoli in my salad.

About this time I was two months into my transition and I really felt that my food choices were dwindling. My friends were very supportive, though, so that helped me quite a bit. Plus, for the first time I was losing weight since becoming hypothyroid. But then the painful rash on the back of my head started and I had yet another bout of really bad IBS. I decided to make an appointment with Dr. Doug Graham for counselling because I had so many questions and I wasn't sure if I was eating properly enough for my special health conditions.

My conversation with Dr. Doug really did change my life around. He was so positive and supportive and kept telling me to eat more fruit — which I really didn't like very much. But, thankfully, I decided to take his advice and went to the store that very day to buy fruit.

Following that session with Dr. Doug, my diet evolved into: a fruit smoothie in the morning with salads for lunch and dinner. Later it evolved even more to replacing another meal with fruit.

About this time, it was fall of 2001 and I had lost about 15 pounds or so. I had to give up my personal-trainer work-outs because I hadn't been able to find a job yet. But the one thing that everyone was commenting on was my skin. I was so thrilled to see that my acne was clearing up. I had suffered from severe acne since I was about 13 years old. I had been on every antibiotic and cream treatment for acne that ever existed. One of them made me very ill and didn't even work.

But the holidays were coming up and I was fretting about how to eat and what to do. I finally decided that the stress I was putting myself under to keep eating raw during the holidays wasn't helping any. I decided to just not worry about it. I would have raw food around and if I wanted to eat cooked food then so be it. Needless to say, I didn't lose any weight over the holidays but I do feel that I made decent choices as far as eating cooked food goes. I kept it vegetarian and brought raw desserts to the family gatherings.

Getting back on track in January was very difficult. I had eaten a lot of garlic bread — which is one of my favourites — and my body didn't want to give that up. I soon learned that garlic is one of my food binge triggers. I took garlic out of my raw salad dressings and found that I was able to get back onto about 90-95% raw without any problems.

About mid January, I went to my allergist for the retesting of my seasonal allergies. In December I'd had bad reactions to the shots and my allergist said that the serum was still too strong and it was obvious that I was far more sensitive to my allergens than I had been in the past. I had to take a break from the shots for a few weeks through the holidays. I was not looking forward to going back on the shots but without them, I was completely debilitated and unable to function because of my allergies. I remember one December I actually passed out because of my allergies, and I never wanted to repeat that again. The doctor told me that I would have to be off of all antihistamines for 5 days before the testing in order for it to be accurate. I was terrified. But when I went off the medication, I found that I could still breathe, even at night — which was usually the worst time for me. The doctor did the skin testing and we waited for 15 minutes. The last time I was skin tested, the doctor became very alarmed because I was reacting severely to the pricks within seconds. Now, after 15 minutes, she and I sat staring at my arms — there were only two reactions: one to Bahia grass and the other to dust mites. We were stunned. She then did a second test and made the serums a little stronger. Another 15 minutes went by and only the same two allergens created a welt. The last time I was tested for grass allergies, my entire arm swelled up — and here was just one coin-sized welt. I looked at her and I said, "But what does this mean?" She just laughed and asked me about my diet.

A few weeks later, I went back for food allergy testing. I was severely allergic to corn and soy — both these allergens would cause my arms to swell to enormous sizes. And I was also allergic to about 7 other popular foods like nuts, fish, strawberries, etc. We tested for all my old food allergens — except fish. It didn't really matter if I was no longer allergic to fish because I would never eat it again anyway. And once again, there was no reaction. And once again we just looked at each other in stunned silence. And once again I asked, "But what does this mean?" And her response was, "What it means is don't go out and eat all these foods at once." But I went to the health food store and bought lots of different nuts and sampled them all and gave myself a tummy ache. The next day I got to eat my very first strawberry!

A month later I was at the gynaecologist's office for my yearly exam. He was thrilled with my weight loss — now up to 30 pounds. As he was beginning his exam I said,

"Remember last year when you found the small fibroid tumour? Well, feel free to tell me it's gone." He laughed and said, "Sure, I'm running a special on that this week." At the end of the exam he was discussing what he had found and then he said, "And remember that special I told you about? Well, you got it!" I was so happy! We were both laughing. So of course he wanted to know all about my diet.

It is now about 17 months since I started eating raw and I maintain about 90-95% raw foods fairly easily. During this time I have seen these health changes:

1. Loss of 42 pounds.

2. Muscle definition from my work-outs that I didn't have before I went raw.

3. IBS is gone! I have had this since high school.

4. Acne is gone! Though I still break out when I eat nuts.

5. Fibroid tumour is gone!

6. Seasonal allergies are gone (with the exception of bahia grass and dust mites, but in six months perhaps those will be gone as well).

7. Food allergies are gone!

8. I cut my second thyroid medication daily dose in half because I was no longer falling asleep in the middle of the afternoon.

The only thing I have not seen a huge improvement in is my thyroid and my cholesterol. My thyroid doctor was thrilled with my diet and my weight loss and the results I've achieved so far. He told me not to worry about my cholesterol because I was obviously eating correctly. I had hoped for another thyroid medicine reduction but perhaps that will come next year.

I am so happy that I realised that good health was attainable through a raw food diet and I'm so happy that I have stuck with it. I no longer fear bringing my own food to restaurants! I just walk right on in with my oranges and bananas and no one complains at all. And I thank the Internet for putting me in touch with wonderful support groups and doctors in the raw food movement.

Jatinder Daniels

Jatinder lives with her husband Derek and children Raman, Priyanka and Mohan. Her incredible story might bring tears to your eyes, but they'll surely be tears of joy.

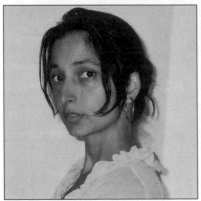

Jatinder, aged 42

For many years, I believed detox was something Hollywood stars did to attain clear skin and recover from drug abuse etc. How could detox serve me? I didn't drink, smoke and ageing at the speed I was ageing was part of the cards life dealt out. I didn't have a choice. C'est la vie! However, as the years went by circumstances drew me to the conclusion that I did have a choice. And when that choice was exercised, I got mind-blowing results for me and my family!

In January 1998, we discovered our close friends' 3-year-old son had cancer. Derek spent many nights looking for alternative cures and one night found David Klein's Living Foods web site. Two months later I became pregnant with Mohan, our youngest child. Having suffered from crippling arthritis since I was a teenager, I felt emotionally and physically weak. How the hell was I going to cope with another child? We both knew we had to do something different in order for me to be able to get through this. One day Derek came up to me and said, "Do you want to try going raw?" I laughed and said "Yeah in my next reincarnation!" But somewhere deep within I was ready to detox.

My health was at a lifetime low and I knew it was make or break time for me. Our whole family had health hurdles to leap over.

So, we all reincarnated without dying!

At the start of this journey, I had the following health challenges:

- Chronic rheumatoid arthritis for twenty-two years

- Hay fever for twenty-two years

- Continuous sore throat (especially right tonsil) for eleven years

- Continuous feeling of tiredness, headaches, runny nose and a "heavy" feeling in the head for twenty-six years

- Right nostril swollen for eleven years
- Many allergics
- Stomach ulcers due to anti-inflammatory drugs taken for rheumatoid arthritis
- Beginnings of asthma symptoms
- Spiritual negativity
- In truth I cannot even remember all the problems I had! In reality I believe this list would be longer!!

Derek was outwardly the healthiest out of us.

Raman was ten years old and was suffering from the following health challenges:
- Asthmatic, having to take steroids to control his "condition"
- Prone to eczema
- Hay fever
- Many allergies
- Overweight

Priyanka was six years old and had spent those years in immense suffering. Her health challenges included:
- Chronic eczema. She smelt of rotting flesh and blood most of the time. Her skin was discoloured and some of it thin due to the use of topical steroid creams for the eczema. She would cry for hours because of the pain. Sleep was a luxury in very short supply for her and us.
- Asthmatic. Like Raman she had to take steroids to control her asthma.
- Chronic allergies to many things.

So how did we end up in this sorry state? Well, in Priyanka's case and mine it is blatantly obvious to me that the main culprit was vaccination. The German measles vaccine in my case and the Hib vaccine in Priyanka's case.

Both of us reacted severely straight away. I had a very high temperature the night after my vaccination and I was ill and in pain with one thing or another then two years later the label of rheumatoid arthritis was placed around my neck like a noose. And in my opinion, the twelve amalgam fillings I was given during this time didn't help. In fact, my first severe attack of rheumatoid arthritis was a few days after the twelfth amalgam filling and a tooth extraction!

In Priyanka's case the injection "site" became hard like a stone and then red. As the weeks went by the red skin spread all over her body like wildfire which she scratched and clawed with clenched teeth. It was a horrific experience to watch our perfect at birth, content child turn into a mass of screaming pain.

I believe that Raman's symptoms were also caused by vaccinations. I feel that vaccination chisels away at the healthy immune system breaking it down. Sometimes this process is rapid and sometimes not so rapid but the results are equally devastating.

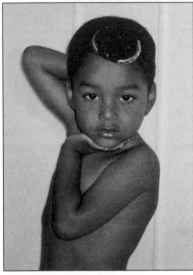

Mohan, aged 4

Mohan arrived in December 1998. We steered clear of vaccinations and he remained healthy! I believe that the fact that he was being breastfed (and currently still is at the age of 4) also greatly contributed to his wellbeing.

For me this was a most challenging time because my new knowledge (remembering) was shouting at me "time to change your core beliefs in nutrition!" It made absolute perfect sense to eat natural unadulterated food. However the pillars of society seemed to be screaming to me "How dare you have the audacity to go against and question what mankind is doing, and has been doing for centuries!" I had been down this road before in my choice of marriage partner. The pillars had screamed then too. But I had to be true to myself and do what I believe is the best.

Here we were ready to create our experience. Create ourselves anew. We had gone along with the experience humanity has created around nutrition (and other matters but that's for another book!) and I felt it had not served me or the rest of humanity well. Just looking at all the obese and ill friends, relatives and pillars of society telling us we are wrong made me reflect and even laugh on many occasions!

We had enough faith in ourselves to recreate ourselves and with a little help from our friends we did! Well who were they? They were and are the various raw web sites, the books, the lecturers, the other people on this journey of discovery of health and all the doubters. **We thank all of you.**

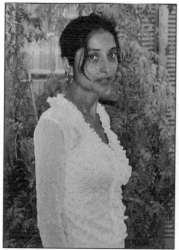

Also in my case I had immense faith in the raw diet because I knew the yogis in India had practised this way of life and many of them lived for hundreds of years. In fact my mother and father told me this when I was very young. I interpreted this as something that mere mortals like us couldn't do. It was the way of gods!

However, our children were old enough and had suffered enough to understand the possible benefits of this diet so we were all ready to sit on the same platform as the gods!

The first year we transitioned to a vegan diet, we were already vegetarian at the start of this journey. Then in June 1999 we attended an all day lecture by David Wolfe and it speeded up our raw journey immensely! By October 1999 we were eating mainly raw and organic food. Cooked food was eaten about once a week. We started to detox almost straight away, diarrhoea being the main symptom. Priyanka's eczema disappeared within three months! Both children didn't need any inhalers for asthma either at this point! I had less pain in my joints. It was amazing the speed with which healing took place.

We all lost weight too, and the doubters (while coughing and spluttering) told us that it was a sure sign of bad health! We remained calm despite the fears written over their faces. I think their fear was a double-edged sword. The fear that they may be wrong. On the other hand we all had lost weight and there was genuine concern too. It was a great experience for us as well as those who looked upon us with fear and doubt.

All my life I weighed around eight stone (52kg) and at this point my weight came down to seven stone. Raman lost a lot of weight too. His diarrhoea was the worst. My parents expressed concern over his frail looking body. Priyanka and Derek lost weight too but neither reached a point where they looked gaunt like Raman and me. Throughout this, Mohan looked great!

The following is a list of the detox symptoms I had that I am aware of:

- Severe teeth pain in March 2000
- Black faeces in the initial detox stage
- White pus spots round my right tonsil
- Dizzy spells

In November 2001 I had a massive detox and my weight came down to 6 stone. At the time I felt I was sitting in a car whose brakes had stopped working. My health seemed out of control and I momentarily doubted what I had started. But seeing and focussing on all the health benefits I realised I was simply scared by the detox process I had gone through. Diarrhoea was accompanied by dehydration. (Mohan was still breastfeeding.) This bought on buzzing in my ears and a severe drop in blood pressure. No one else in the family had severe detox symptoms like this! Luckily it wasn't to last for ever...

After four years of recreating ourselves I am experiencing amazing good health. However, I have every wish to continue creating myself anew for I know even better health awaits my family and me and I can't wait to experience that!

Here are a few of my health improvements:

- I NO LONGER LIVE IN PAIN!
- No sore throat
- No continuous runny nose
- No headaches
- I have bags of energy
- I feel much happier and positive about life
- I have softer skin and hair
- The very dark circles around my eyes have gone
- I need less sleep and food
- I feel and look great compared to how I felt and looked four years ago
- I can walk for miles. Four years ago walking twenty yards was often excruciating!
- I don't want to sound cheesy but I feel fabulous! Recently a friend said to me "you must feel like you have got your youth for the second time." (I am 42 years old) I replied "No, I feel like I have got my youth for the first time. I never knew a pain free, healthy state of being all my adult life."

Since 2000 we've all just steadily been improving. We all have a much more robust immune system. We don't get colds and flus like most other people around us! Derek has good health. Raman is fourteen now and looks good, his health is great. Priyanka is ten and well too. Mohan is four years old and still doing great.

So far I have only spoken about physical detox. However, for me the notion of detox on a purely physical level is insufficient. I previously felt that detox was about clearing an unhealthy human body. Now I feel that to truly detox, my lifestyle has to help detoxify the body of this planet too, otherwise I cannot be toxin free. And the story for me doesn't end there either. For me, detox ends at my spiritual being. My thoughts, words and actions have to stem from love — love for my Self and this beautiful Universe and all that vibrates in it. To this end I thank all the spiritual masters of many religions and many spiritual people alive today. With so much love and dedication, they remind us of the almighty creative power that we all have at our disposal and for us not to fear to use it for that is what it is there for.

> I MUST RECREATE MYSELF ANEW
> IN THE GRANDEST VERSION OF
> THE GREATEST VISION I
> EVER HELD ABOUT
> WHO I
> AM

Jatinder Daniels, Spain/UK

In her story, Jatinder mentions that David Wolfe helped her.

You can learn more about David Wolfe at **www.davidwolfe.com**. He lectures all over the world, so find out when he's next at an event near you and get inspired to make those changes which could set you free.

Jay Banks

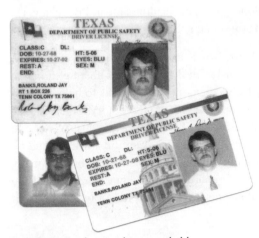

Jay's licenses, showing his remarkable transformation. He is 27 on the one at the back, 29 at the top and 34 on the front license!

Here, Jay tells his story of how he lost sight of all his illnesses when all he thought he was doing was going on a diet!

In February of 2001, a co-worker mentioned the Hallelujah Diet to me. Since I had once been a strict vegetarian (well, basically a meatless-version-of-the-SAD) for well over a year, back in my early twenties, I was intrigued by the Hallelujah Diet enough to give it an honest try. At that time I had a list of health problems: quite overweight, general lethargy, slept too much, terrible allergy and sinus problems that had plagued me for years, fungal problems, several bouts with suspected kidney stones, chronic constipation and irritable bowel syndrome.

I have really been into alternative medicine since my late teens and have taken supplements off and on for most of my adult life (I'm 34 now). At the time I heard about the Hallelujah Diet, I was taking huge amounts of vitamins and supplements, most of which were very expensive. After reading Reverend Malkmus's "Why Christians Get Sick" and viewing some other material, I gave away or threw out all of my supplements except B12 and never looked back. I purchased a juicer and started drinking fresh carrot juice 1-2 times per day and tried to eat the best I could — eating anywhere from 75-85% raw to 100% at times.

Coming from someone who has pretty much covered the spectrum of diets from junk food to eating healthy, or what I thought was healthy, from no supplements to large amounts of supplements, I can honestly say that under the Hallelujah Diet, I have felt about the best I can remember — probably since my childhood or early teens!

My energy increased, I can breathe through my nose now, and, although I hate to use the term "cured," I would say my irritable bowel syndrome and chronic constipation are at least between 75-85% better. I went from having a horrible time going to sleep and then not being able to wake up once I did, to being able to go to sleep quickly and waking up much more easily, and actually feeling refreshed (most of the time). And perhaps one of the biggest changes is that exercise went from something I had to force myself to do, to something I actually wanted to do!

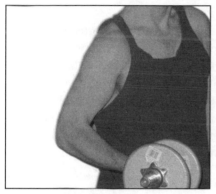

And in the exercise area, although I went on the diet to improve my health and not really to lose weight, I started an exercise program I saw on a late-night infomercial and was actually able to stick with it consistently, even while having a newborn in the house. Based on my medical records, my highest recorded weight was 253 pounds (about 18½ stone). My weight now is 144 pounds (just over 10 stone), making for a total loss of 109 pounds (about 7½ stone). And again, I consider that to be more of a bonus than what I was trying to do, which was simply to feel better.

I must admit that I was sceptical of the Hallelujah Diet when I first heard about it, but I felt like I was going downhill fast and had nothing to lose by trying it. After all, all Rev Malkmus was asking me to do was eat a lot of vegetables and fruits and drink some carrot juice. What a change for the better it has made in my life, too. It makes me think back to the first time I was a "vegetarian" in my early twenties. One of the first books I saw on vegetarianism at the time said there were two ways to go: raw or cooked. At the time I chose cooked and never gave it a second thought. Now I wonder what a difference ten extra years of feeling better would have made in my life?

Jay Banks, Texas, USA
www.roadtowellsville.com

___

You can see more of Jay's photos at **www.roadtowellsville.com**.

For information on The Hallelujah Diet, please visit **www.hacres.com**, where you can see more testimonials, recipes, programme information and event listings.

Michele Déradune

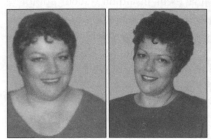

Before detoxing   7 months later

Michele, aged 49, had been on and off the road to wellness and weight loss several times, before finally working out how to get there permanently and safely.

I am so happy to have the opportunity to share some of my story with Shazzie's readers. As a matter of fact I am a lot happier these days in general, since switching to raw diet. Where I have been dreading the near future and increasing ill health for years, now I am much healthier and have much more energy than I did just six months ago before going onto raw (mostly vegan) diet. And now I can look forward, God willing, to a hopeful future in regard to my own body's ability to keep up with and enjoy doing all the things I want to do.

Not so long ago, gloomy images of the future held me captive. I could see myself becoming less mobile, gaining more weight (though I was already what is medically termed as morbidly obese) and just becoming decrepit in general. With aches, pains, insomnia and blood pressure on the rise and having gained yet another 20 pounds in the past year, I knew I already had a head start to just such a future. Now, thanks to my raw diet and a little bit of mild exercise (I take long morning walks), such dread is a thing of a past.

Most of my life I was "just a little" overweight, in between times of calorie-restricted diets and getting thin and then gaining it back. I used to feel absolutely huge when I was 20lbs overweight. Little did I know that one day I would grow to be a hair's breadth from a total of 300lbs (over 21 stones) in weight.

Fortunately for me, long before that happened I learned that my size was not the most important thing in life. I was lucky to find Prem Rawat (referred to as Maharaji by most of his students), my Teacher and Mentor, at a young age, and by his grace I learned to truly appreciate the life I have been given — and to feel very fortunate indeed to have a human body at all, never mind the size, looks or condition. At the time I found him he was only 14 years old, and truly had I not come to realize the importance of the life within my body, I don't believe I could ever have come to accept and love myself — and life. I needed that first and foremost — especially the self-acceptance.

Today, even as a vegan raw foodist, I do not feel judgmental of others who eat differently. I can totally relate to the addiction to cooked foods, especially the meat and the junk! There were many years of my life that a meal just didn't seem complete without an animal product. If there was no meat in the menu, I looked for cheese or some other dairy product. I really could not fathom eating any other way. Surely it would make me feel deprived, empty, weak and hungry. Or so I thought. Some people have told me my story is inspiring to them, and I figure that is because they can see nearly all their own weaknesses in me, and they figure that, "If she can do it, I can too!"

By the time I was thirty years old, I got fed up with dieting. I had dieted, and fiercely, for much of my life. I had to work very hard to keep down to medium weight by then, never mind slim. I noticed that to stoke the fires of my motivation to diet, I had to become more narcissistic and vain. I was constantly looking at my reflections in the mirrors, windows and shiny buildings I passed. Every time I was tempted to eat something fattening and delicious, I had to replace thoughts of eating that with thoughts of how much better I was going to look by staying on my diet. Think the last straw was when a guy I was keen for fell head-over-heels for a fat girl. It seemed so unfair — here she got to have her cake (him) and eat it too (chocolate, whipped cream and all). In an effort toward self-improvement I decided to focus the enormous amount of energy that had been going into losing weight toward more worthwhile pursuits. I was still young enough, and thin enough, that health matters were the last thing on my mind. Within six months, I had gained a good 40 to 50 lbs and stayed there at 190lbs steady for the next year or so.

Then I had a baby. By the time my son was three years old I weighed in at 220lbs (15½ stone). Weighing myself for the first time in years, I was shocked and dismayed. Anything over 200lbs sounded truly frightening to me. So I went on another diet, again cutting calories, and after losing 20lbs the scales would not budge and I was very cranky. I threw up my hands in dismay and disgust, and went back to eating anything I wanted — and then some. By the time my son was five years old, I weighed in at about 300 lbs (over 21 stones).

Then a new "health fact" which turned out to not be a fact at all, was all the rage in the mainstream media: Eat pasta to lose weight! Oh boy, I jumped on that one! Pasta with spaghetti sauce, pasta with white sauces, pasta salads. I ate them all eagerly. After just a few weeks of this I found myself one evening in the kitchen eating a third or fourth helping of pasta salad, and suddenly I saw that what I was doing terrified me. I was shoveling this food in my mouth as if I were crazed with hunger, and yet at the same time my tummy was totally full and even aching from what I had already eaten. To be still hungry while full and still shoveling it in, I have often reflected, is a pain that perhaps only the obese truly know. I "hit bottom" and became truly desperate. I knew I needed help, and I knew that things just had to get better. I knew I had to do something.

Luckily, I had over the previous few years taken an interest in raw food diet. Though I had never practiced it much, what I read in a number of books intrigued me. They sounded so right and true, and when I would test the waters of the raw food diet (with just the little toe mind you) it really seemed like a great way to eat. I was also fortunate in that I had met one person who had been eating only organic raw vegan diet for 8 years a year or two previously. He told me that 8 years earlier, diagnosed with a crippling disease, he had been told by doctors at the age of 17 that he would never walk again. Not willing to face such a fate, and having eaten a junk-food-oriented diet up to that time, he turned to many books and many diets before he found the one that began to erase all symptoms of his disease. Macrobiotic diet did not work for him, but raw diet did. More importantly for me, I felt that raw diet would help me in my own very different case. I had read about how the body continues to feel hungry and crave food even when eating due to lack of nutrients and/or lack of nutrient absorption. And I had read how easily one could lose excess weight on raw diet. And thus I began.

I started with an 80% raw diet right away, and read every book about the raw food diet that I could get my hands on. I started a small press newsletter, and also a local raw food support group. I began by eating fruit for breakfast and tossed green salads for lunch and dinner. In the first month or so I would also have some steamed vegetables, dressed with olive oil rather than butter, and sometimes some baked or steamed potatoes. I had read about the detoxification that happens when switching to a raw diet, and I wanted to slow down the detox. Looking back, I am not at all sure it really helped, but it was all right anyhow.

Sometime in those first few weeks I had a terrible ongoing headache, but I knew this is common among those transitioning to raw diet and I held on. I did a lot of enemas at that time, thinking it would help. Anyhow, after about a month I got symptoms that seemed a lot like pneumonia, but after visiting several doctors it was clear that it was not. In fact, no cause was ever found, but I know what it was: Detoxification! Looking back I see that my discomfort would have been lessened immensely, had I been drinking plenty of water.

Once I got through those first initial and more intense detoxification periods, nothing very uncomfortable ever really happened again.

After nearly 2 years eating 80-90% raw diet I lost 120lbs (over 8 stones). I still had more to lose, but unfortunately at that point other things in my life converged and old habit patterns of eating wrong foods and giving in to a feeling of helplessness re–emerged. I began more and more to look forward to that cooked (and processed and junk food) 10-20% of my daily diet more and more.

I got divorced. I felt sorry for myself. I started reverting more and more to my pre-raw diet patterns. The first 40lbs I regained were the fastest. It took me another 6-7 years to regain the other 80lbs. All during that time I wanted to return to the good health and energy I enjoyed with raw diet, but was emotionally crippled by giving in to the shame and humiliation I felt at having achieved so much and thrown it all away. I didn't want to face old "raw" friends and avoided seeing most of them any more, and really tried to block the matter out of my mind. I pretty much succeeded in doing that, in fact, until poor health and feeling so tired that sometimes I just wanted to cry came knocking at the door. I had a health scare in March of 2002 and really woke up to the fact that I was getting in worse condition and was not going to get any better without a true and conscious effort.

I started eating 80-90% raw diet again in early April of 2002 — aged 49. After one month at that percentage raw, taking heed to the experience of others, I decided to go 100% raw. This is a personal choice not so much because it is healthier to eat an all-raw diet (even though it is!) but because I don't ever want to do that regression thing again like I did before. Cooked food, for me, is very addictive. As long as I don't eat any of it at all, I feel a freedom from food cravings like I have never known. And it makes staying on raw diet much easier. My son still eats cooked foods, and where I sit to do my work at home I am right next to the kitchen. I smell those old familiar smells of foods I once enjoyed in the mouth (but did not enjoy in the stomach) just about every day. Since May 9, 2002 I have been on all-raw diet, not just 80% or 90%, and I can tell you for sure that it is much, much easier for me now. I try to walk most mornings, and walk on average from 30 minutes to an hour daily.

Combined with raw diet of mostly fruits, vegetables, seeds, nuts, leafy greens and sea vegetables, I am feeling great. I have lost all the weight without any concern for limiting (raw) fat intake. Some days I even eat as much as 4 avocados plus other fatty foods. Yet still, at 100% raw, I have lost an average of 8-10 pounds every month. Some days when I feel more tired I come to discover it is yet another little detox, and I up my water intake to help out. Several of my friends have begun eating more raw foods in their diets. I know it is not because I talked them into it (because I didn't), but because they think I look so much better. And that feels good too. I have lost a little over 60lbs in the past six months and still have a way to go before I am down to size, and I can tell you I am enjoying the process very much, especially nowadays with recipes such as those Shazzie has to offer, my food never needs to be boring — although I find more and more, to my surprise, that often a simple meal with no real preparation involved satisfies me just fine, and is most appreciated on days when I am on the run all day with no time to throw anything together.

My son (now 16 years old) is getting serious about wanting to eat a high percentage of raw food too. I just share with him when I fix something he might like, but I know he will have to find his own way with raw food diet.

I'll be there to support and encourage him and give any guidance I can, but I know that it is his own journey, and it makes me feel really great, as a mom, to know that my example is helping my child to make wise eating choices.

Thanks for reading my story.

Michele Déradune, Texas, USA
www.deradune.com

Tony Thorpe

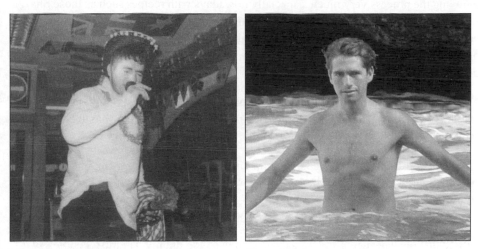

Tony before detoxing   Tony after detoxing

In January of 2000, I played golf with my golf teacher, Ken Martin. Afterwards, we had a discussion about diet and health. I had been a vegan for seven years, and vegetarian for ten. The subject of raw food came up, and I told him.

I had heard of people curing themselves of serious diseases by not eating cooked food. I thought it was only the chronically ill and people with cancer who needed to eat raw. He went on to tell me that there are healthy people all over the world who were eating raw foods. Ken used to live in San Diego and he told me about Nature's First Law and David Wolfe who has eaten raw for many years. A light went on in my head and I knew that the raw-food diet was man's correct diet. I immediately stopped eating cooked food.

It was easy for me to immediately change my diet because I knew I was doing the right thing. I had no desire for any cooked food at all. The only thing I craved was beer. It took me a couple of months to let go of it completely.

Each time I craved beer I had one and immediately felt ill. I got the message eventually. I had a couple of cooked meals too, but each time they made me feel sick. After being raw for six months, I decided to go out for a drink and a meal with my brother Ged, in England. After my third drink, my body shut down completely. I couldn't even sip the next one. Later on, I had a vegetable curry. It had a terrible effect on me. I felt like my stomach, chest, and head were about to explode. I decided to go lay down and hope for the best. The next morning I awoke and vowed to never eat cooked food again.

When I returned to the US, I visited my friends in Daytona Beach, Florida. My friend Amy had made some vegetable soup for me. Not wanting to be rude, I had a bowl of it. As I left in my car I almost fell asleep at the wheel. It was 11 am. That was finally the end of cooked food for me.

There have been several physical and emotional changes for me since I became a raw foodist. I was always athletic, but no matter how much I trained or how many abdominal exercises I did, I always had flab around my midriff. After a few weeks of raw food, it was gone.

I always had dry skin on my face which required daily moisturizing. I had been using moisturizer for 15 years. After going raw, my skin became soft and supple, and I have no need to moisturize it any more.

I found that the bags under my eyes disappeared, so too did my dandruff. People say my eyes now sparkle and I have a vibrant look about me.

Since I was a baby I had chronic sinus problems. I can breathe clearly now. It's wonderful to be able to breathe through my nose.

For five years I had been getting more gray hairs. They not only stopped in their tracks, but they are even turning back to their original color. Friends who haven't seen me for a long time wonder where my gray hairs have gone. I told them the secret.

Going raw eliminated my body odor too. I don't have to wear deodorant any more. I don't even smell after playing soccer or basketball for hours. For years I had a bad case of athletes foot. It too disappeared. I now hold a tan amazingly well and am less prone to sunburn.

Mentally I am in a much better state than before I went raw. I used to suffer from depression, and I worried so much it made me sick. Now I'm very much on top of the world. Everyday is a delight! My thinking is clearer, and I am able to make better decisions. I am much happier knowing my food choices are not adversely affecting anybody else, or anything on the planet.

In terms of physical activities I have had a rebirth. I'm as fit and as active as I have ever been. I play basketball for hours at the gym and feel energized by it, not tired. My stamina on the soccer field is amazing. I can't get tired no matter how much I run. After getting slower and slower with age and increased weight, I have completely turned it around. I feel like I can do anything.

My strength has increased dramatically since I've become raw. When I ate cooked food, I could do only one or two pull-ups. The other night I did 14 in my first set. I could only curl 50 lbs. with a barbell, now I do 80 lbs., same reps. I used to struggle to do 20 push-ups, now I can do 100.

I moved to California and helped form The Healing Waters Band, an all-raw rock band. We spread the message of how raw food raises consciousness and helps solve a lot of the world's problems. Here are the lyrics to a song I wrote about me called **Tony's Story**.

Tony's Story

I came down to earth in my chariot of light,
From my home in the heavens one dark winter night.
I was handed my mission, at first it seemed frightful.
But now I'm aware that it's one most delightful.
They filled me with drugs, cooked food and red meat.
It didn't take long to be knocked off my feet.
I spent my childhood in hospitals dying,
But nobody blamed it on food we've been frying.

With adenoids out, tonsillectomy too,
Thirteen rotten teeth and unable to poo.
Pneumonia set in, they believed I was stewed.
They never suspected it might be cooked food.
Unable to breath through my nose for ten years,
They flushed out my sinuses, rinsed out my ears.
But just when I thought that it couldn't get worse.
I had my appendix turn gangrene and burst.

Chorus

So look now and see the reason why we cook food,
Then waste away and die.
Eat all raw or you could live your life in sickness,
Under a surgeon's knife.

The science facts have been overlooked.
White blood cells attack the food that's cooked.
My Story, for you has now been told.
I'm well now, and I'll never grow old.

During adolescence I got into drinking,
threw up every time, don't know what I was thinking.
You're offered a drink? I suggest you don't grab it.
It took me fifteen years until I kicked the habit.
But one Christmas Day when I ate a pork pie,
I got so violently ill that I thought I would die.
Then I realized that each time I eat meat,
Could be the last time I'm seen on my feet.

Chorus

If you use your senses with your intuition,
And inside yourself fill with rawfood nutrition.
You'll find you've stacked all the odds in your favor,
And raw food tastes better cause' it's got more flavor.
With every hardship comes benefits too.
I gained priceless knowledge from what I went through.
The medical research in Britain and Sweden says
Cooked food is poison, so watch what you're eating.

Chorus

(End of song)

Sometimes the truth is quite shocking. Thankfully I've had the most wonderful transformation. I feel so fortunate that I discovered raw foodism at a relatively young age. I'm getting younger too! This is absolutely the best thing anybody can do for themselves if my experiences are anything to go by. One day everybody on the planet will eat a raw food diet. Until then, I'm going to keep having fun while getting younger everyday.

Shazzie

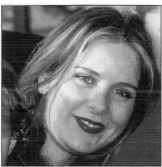

Me before I detoxed my world

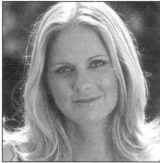

Me after I detoxed my world

I wrote this story so you can find out how my personal journey to health began, and how it changed my life. I want to show you that this self-help book comes from a place of great experience and adventure! I hope that by sharing my triumphs as well as tribulations, you are ever more encouraged that this magical life can touch you.

I hope you enjoy the final success story in this book, as I certainly enjoyed the process of getting here.

As a child

Sadly I wasn't given the best start in life. As I grew up we were literally fed the same lies as everyone else in our world. My diet consisted mainly of roast beef, Yorkshire puddings, cod and chips and bread and dripping. I remember having salad, meat and chips on a Monday. I didn't like vegetables (who really does like boiled cabbage and carrots?), and I always wanted to eat bananas.

I remember once when I must have been about five asking my mum for sandwiches with cress in, but I didn't know what cress was exactly called so I kind of mouthed it and she thought I meant crisps, so that's what I got. Bless me for trying to go the sprout way at such a young age!

Because I hated vegetables so much, my mum was worried I wasn't getting enough nutrients, so she'd give me this horrible tasting green supplement. She would also hide baked beans under my Yorkshire puddings to try and get me to eat some by accident. Looking back, it's funny how she thought baked beans were healthy and I was missing out if I didn't eat them.

As a teenager

My diet changed radically after I'd been through a major trauma. At that time I realised that I would never want to inflict suffering on another being, especially one who couldn't even defend itself, so in 1985 at the age of 16, I became a vegetarian. As I stopped eating meat I started eating cheese, cheese and more cheese (as well as crackers and pasta). Then I realised that although I didn't feel any worse on this diet, it just didn't feel right and I couldn't live on it for long. I didn't know anyone else who was a vegetarian so I read some magazines and experimented a bit. My family had a restaurant at the time and I persuaded them to sell vegetarian or vegan specials on the menu. No one bought them!

A year later I gave up eggs. I tried to give up milk but soya milk gave me a terrible

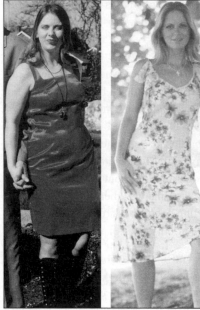

Before   After

tummy ache, and my three Shredded Wheat for breakfast was my one remaining pleasurable link with my food past. Six months after giving up eggs, I finally managed to give up milk. I desperately wanted to be a vegan but had to overcome the cheese addiction. I managed it two years after first turning vegetarian. So by 1987 I was an alienated vegan who was relieved that I'd removed as much suffering of others from my life as possible.

I heard about raw food

After becoming vegan, my diet and my state of mind didn't alter for a few years. I slipped in and out of depression (concealing it very well from those around me), and started putting on a bit of weight. While at college in 1992 I picked up raw food leaflet. I read about some bloke who lived on fruit. He said he had lots of energy and that he did a stack of skipping in his spare time. I thought "What a waste of a life, skipping". Interesting though the leaflet was, it didn't rattle anything in my head — although I now realise that was the planting of my raw seed, destined to grow many years later.

I muddled my way through college, leaving early yet still finding some excellent jobs which took me through design and corporate identity. One thing I did know was how to turn on the charm at an interview! Remembering the many poverty-stricken years before, I ploughed much of my energy into work as I was determined to live a better life, at least materially. Men came into my life and went again — they didn't keep me happy for long. The only real identity I felt I had was being vegan — being kind to our Earth through my love of animals. I sometimes wanted to leave this society and live in a community, but I didn't think I'd fit in — I'd never really fitted in anywhere. In any case, I was so stressed out about having the security of a home and job, because I didn't want to be poor ever again.

As time went on I found myself a social life, did a lot of dancing and started drinking alcohol at the age of 25. Isn't this when people start to think about giving it up? Well, I never did follow convention. My diet remained vegan, but as more vegan convenience foods were being developed (soya cheese, soya meat, burgers, grills etc), my diet became worse. Eventually, most of the food I ate came out of tins or packets, which was reflected by the cellulite, puffy face and ever-shortening temper I was cultivating.

I met a raw person

My first meeting with John Coleman was in 1996. At that time he was eating a high-raw diet, with the intention of soon eating all-raw. He bought me a book called **What Doctors Don't Tell You** by Lynne McTaggart. While reading it I nodded my head in agreement that the medical profession is there to mask symptoms, not cure diseases. Even at that time when I had little confidence, I wouldn't have trusted my life with the medical profession. I hadn't taken many tablets in my adult life, because I was so against animal cruelty. I'd frequently get bronchitis and cough up blood, but I only went to the doctor once about it. I mostly just suffered, thinking that this was meant to be because I was inherently weak and couldn't change that. Meeting John was like pouring water on my raw seed that was planted several years before. But only a bit of water.

Over the next few years, I started reading some raw stuff on the web — mainly recipes but the odd fact here and there came up. I'm staggered now to think that I didn't look for more raw stuff on the web, as I had full access to it and looked for everything else on there. In 1997 I even bought my house on the web!

As my mental and physical health deteriorated it seemed that it still wasn't the right time for my heart to embrace living foods. I was obviously not prepared for the massive changes it would impose on my life.

Everything started deteriorating

I know I'm not alone in this: as time went on I just started getting more and more things wrong with me. I'd suffered some of the symptoms for years or sometimes as long as I can remember. I'd always felt that I was runt-like but I'd started to find survival on a day-to-day basis increasingly difficult.

The health of my family was no better, and whenever I looked at them to see how I'd turn out in 20 years I was truthfully horrified. Close members of my family suffered heart disease, arthritis, cancer, diabetes and all the other diseases that are accepted as normal but unfortunate these days. I didn't want to end up like that but as I was related to them, what chance did I have? Without radically changing something in my life, I don't think I had much of a chance at all. After all, I was a next-generation runt, my illnesses were bound to have been bigger!

So without detailing everything that was wrong with me (and there was a big list building up) here's the abridged version. See how many of these symptoms you recognise in yourself:

- Constantly tired: unable to sleep, but then unable to wake, felt jet-lagged all the time.

- Colds and flu: I had always suffered two week stretches of colds or flu about four to six times a year, regularly coughing up blood.

- Emotionally unbalanced and depressed, feelings of hurt, anger, disappointment and apathy.

- Difficulty breathing, a really runny nose, cellulite, overweight, whole right hand side aching, cystitis.

- Short attention span (daydreamer), difficulty understanding simple stuff such as left and right and map reading.

- People took my energy and I was powerless to stop it, feeling exhausted and even ill in the presence of some. I also felt the pain of others so much it hurt. Leaking my energy and absorbing the energy of others in totally inappropriate ways.

To the outside world I seemed fine — I could laugh and joke with the lads in the pub all night. But on the inside I was dying — I could feel my life force slipping away. Sometimes I don't know how I got through the day, sometimes I didn't get through the day. I would come home at night and cry and cry and cry. I told my boyfriend that I couldn't cope with the stress of work and wanted to be a housewife but the reality was that I often couldn't stay awake for a whole day — if I did I was so depressed that I wanted to be asleep. I was living in a vacuum waiting to be sucked away.

I reached rock bottom

The lowest point in my adult life was just around the corner. In 1998 I'd been very stressed for about a year. I was even more tired than usual. Work was taking its toll on me, I was working about 12 hours a day most days and getting no thanks for it. I had a permanent pain in my stomach which I'm sure was an ulcer (but I wouldn't go to the doctor). I constantly wanted to throw up and most days could only eat boiled rice with vegetables. I was really scared, and couldn't understand what was happening to me.

After gradually putting on weight over the years, there was now a surprising 11 stone (154lb) of me struggling to fit into size 12 (UK) clothes. I flatly refused to ever buy a size 14 — that would mean I'd been defeated. My thighs were like two sea lions — my friend Chef said I had "Cider thighs"! I had a permanent frown, my face was baggy and puffy like a Yorkshire pudding with jowls. In fact, I was puffy and squashy all over. Internally I was no better — I had a pulse of about 90 and my blood pressure had started creeping up. I wondered how I got like that, and whether it was my destiny. I thought about most other women, and how overweight they are — and thought maybe that's just what happens to you as you get older. At the age of 29 everything was heading south — my skin, my chin and my spirits.

One day towards the end of this very stressful year, I think I had a nervous breakdown — how exactly do you know when you won't go to doctors? I even resigned from my job (which I didn't end up leaving). Nothing was right. Yes, I had a nice house, a lovely boyfriend, a well paid job, some very dear friends and a family who loved me, but nothing was right. Why, when I had so much, did I have so little inside? Why was my heart and spirit so empty? I didn't even understand how these problems were real — after all, I wasn't in a wheelchair or an asylum, but I truly felt like the world had ended. I couldn't get any lower. One day I was standing in the car park at work crying and my boyfriend at the time said that he couldn't take much more of this as he didn't know how to help me. The truth was, I couldn't take any more either. I gave myself a good talking to: "Either do something about this state of your life or kill yourself. You are not going to continue living like this any longer" Well, I didn't kill myself...

I picked myself up off the floor and picked up a book

Shortly after that time I spotted **The Optimum Nutrition Bible** by Patrick Holford in a bookshop. As I flicked through it I noticed he mentioned depression and stress. He also seemed to advocate or at least condone a vegan diet, so I bought the book. I read it twice and did the test to see what I was deficient in (the test asks you a long series of questions and from that you work out how deficient you are in certain vitamins, fats and minerals). I wasn't surprised to find out that I was deficient in almost everything. I was on a vegan diet because I didn't want anything to suffer just so I could have a life, but I was suffering so much. I thought about it and realised that I might have been even worse off on an animal-based diet — I was a runt, remember. It then made sense that my body was puffy — there was no good stuff holding it together. I decided to change my diet and take mega supplements immediately. I also took St John's Wort for the depression. I was determined to get out of this slump. I really wanted to start living.

At work I went on confidence and assertiveness courses. People laughed at me going on these because they didn't distinguish confidence and assertiveness from the aggressiveness and loudness which I previously displayed. I also bought tapes on how to deal with difficult people — I needed these social skills because whenever I got attacked at work I'd attack back which was both unprofessional and unproductive. These positive actions did me so much good. Coupled with the supplements I was taking, I could see an improvement. Also, because I'd reduced my coffee intake to just one cup in the morning, I was sleeping a tiny bit better.

In that year, I also had reflexology, lots of massages, acupuncture and osteopathy. This very tight ball of wool was slowly beginning to be unravelled.

I did think about how unnatural (not to mention expensive) taking mega supplements was. I'd always tried to look to nature whenever I questioned human behaviour but I was now popping pills morning noon and night. In hindsight, it's very odd how the penny still hadn't really dropped about eating natural — uncooked — food. I believed that food must be so deficient these days due to modern farming methods that we all had to take supplements. I believed it was an unfortunate modern-day necessity. Of course, that's what many people would like us to believe, so we can then buy their essential pills and potions and get locked into society. I read a few more of John's raw emails and got turned off soya but then turned on it again when I missed it.

I decided to lose weight

As I'd seen an upturn in my mental state, I decided it was time for me to go on a diet ready for Christmas of 1998. I told myself that if I turned 30 and was still fat then I was a failure and must remain fat for the rest of my life — how horrible are we towards ourselves? We wouldn't talk to our friends like that! I found a vegetarian weight loss diet, which I easily converted to being vegan (I was an absolutely amazing cook by this age!). I went on the diet and lost about a stone (14lb).

That Christmas I got the flu and had to cancel the whole day. I couldn't eat for about a week and questioned why my supplements weren't being as miraculous as they seemed to be at the start. I thought maybe I was so weak that even supplements couldn't help me. I lost another 7lb that Christmas because of the flu. I was down to 9½ stone (133lb), and almost happy with that weight.

I started eating fruit, my family got more ill

I had no New Year resolutions for 1999 but something inside me pushed me towards eating more fruit. I made loads of salads, too. I reduced my coffee to about half a cup every other day. I was hooked on papayas, tomatoes, avocados and melons. I didn't think too much of it, but I noticed that I felt happier. Though I was eating more raw food than ever before, I still ate lots of cooked food. I ate fried breakfasts every Sunday, and made full use of stews, bread and pasta. Because of my stomach pain, I hadn't eaten breakfast for several years, so my first meal of the day was often fruit during the mid-morning while sitting at my computer. I didn't think I was preparing to turn into a raw foodist, it just made me cope with life and prevented me putting on weight.

I also experimented with wheat products in this year. I'd read a lot of information on how wheat is not an optimal food choice. During the times I stopped eating wheat, my mood was lighter, as were my sleeping patterns. My bloated tummy deflated, too. During this year I was a UK size 10 (but still with womanly thighs!). I naturally bought many new clothes to celebrate!

My boyfriend at the time said that for most of this year I talked non-stop about raw food and how good it was supposed to be. On a visit to the States, I bought an uncook book which really didn't inspire me, but I knew I wanted to believe in the power of raw — I just needed the right words.

Early on into the new year my mum was diagnosed with spondylitis, her vertebrae had fused in her neck and she was in agony. She had about six months off work. I looked into ways of helping her but she was frightened and confused by what the doctors had told her. My sister also developed back problems. I was concerned about my back (I'd been crashed into a few times and two vertebrae were out of place) — my osteopath wasn't improving my back, and I really didn't want to end up like my mum.

Then one day in 1999 I heard that my lovely uncle Ray had cancer. I'd read and been impressed by **The Cure for All Diseases** by Hulda Clarke a few months back, and so when I saw **The Cure for All Cancers** by the same author in a shop in the States I bought it for him. But when I went to visit him, and gave him the book, I could see the confusion in his face. This wasn't where his head was, and besides that, the surgeons had already butchered him. I thought about these times when I tried to help others with their health issues but I would always find something too "radical" for them to believe in or trust. Then I thought about me, slowly getting back on my feet but still not feeling anywhere near well or right. I wondered when I'd be shown the way. I wondered when

I'd get shown something radical which I could believe in.

I looked at the statistics for cancer in the UK — something like 1 in 11 women will get breast cancer at some time in their lives. That's too much of a risk. I questioned why so many people get cancer. I looked for information and realised that out of all the scientific research there was one thing standing out head and shoulder above the rest. Only humans have these massive odds stacked against them. This is the same for all diseases: arthritis, diabetes, heart disease, obesity — only humans suffer so much with them. At that time I didn't make the connection (and it hadn't been pointed out to me) that only humans (and their "pets") eat cooked food.

I thought about burning causing toxins — I wasn't sure how but I thought cooking and cancer were linked. I thought about this feeling, as I'd thought about raw food before and filed it under "Yes, sometime in the future or in another life, maybe". When I was making my "healthy" stir-fries, I'd look at the bright crisp and flavoursome vegetables as I was chopping them, and then I'd see them wilt and wither in the wok and I'd have to add a sauce to replace the flavour that they'd just lost. I wondered "What is cooking doing to these vegetables? It can't be adding any goodness to them".

I imagined what I'd do if I got cancer, then I thought "I don't want cancer. I don't want arthritis. I don't want diabetes." Why should I get these illnesses? Though the odds were stacked against me, I'm not a statistic, and won't be ever counted in this medical charade. I knew I wasn't going to be a victim to anything ever again in my life, I was going to be strong. But I still didn't really know how. I just felt some real optimism for the first time in my life.

At the National Vegan Festival that summer, I took a raw food booklet to read. I read it a few times. I wondered. Could I live on raw hummous and cauliflower?

Some time that year my weight started creeping up, only by a couple of pounds. I thought exercise would take care of that in the future as I was too tired to do any now. I'd been a member of a gym for the previous three years and hardly ever went due to tiredness and apathy.

Towards the end of this year, I was more or less happy with my life — some things weren't right, but on the whole I'd had a better year than ever before and was really pleased with my progress. I was standing in light for the first time in my adult life. And I wanted more. *I knew I was ready.*

A book changed my life

That Christmas, in 1999 my boyfriend at the time bought me **Nature's First Law: The Raw-Food Diet**, by Arlin, Dini and Wolfe (now deleted). I read it while we were in Scotland, and as I turned every page I was saying "Blimey!", "Cor!" "F*** me!".

Finally the penny had dropped. How long did it take? For four years I'd been looking at raw food information, and finally, something made sense to me! It was telling me what I felt but I could never make sense of these feelings as I was so fogged up.

The one thing that stands out in the book is the final sentence at the end of each chapter: "Cooked food is poison." As soon as I saw it, I knew that was it — I was being poisoned! No wonder I felt like I was dying. I was toxic since before I was even conceived, even since before my mum was conceived! Every cell in my body was made up of substandard material and with these shaky foundations there was no wonder I'd been crumbling.

I understood

Finally, I understood why my life had been such a struggle. And I understood about generations degenerating — I was from weak stock and had been fed dead food since before I was conceived. No wonder I felt like such a runt. I immediately understood the importance of raw mummies and raw daddies making raw babies. I understood that even the most unhealthy people could turn their life around a long way by being raw. I knew I'd never be the fittest, healthiest person in the world, but I could rejuvenate and remove the toxic cells in my body and replace them with healthy raw ones.

I knew this raw food natural law was right — it hit me in the gut as if it were a brick. I understood. I finally understood. I can't begin to say how humbly grateful I was at having this life saving book come to me at a time when I felt strong enough to fully digest the information.

I wanted to be raw

This was the key to the door that I'd always found locked, no matter how much I'd batter and kick it. I can't say how relieved I felt just by reading this book — it also proved to me that I wasn't mad in looking to nature for the right way to live, but I was just so messed up that I couldn't think or trust myself to look to nature regarding food.

As soon as the shops opened after Christmas, I went and bought a load of salads and fruit. I preferred them over the fake turkey dinner which I had a couple of days before, and the soya cheese on biscuits which I'd been eating to pretend like I was having a pigging-out Christmas just like the meat-eaters. I ate my salads and thought about the different tastes, textures and feelings between the raw bits and the cooked bits. I read my golden, beautiful book at every opportunity that holiday. It went everywhere with me. I carried it around as if it was a bible, and I read it at every opportunity — unsociable woman that I am.

I tried a whole raw day as soon as I got back home, and wanted to put the raw diet into practice straight away. However, it was almost the year 2000...

Happy new Millennium

We spent New Year's Eve in Hull at a house party. There was meat in all the salads! I was trying to eat as much fruit as I could when I was in Hull but the shops were either closed or only sold something like one mouldy apple. I resorted to Pot Noodles and jars of baby food. In hindsight I think I'd probably rather have gone hungry but people question you too much when you don't eat three square meals a day.

I talked to my parents about going raw, and told them why. I remembered back to when I was 16 and my dad thought I'd only be a vegetarian for a year so I expected him to think this was a phase, too. My mum said that I can't just live on raw food: where would I get my protein, my B12, wouldn't I get bored, and can't I just be normal? I just trusted this way of eating, I didn't have any questions myself because it felt right. I didn't think about how many greens I'd need, or how much fat or what type of fruit, I just knew that from now on, while living according to this natural law, I'd be guided and protected. But I also knew that I had to find out all the questions and answers because I'd get bombarded with them — and I had to be prepared for that. I knew that saying "Well, animals don't ask all these questions and they're healthier than most humans" wouldn't satisfy people. I also wanted people to know this was the only real true way to eat before I'd even tried it — what faith!

Happy new life

After reading and re-reading my-life saving book it didn't occur to me that I should gradually go into raw food: 50, 60, 70, 80, 90, then finally 100% raw. If cooked food is poison and I wanted that poison out of me then it was all or nothing. I suppose I'd just had enough of hanging around. I don't know how much raw food I ate the previous year, I was only semiconscious about it. However, that year had been good enough for me to realise life could be OK and I wanted it to be great. I wanted it to be fantastic. I wanted it to be perfect. I wasn't yet blessed with any other raw information except a half-raw recipe book and my old uncook book, but on the 3rd of January 2000 (the first normal day of the year), I stopped taking my supplements and thought I'd try a little experiment, just to see how I felt...

Changing times

Over the next few years, everything in my life changed. My illnesses disappeared. I finally got rid of my crippling period pains! Little nagging things like tinnitus, a runny nose, cellulite and those white spots called milia on my face went away. Big nagging things like depression, negative thoughts, weight control problems, achy bones, insomnia, and so much more, all disappeared.

For a while, I didn't know who this new me was. In some ways I felt like an alien, and I was experiencing everything around me with new senses. Nothing looked, felt, tasted, sounded or smelled the same! I would put on music which I'd had for years, and my new detoxed ears would hear completely new sounds in the music and understand more lyrics. I would walk across parks and purposely brush my face across hanging leaves on trees. The sensations I was feeling were truly out of this world, yet totally in it! I was loving every second of discovering the new me, and once likened it to having an affair with myself.

These changes were reflected in all aspects of my life. I moved to Spain and spent five months staring at a mountain, nearly non-stop! I lived in Spain for 18 months and when I came back to England, I knew I was ready to face a new set of opportunities based on the person I'd become, not the one I'd left behind. I was only able to write this book because I made those changes. Before that, I wouldn't have had the experience or the continuous connective flow that comes with tapping into the natural way of things.

I'm so glad that I kept notes of how I felt before and during my life changes, as I had forgotten the deep despair I used to feel. Looking back, it's like reading about someone else. I really don't feel like I have it in my cellular memory any more that I ever felt that way. I do remember feeling depressed, but that enormous black cloud which used to engulf me had long gone from every part of me. It still seems like a dream that I don't have to sleep in the middle of the day, and my aches and pains are barely there. When I treat myself correctly — when I get enough sleep, do yoga, meditate and eat lightly — I feel fantastic. It does take time and practice to get used to that fantastic feeling, but it's so worth persevering.

I can't imagine how I would feel right now if I hadn't detoxed my world. Everything

I've experienced in the last four years, when I first started taking control of my life, has been nothing short of magical. This is a different life. It's real. It has to be experienced...

2007 update

My life continues to be wonderful and inspiring. I've been faced with many opportunities for growth since writing my story here. My company has an online shop, www.detoxyourworld.com. We sell over 700 hard to find health-giving products. We are now the UK's number one importer of some of the best certified organic raw superfoods that this blessed planet has gifted us with. I have some amazing employees, including my family! I feel ecstatic that we are positively affecting the health of the nation.

I'm now a mummy to Evie, my two year old raw vegan toddler. I have brought her up as naturally as I can in the modern world, and she's a constant source of amusement and light for me.

In 2005 I co-wrote **Naked Chocolate** with the US raw food guru David Wolfe. This started The Raw Chocolate Revolution which is currently shaking up the UK's health food industry!

Finally, after seven years, I decided to hang up my online journaling hat. This is the one of the world's longest online journals, and I'm so happy that it's altered the lives of millions of people. Yet now is the time for me to become more private and to live my life in a new expression.

As I mentioned at the beginning of this book, detoxing your life is just the start, so things haven't stopped and will never stop being a whirlwind of wonder for me. The one thing I notice above all else is that when I go with change, accept newness and face my fears, I make massive leaps in every area of my life. This is why I can advise you to do the same — I know it works!

Because my life alters at such a fast pace, you can visit my up-front and personal web site at **www.shazzie.com** to find out up-to-the-minute information on my products, events and services.

Bless you for your time. I wish you all the love in the world.

The recipes

When buying or growing food, remember this: as you eat the item, you assimilate it and it becomes you. Do you want to be made of the best unprocessed ingredients in the world? Do you want to be full of enzymes, life force, vitamins and minerals? If you do, then buy or grow the best food that is available. Make a pact to never compromise on your health.

When detoxing, it's important that you really enjoy the process. As you become accustomed to the recipes, you will notice how easy it is to alter them and create new ones. Let your imagination run riot in the kitchen! Play with the recipes and offer them as gifts of love to your nearest and dearest.

There are over 100 original recipes here, which will give you some idea of how interesting, versatile and delicious a lifetime of eating this way can be. Not only do you fulfil your taste buds' dreams, you become healthy in all areas of your life. However, if the recipes here leave you gagging for more, discover my recipe book, **Detox Delights**. It's the perfect companion to this recipe guide and can also be used when detoxing, or maintaining a detoxed body. In fact, I've included here a select few recipes from **Detox Delights**. This will give you a feel of the book, so you can decide if you want to buy it and fall in love with it, just as thousands of others have!

Because of space restrictions I can't put photos of the food in this book. However, you can check some of them out on the web site, **www.detoxyourworld.com**!

Food notes

These recipes sometimes call for ingredients such as oils, nut and seed butters, carob, olives etc. Make sure that you buy these products unpasteurised, organic or wildcrafted and raw. This will ensure you are buying the highest quality foods containing the lowest amount of toxins. These products may be hard to find in the shops, so check out the *Resources* chapter for convenient mail order services.

Carob powder

Carob is a protein-rich chocolate-tasting pod which grows on trees. When ground into a powder, it makes a great chocolate substitute for drinks, cakes and puddings. Most carob powder is dark, which indicates that it's been roasted. The lighter carob powder is often toasted. There are very few outlets which sell really raw (and therefore less toxic and more nutritious) carob powder. Suggested outlets are listed in the back of this book.

Nut or seed milk

Where I mention the use of nut/seed milks, it's useful if you already have it made up. Try to make a fresh batch to last you two or three days. Store it in the fridge and shake before use. Add a dessertspoon of ionic silver to keep it fresh. I find the best milk is almond and hemp milk, as it's the easiest to digest and has a lovely sweet flavour.

Oils

As with all fractured (non-whole) foods, use oils sparingly, especially when on a detox plan. Though I don't use oils much, they are in some recipes. All oils should be cold-pressed or stone-ground, organic and stored in dark bottles. Please check out the resources at the back of the book for more details on where to buy trusted oils. Ones to look out for are olive, coconut, hemp, sesame and flax seed. I also use Udo's Choice. Olive oil gives its oil very freely, and is a fruit oil, so it's very unique in the world of oils.

Olives

Olives are best if they are not preserved in added salt. If they are, soak them in water before eating them. All olives in cans are cooked, so it's best to stay away from them as they are nutritionally inferior. The best olives are the ones you eat off the ground, which are black (ripe) and sundried. You can now buy these from www.detoxyourworld.com, and they are called Peruvian Olives. Green olives are unripe olives, and although they taste good when processed with salt, water, garlic and herbs, they aren't palatable in their natural state, so limit the amount of time you give to them!

Salt

Table salt is toxic to the body. If you want to use salt to slow down the detoxification process or to increase trace mineral intake, use sea salt or Himalayan crystal salt sparingly. Also make use of more salty foods such as celery and seaweeds. Try making **Fake salt**, as described in the *Food for thought* section.

Seaweed

Black nori sheets are sometimes uncooked, which is more natural than the green toasted variety. It is made from seaweed, which is ground and then pressed into squares which measure about 20 square centimetres. As well as making **Easy sushi**, you can make satisfying nori wraps. Look for black nori in your health food shop or use the resources in this book.

Thick seaweed such as dulse is great soaked and added to many dishes or eaten alone. If you can get Atlantic sea salad, it makes a great addition to salads — I just sprinkle it on top straight from the packet.

Organic or wild

As mentioned previously, try to ensure organic or wild food makes up the highest percentage of your diet as possible. If you buy non-organic, wash the produce thoroughly and be prepared for the meal not to be as toxin-free and tasty as it could be.

Transatlantic translations

Because Americans wear their pants on the outside, they also use some other words differently. Here are the common food words which differ between us.

coriander = cilantro	punnet = plastic fruit basket, about 2-3 cups
aubergine = eggplant	dessertspoon = 2 teaspoons
sharon fruit = persimmon	little gem = tiny lettuce, like a mini-romaine
courgette = zucchini	rocket = arugula
beansprouts = sprouts	sweetcorn = corn/maize
spring onions = green onions	crisps = chips
chips = fries	beetroot = beet
chick peas = garbanzos	pepper = bell pepper

Baby sweetcorn isn't used very often in the USA, so normal sweetcorn, cut from the cob, is a sufficient replacement.

Water

Where water is mentioned, you can either use your preferred water (I use mineral water) or the freshly squeezed juice of a cucumber or celery or the water from a young or old coconut, depending on whether the dish is sweet or savoury. If you find organic coconut water hard to come by, try Dr Martin's Coco Drink and Milk. These products are both now available in the UK, and they're 100% raw.

Equipment notes

Heavy-duty expensive equipment is lovely to use, but it's not totally necessary. In the recipes, I always offer alternatives to the expensive equipment route. Here's a list of equipment commonly used in these recipes. If you can't find these items in the shops, have a look at the resources at the back of the book.

Spiral slicer

This is one of the best gadgets that I've come across. It's also known as the spiraliser and the saladacco. In the years I've had mine I haven't got bored of it, so I know it's not just a gimmick! It creates angel-hair pasta out of courgette, and noodles out of squashes. It changes the taste, texture and chewability of every vegetable it touches and it's manual, so there are no electric noises or energy issues to contend with.

Juicers

Juicers can range from the £40 centrifugal variety, to the £400+ masticating variety. I always advise people to start off with the centrifugal one, and when they want to move on, they have a gift so a loved one can get started on this path. There are also citrus juicers, and I'd advise that you get yourself one of these if you juice a lot of citrus. It means you don't have to peel the fruit first which saves you a lot of time.

Mandoline

Another manual gadget; this slices, chips and juliennes. It's great if you have a family, as it can whizz through vegetables at a very fast rate. Some food processors work in a similar way with their various attachments, so check the backs of your cupboards first.

Blender

A normal blender is capable of doing most things you want it to, such as blending soups, smoothies and dips. However, the high-powered Vita-Mix really comes into its own when you want to blend thicker, harder items. It can pulverise carrots and make a "juice" out of the whole vegetable. It's my favourite blender! Because it's a commercial blender rather than a domestic one, don't be surprised at the £400+ price tag.

Hand blender

Also known as a liquidiser, this is the type that you hold and push into the food, whizzing it up in the process. Americans sometimes call it a wand blender. It's great if you don't have a Vita-Mix, as it will blend thicker food than your average blender will manage.

You can buy them for about £5, but that type seem to have a tiny blade which doesn't do the job very well. Go for the ones which are about £20 and have larger blades that point both up and down.

Food processor

This machine revolutionises the preparation of raw food. Make pies, crackers and pâtés in minutes. With the many types on the market, look for one with a large basin and a fast speed, as it will make a difference to the convenience of your food preparation. I personally prefer the Kenwood Chef, as it's very reliable. Mine is now ten years old and I use it most days!

Spice/coffee mill

If you have a food processor with a blender or a solo blender, you might already have one of these. If not, you can buy them quite cheaply. They are fantastic for making small amounts of really smooth dressings, and for milling dry seeds and raw cacao nibs.

Dehydrator

A few of the recipes here call for a dehydrator. This is a machine like a cool oven, that blows warm, but not hot, air over the food. The food changes in structure as water is removed, but enzymes and other heat sensitive nutrients aren't lost in the process. Dehydrating the odd meal acts as a good bridge when starting out, and it's also a nice treat every now and then. If you don't have a dehydrator, you can achieve similar results by putting your oven on its lowest setting and leaving the door open, or using an airing cupboard or the sunshine.

Cups

You'll see that I use cups instead of weighing. This is a much quicker way of working. You can buy inexpensive measuring cups from all good supermarkets and cook shops.

Smoothies

A smoothie is a mixture of fruit and other food which is thin enough to drink. If you wanted a smoothie but get a pudding add more soft fruit, water or freshly made fruit juice. In addition, all the smoothies can be made into puddings by using less soft fruit or adding nuts or seeds. I find that my blender prefers to get started with the soft fruit and liquid, and then I add the banana or harder fruit.

When on a detox plan you'll normally have these for breakfast, as they're your main fruit meal, and fruit is the best thing for you in the morning. But if you want to eat them at night, then that's fine too!

Coconut drink

Serves 1-2.

1 banana

½ old (brown) coconut and all its water or ½ carton of Dr Martins' Coco Drink

½ lime, juiced

½ teaspoon of spirulina

2 oranges, juiced

Add all the ingredients to the blender and blend until smooth. Either strain or drink as is. If you want a medium consistency, strain it all and then stir some of the pulp back in.

Celery

Celery is a great source of organic sodium. It's even reported to lower blood pressure. This is great news for those suffering from high blood pressure who are following a low-sodium diet!

Celery is also a good source of bioavailable calcium.

Blue Manna contains lots of B12!

Seaside smoothie

The celery in this smoothie makes for a really rounded taste. It's great for feeling like you're swimming in a blue ocean. Serves 1-2.

3 bananas, peeled

2 stalks of celery

1 teaspoon of green superfood

2 pears, peeled

¼ litre of water

½ teaspoon of Blue Manna (AFA algae extract)

Chop the celery quite fine. Add the water, bananas, pear and celery to the blender and blend for a few seconds. Then add the superfood and blend until smooth.

Big green

Serves 1-2.

3 bananas, peeled

1 avocado, peeled and stoned

A pinch of fresh lemon rind

¼ litre of water

2 teaspoons of green superfood

Add the water, bananas, avocado and lemon rind to the blender and blend for a few seconds. Then add the Superfood and blend until smooth. If too thick, add more water.

Mangos and antioxidants

Mangos are rich in vitamins A and C, beta carotene and fibre. All of these nutrients help fight off nasties in your body.

They also happen to be one of the most delicious foods on earth.

Chocolate orange smoothie

Serves 1-2.

4 oranges, juiced

1 teaspoon of green superfood

2 dessertspoons of really raw carob or raw chocolate powder

2 bananas, peeled

1 mango, peeled and stoned

Pour the orange juice and all other ingredients into your blender. Blend. If desired, add more juice or water to thin the smoothie.

This is where the sun got to

Serves 1.

2 oranges, juiced

1 mango, peeled and stoned

1 banana, peeled

1 inch of vanilla pod

½ inch of ginger

Pour the orange juice and all other ingredients into your blender. Blend. If desired, add more juice or water to thin the smoothie.

There are many more smoothies in **Detox Delights**!

Juices

You don't need expensive juicers to get the benefits of juicing. A small centrifugal juicer will do juicy fruits, some greens and even hard carrots. Just in case you don't have a super juicer, I've given alternative methods of making each juice where appropriate.

Remember to drink your juice immediately, chew it in the mouth to ensure correct digestion, and finish it within 15 minutes.

The candy floss tart

This is such a sugar pink colour, it glows! Don't mess with the sweet sugary vixen lurking at the bottom of this drink — she might just turn around and bite you! Serves 1-2.

3 pink grapefruits

2 limes

2 ripe soft pears

2 cups of melon

Remove the citrus peel and juice all the ingredients. Add everything to a blender and blend (you can strain this if you like).

Bottoms up

This sweet juice is so smooth, it goes down almost without you knowing. Serves 1-2.

1 cantaloupe melon or ½ piel de sapo, removed from peel and seeded

3-4 peaches, skinned and stoned

Juice both ingredients — add some ice if you like. Serve in a late summer English garden. If you don't have a late summer garden to hand, close your eyes and think of England!

Wake up, ginger

Serves 2.

2 inches of ginger

4 oranges

1 cup of berries, such as redcurrants, strawberries, or blackcurrants

Juice all the ingredients and serve immediately.

Hopping wild

Now we start getting into the serious juices. Green juices deliver much needed nutrients quickly and easily to wherever your body needs them. Serves 2.

10-20 big wild leaves from your garden (such as dandelion, dock or plantain)

2 apples, peeled and cored

5 stalks of celery

Juice all the ingredients, mix and drink. As you get used to the strength of the wild greens, increase the amount. If you find them too strong to start with, use only five leaves and gradually build up.

Variation

If you don't have a garden, and there are no wild plants near you, use kale, spinach, watercress and herbs instead of the wild garden greens.

Brutus is scared

This will turn you into no ordinary Popeye! Serves 2.

4 cups of spinach, packed tightly

2 large carrots, topped

4 tomatoes

¼ lemon

1 cucumber, skinned if not organic

Juice all the ingredients, mix and drink.

Fractal fortnight

Honestly, do this juice regularly for a fortnight (that's two weeks to you Americans!) and every perception in your head will have shifted. The E3Live forms beautiful shifting fractal patterns when you look closely at it, it's a kaleidoscope in a cup! Serves 2.

2 teaspoons of E3Live

1 cup of kale or savoy cabbage, tightly packed

4 pears, peeled and cored

4 stalks of celery

Juice all ingredients, mix and drink.

Cucumber number

Serves 2.

1 cucumber
1 teaspoon of lemon peel
3 apples, cored

Juice all the ingredients and serve immediately.

Apple and orange

Serves 2.

4 apples, cored
4 oranges, peeled

If you keep a tiny bit of orange peel on, it adds a lovely flowery flavour. Remember to keep the pith on. Juice both ingredients, and serve immediately.

Spicy pear

Serves 1.

4 pears, cored
4 stalks of celery
¼ teaspoon of cinnamon powder

Juice all ingredients and serve immediately. Note: You can run the powder through your juicer in between ingredients, or you can stir it in afterwards.

Supercharged celery

Serves 1.

8 stalks of celery
1 teaspoon of E3Live
2 apples

Juice all ingredients and serve immediately. If you don't have E3Live, use another type of edible algae or pick a handful of edible wild leaves from your garden.

The lady juiced her fingers

Serves 1.

10 okra (ladies fingers), topped
1 yellow or orange pepper, de-seeded and destalked
2 tomatoes, destalked

Juice all ingredients and serve immediately.

Rocket fuel

Serves 1.

2 cups of rocket
4 stalks of celery
1 yellow or orange pepper, de-seeded and destalked
2 pears

Juice all ingredients and serve immediately.

Cherry chaser

Serves 1. Really, don't share this with anyone else!

1 cup of cherries, lovingly stoned
2 apples

Juice both ingredients and serve immediately. Note: Cherry juice stains, so wear an apron when juicing!

Sangria Maria

Serves 2.

8 tomatoes, destalked
4 stalks of celery
1 red pepper, de-seeded and destalked
½ medium chilli (optional)

Juice all ingredients and serve immediately.

Strawberry patch
Serves 1.

4 cups of strawberries

1 little gem lettuce

2 cups of blueberries

Juice all ingredients and serve immediately.

Cucumber and apple
Serves 2.

1 cucumber

2 apples, cored

A sprig of fresh mint

Juice all ingredients and serve immediately.

Cabbage and carrot
Serves 1.

4 outer or 6-8 inner cabbage leaves

6 carrots, topped and tailed

½ inch of ginger

Juice all ingredients and serve immediately.

Give your heart to ginger

Ginger offers protection against strokes and heart attacks. Ginger fights off bad hormones and helps good hormones in the heart battle. The result is less pain, less clotting, less constriction of the blood vessels and less inflammation.

Hot orange
Serves 2.

4 oranges, peeled

½ inch of fresh ginger

If the oranges are organic, add a little of the orange peel to the juicer. Juice both ingredients and serve immediately.

Carrot top-up

Serves 2.

8 carrots

4 dark cabbage leaves

Juice both ingredients and serve immediately.

Runny romaine

Serves 1.

10-15 romaine leaves

1 large mango, peeled and stoned

Juice both ingredients and serve immediately.

Detoxing with grapefruits

All citrus fruits are great for detox, but pink grapefruits have that special something!

Adding the juice of half a lemon to your grapefruit drinks will cause the mucous in your body to be dissolved.

Sweet grapefruit

Serves 2.

2 pink grapefruits, peeled

2 cups of melon

Juice both ingredients and serve immediately.

Drinks

Melonlemon

Serves 2.

You wouldn't believe how a little bit of lemon peel can turn a juice into a divine cocktail.

1 cantaloupe melon

About ¼ teaspoon of lemon peel

Cut the melon in half, scoop the seeds out, and add to a blender with the lemon peel. Drink!

Variations

To make this drink totally different, use a honeydew, a galia or a piel de sapo. Add the peel of lemon as above or the peel of lime or orange. Combining the different melons together also gives a lovely refreshing drink.

Warm apple punch

Serves 2.

8 apples

½ vanilla pod

A cinnamon stick

4 slices of lemon

4 slices of orange

1 teaspoon of five spice

Juice the apples and place in a serving jug. Roughly chop the vanilla pod, and break up the cinnamon stick. Add all the other ingredients to the juice, and allow to marinade for 1 hour in the sunshine. If you don't have the sunshine, place in an airing cupboard or somewhere else warm (but not hot).

Cardamom cooler

4 cardamom pods

1 pint of almond milk

1 papaya, peeled and de-seeded

Split the cardamom pods open and scoop the black seeds into the blender. Add the papaya and almond milk. Blend all the ingredients. The little black cardamom seeds are full of flavour, and make this drink really special.

Chockie milkshake

This is the smoothest, best chockie milkshake in the world. Serves 1, because you won't want to share it!

20 brazils, soaked at least 2 hours

¾ pint of water

1 banana, peeled

1 inch of vanilla pod

2 medjool or 4 smaller dates

2-4 teaspoons of raw carob powder (depending on taste)

Blend the brazils and dates with the water, and strain. Use the nut fibre for another recipe such as rissoles or burgers, and add the milk back to the blender. Blend all ingredients together and serve.

Variation

For a thicker shake, use a sliced, frozen banana.

Red whine

Serves 2.

This version is so much more healthy than that alcoholic tripe. You get the goodness of the red grapes without the hazards or headaches of the alcohol. This is perfect for the long summer days when you want a relaxing drink to chill you out.

1 bunch of red grapes

2 oranges, peeled

Juice all the ingredients. Clink "Cheers" and drink!

Sunrise

Serves 2.

This is such a lovely drink to wake up to. Make it when you know it's going to be a hot day, take it to the beach or to a lovely green hill, and sip it as the sun comes up...

2 Pakistani or Indian mangoes (other mangoes will do, but you may want to add a couple of dates for sweetness)

Liquid of one young coconut

Jelly of one young coconut

1 banana

Blend all ingredients together. Pour into long glasses, decorated with a slice of banana. If the coconut jelly is a bit meaty, and your blender isn't super-strong, then omit it.

Quick chockie thickshake

Both children and grown-ups love this, so make lots! Serves 1.

15 macadamias (they don't have to be pre-soaked)

¾ pint of water

2 frozen bananas (you can use fresh if you don't have frozen, but it won't be as thick)

1 inch of vanilla pod

2-4 teaspoons of really raw carob powder (depending on taste)

Blend all ingredients together and drink. If you don't have a tough blender, such as a Vita-Mix, make sure you slice your bananas before freezing and let them thaw for just a minute or two before blending.

Vanilla pods

Vanilla is the pod of an orchid plant called vanilla planifolia. Though there are over 20,000 varieties of orchid, this is the only one to bear an edible pod.

Green hemp milk

4 carrots

4 cups of spinach

1 orange, peeled

2 sticks of celery

A sprig of rosemary or sage

1 cup of hemp seeds, soaked overnight

Finely chop the celery and add all the ingredients to your blender. Blend really well. Place a clean cloth such as muslin inside a strainer, and place this over a bowl. Pour the mixture out into the cloth, wrap the cloth up and wring it to get all the juice out. There's something lovely about getting your hands into this one. Must be something to do with the love vibe!

Soups

When detoxing, you might sometimes feel cold. You can warm quite a few of these recipes up, and soups are the most successful for this. To warm up your soup, pour it into a ceramic bowl which is sitting in hand-hot water, then cover the whole lot. Stir it every now and then, and wait for about 10-30 minutes before eating. The soup will be a lovely temperature and you can wrap your hands around the bowl.

These soups are all very quick to make, as they aren't cooked. It means you spend less time in the kitchen, and you get more nutrients, antioxidants and water. Serve with **macadamia cream**, an avocado, some sundried olives, a few nuts of your choice, or some raw breads or crackers for a filling meal.

Sweet beet

Serves 1.

1 beetroot

3 strawberries

1 tomato

2 cups of water

5 spring onions

Chop all solid ingredients and blend with the water. If you like, you can strain it and add some of the pulp back in to get the consistency you like.

Cream of pepper soup

Serves 1.

1 red pepper

4 sundried tomatoes, soaked for at least 2 hours

4 tablespoons of **Macadamia cream**

1 orange

2 dried apricots, soaked for at least 2 hours

1 teaspoon of acai powder, optional

Juice the orange, and add the juice to the blender. Chop all other ingredients and add to the blender. Blend until it is liquidised.

Squash and kumquat soup

Serves 2.

½ acorn squash (or whatever squash you can find)

6 kumquats

1 carrot

1 yellow or orange bell pepper

1 teaspoon of freshly peeled lemon rind

1 small hot chilli

1 tablespoon of fresh coconut meat

1 clove of garlic

5 dried apricots, soaked 2-12 hours

1 sundried tomato

1 cup of sunflower or almond milk

2 cups of water

> ### Kumquats
>
> Kumquats look like tiny oranges. The skin is sweet and full of flavour, but the flesh isn't very nice!

If you have a juicer: juice the kumquats, bell pepper, coconut meat and apricots, then add everything to the blender and blend until liquidised. If you don't have a juicer: chop all solid ingredients and add everything to your blender, blend until liquid and then strain the soup. If you want a thicker soup, add some of the pulp back in.

It's nice to serve this with a little grated squash, some sunflower seeds and some chopped spring onions on top.

Cream of orange soup

This is a simple, yet very tasty soup. Serves 2.

2 avocados, peeled and stoned

8 oranges

1 teaspoon of grated lemon peel

½ inch of ginger

Juice the oranges, discarding the peel and pips. Finely chop the ginger. Put the juice in a blender with all the other ingredients and blend. If this is too thick, add more orange juice. Serve in bowls.

Cream of shiitake soup

Serves 2.

1 cup of fresh shiitake mushrooms

1 tablespoon of raw almond butter

2 cups of almond milk

½ red onion

Dried mushrooms to garnish

1 cup of celery

1 teaspoon of sesame oil

½ cup of spinach, tightly packed

Clean the shiitake mushrooms and remove any really hard stalk bits. Add them, the almond butter and the almond milk to the blender and blend. Finely chop the onion and the parsley, and stir this into the soup. Pour the soup into serving bowls. Very finely chop the celery and spinach, and mix together with the sesame oil (and a little sea salt if you like). Pile this mixture on top of the soup, and sprinkle some dried mushrooms all over the dish. If you are going to serve this warmed, add the spinach and celery afterwards. Chinese leaves make a great "bread" for this soup.

Yellow pepper and almond soup

This is lovely and creamy. Serves 4.

1 pint of almond milk

4 yellow peppers, de-seeded

4 sundried tomatoes, soaked

Pinch each of cumin, turmeric and coriander powder

½ cup of fresh coriander

1 small onion, peeled

Finely chop the onion and coriander. Set aside the fresh coriander, a couple of teaspoons of onion and one sundried tomato. Put all other ingredients in your blender and blend thoroughly. If desired, you can strain the soup before serving. Add the chopped coriander and mix well. Serve in bowls. Dice the remaining sundried tomato, mix with the remaining onion and top the soup with this mixture.

Jessie's tropical soup
Serves 2.

2 medium mangoes, skinned and stoned

Juice and rind of 2 limes

1 medium-hot chilli, de-seeded

1 avocado, peeled and stoned

1 passion fruit, scooped out of the shell

1 orange, juiced

10 stalks of coriander

2 juicy dates, stoned

½ red onion, skinned

Ripe limes

When a lime is ripe it turns yellow! The flavour is so much softer and mouthwatering than that of an unripe green lime. Ripe limes are also much more juicy!

Look out for yellow limes in your supermarket!

Add one mango, the passion fruit, chilli, dates, lime juice and rind and orange juice to your blender. Blend until smooth and leave to marinade for half an hour to an hour. Once marinaded, strain the ingredients to remove passion fruit pips and other unblended bits. Discard the strained ingredients and keep the liquid.

Dice the other mango and the avocado into half-inch cubes. Dice the onion into quarter-inch cubes, and chop most of the coriander. Put all ingredients in a serving bowl and top with a few whole coriander leaves.

African spicy sesame soup

This soup is based on traditional African flavours, and is very creamy. Serves 4 as a starter.

½ cup of tahini

½ cup of sesame seeds

½ cup of sweetcorn

1 cup of tomatoes

2 stalks of celery

1 dessertspoon of sesame oil

1 large onion

1 inch of ginger

2 cloves of garlic

1 teaspoon each of coriander, cumin and cardamom seeds

1 teaspoon of turmeric

½ teaspoon of cayenne pepper

Open sesame
Sesame seeds are bursting with goodness. They are high in amino acids, calcium, iron, niacin and thiamin.

Using a coffee grinder, grind the coriander, cumin, cardamom and sesame seeds together. This will be the really flavourful base to the soup. Finely chop the onion, tomato, ginger, garlic and celery. In a blender, add the tahini, ground seeds, vegetables (not the sweetcorn), cayenne pepper and turmeric. Blend this until smooth. Pour into serving dishes, and pile equal amounts of sweetcorn in the middle.

Sprinkle on a little more cayenne if you like, for decoration. This goes well with a dehydrated nutty fruit bread.

Golden gazpacho soup

If you can find golden tomatoes, and orange or yellow peppers, this traditional Spanish soup becomes a striking masterpiece. Even if you use red tomatoes, you'll love the cool-as-a-cucumber taste on a hot sunny day. Just make sure you make enough! Serves 4.

8 really juicy ripe tomatoes, yellow if you can find them

1 onion

1 cup of cucumber

1 clove of garlic

2 yellow or orange peppers, destalked and seeded

2 stalks of celery

1 medium red chilli

¼ lemon

A bunch of chives

A bunch of coriander

Juice 7 of the tomatoes, half of the cucumber, half of the onion, the herbs, the lemon, the celery, the garlic and the peppers.

Put the juice into serving bowls.

Finely chop the rest of the ingredients, but keep them all separate from each other. Place in piles or separate little dishes to serve, and chill.

To eat gazpacho, pour helpings of the chopped vegetables into the centre of the soup, according to your taste. Add some crushed ice if it's a really hot day.

You can also serve this with a wedge of lemon and some savoury **Vanilla créme**.

Pulp

What do you do with the pulp after you've strained the soup? I like to make pulp into little burger shapes, dehydrate them out in the sun for a day or two and eat them as little biscuits with the next day's soup! If you don't have the sunshine, you can always use a dehydrator, an airing cupboard, the top of a radiator or an oven on its lowest setting with the door open. Also, try adding soaked minced nuts, and making loaves out of them, dehydrating in the same way, but until still moist inside.

Salads

Making a salad is nothing like cooking a soufflé — you don't need exact amounts of anything. Just experiment with whatever you've got and whatever you fancy.

All the recipes in the *Dips, dressings and pâtés* section complement these salads but remember that the key is to eat simply. You'll naturally do this as you progress, anyway. Try some of these salads on their own in a lovely quiet place and see how you feel when eating them, chewing them over and over.

It's best to eat a salad as your evening meal. If you are still hungry after eating it, wait an hour or two for it to digest, then have some fruit until you are full.

Chakra salad

This is the best party salad ever! Put this on a big pretty plate and watch everyone dip in (if you let them!). It's also great for making up a big batch all for yourself, then there's always something ready made in the fridge for when you get a hunger attack.

Amounts aren't given in the recipe, because it's totally up to you. Obviously, if you don't have one ingredient, it won't matter either. You can substitute lots in this recipe. What makes it so special is the way the ingredients are cut up — you can take in a great volume of vegetables without wearing your jaw out!

Courgette

Yellow pepper

Pumpkin or other squash

Carrot

Broccoli

Tomatoes

Red cabbage

Beetroot

Using the "s" blade of a food processor, process each item separately, until kibbled. Take it out and put it on a big plate in a mound. To preserve the colours, do it in the order listed above, courgette first, beetroot last. For added variety, use your spiral slicer to slice the courgettes, carrot and pumpkin, and use a mandoline to slice the beetroot and red cabbage. Use **High vibe** dressing as a dip, placed in a bowl in the centre of the salad.

Romaine roll-ups

The herbs and spices are used for flavouring, as your taste buds may be a bit sleepy from eating too much toxic food. As you progress, you'll naturally want less and less complex flavours. If you can't get romaine lettuce, use another large-leafed lettuce such as iceberg. Serves 2.

1 big romaine lettuce

3 large tomatoes, finely chopped

1 avocado, peeled, stoned and finely chopped

1 cup of alfalfa sprouts

2 tablespoons of fresh coriander, finely chopped

Any other herbs such as basil, oregano or mint, finely chopped

Onion and/or garlic, finely chopped (optional)

Separate the leaves of the romaine lettuce and put them on a plate. In a bowl, mix up all the other ingredients to make the filling.

Using a spoon, dollop a generous amount of the filling into the centre of a lettuce leaf at one end. Roll the sides over, fold in half and eat like a sandwich. Do this until you are full or until you have finished your filling.

Juicy cukes

The best vegetable source of vitamin E and high in iodine, the cucumber is a top fruit.

Cucumber is great on your skin and can reduce puffiness around your eyes. Blend up some cucumber, put it on your eyes, lay back and relax!

Cucumber salad

This goes really well with Sunflower pâté. Serves 2.

1 cucumber

½ cup of tahini

1 lemon

1 teaspoon of paprika

Juice a quarter of the cucumber and the lemon. Dice the rest of the cucumber and add to a bowl. Blend the tahini, cucumber juice, lemon juice and paprika. Pour the dressing onto the cucumber and mix before serving.

Thai salad

Serves 4, this is a filling and hearty meal. Adjust the spices to how hot or cool you like your food.

4 cups of portabello mushrooms

1 cup of raw peanuts

1 small hot chilli, de-seeded

½ cup of fresh coriander

1 cup of red and orange peppers

4 spring onions

1 tablespoon of fresh ginger

2 tablespoons of olive oil

2 tablespoons of sesame oil

1 clove of garlic

1 cup of fresh coconut meat and all its water

1 lemon

1 stalk of lemon grass

1 lime

1 inch of galangal

A small handful of sea lettuce

Cut the mushrooms so that the stalk and gills are removed, and then cube the remaining flesh. Dice the peppers, mince the garlic and ginger, juice the lemon and finely chop the coriander, spring onions and chilli. Mix the coriander, ginger, chilli, garlic, olive oil, sesame oil and lemon juice together in a bowl. Roughly crush the peanuts then add them and the mushrooms to the mixture and stir thoroughly. Marinade for 24 hours.

Soak the sea lettuce in water for between 2-24 hours, then rinse.

Juice the lemon grass, galangal and the lime. Blend this juice with the coconut meat and enough coconut water to make a sauce. It may need to be processed in a food processor first, and then blended in a coffee mill, unless you have a high-powered blender.

Drain the salad and spoon it on chinese cabbage leaves. Chop the sea lettuce into fine ribbons and spread them on top. Pour the sauce over the top. Finally, zest some of the lime and lemon and sprinkle on top.

The gratest salad in the world

We make good use of grating food for this salad. It makes it easier to get more in, so you're fuller for longer! Serves 1 as a main meal or 2 as a side dish.

1 medium courgette

1 small red onion

1 carrot

1 cup of pumpkin

1 avocado

1 small red pepper

2 dessertspoons of sauerkraut

1 teaspoon of avocado oil or olive oil

1 dessertspoon of dulse or other sea vegetable

A pinch of paprika

Grate the courgette, pumpkin and carrot. Finely dice the red onion, pepper and avocado. Put all ingredients in a bowl, and mix. Serve with romaine lettuce as roll ups, topped onto portabello mushrooms as pizzas, with another side dish or as a main meal.

Lycopene

The antioxidant phytochemical known as lycopene is abundant in tomatoes. However, you can find a more bioavailable source in watermelons. This means your body can digest and use the lycopene from watermelons better than raw tomatoes.

Tomato salad

Serves 2.

4 big tomatoes

2 cups of basil

½ red onion

10 black sundried olives (stoned)

A pinch of paprika

Slice the tomatoes and onion into rings. Layer these and the basil on a plate until they are all used up. Scatter the olives on top and sprinkle with paprika.

I can't believe it's not Waldorf salad

This is soooo much tastier than any other salad, it's really a meal on its own. Just right for when you need to get your teeth into something. Serves 1.

Apples

Eat an apple when you want to freshen your mouth up!

Soluble and insoluble fibre is found in apples.

Pectin is a soluble fibre and it helps to prevent cholesterol build up in blood vessel walls. This can reduce the risk of heart disease and athero-sclerosis.

Insoluble fibre provides bulk and holds water to allow waste to move quickly through your digestive system.

1 sweet dessert apple, cored

5 stalks of celery

½ cup of walnuts

½ cucumber

10 macadamias

1 clove of garlic, peeled

2 dessertspoons of hemp oil

Dice the cucumber, celery and apple, but not too finely, and put them in a serving bowl. Finely chop the garlic, and cut the macadamias in half. Put the macadamias, garlic, a stalk of the chopped celery and about two inches of the chopped cucumber in your coffee mill. Blend the coffee mill ingredients until smooth. Depending on the strength of your blender, you may have to pause for a minute during blending so the dressing doesn't get hot. This dressing goes a beautiful pale green colour and is so tasty. It should be a bit thicker than double cream. If it's too thin: add more nuts. If it's too thick: add more oil or cucumber. Once blended, pour into the bowl and mix so that all the vegetables are coated. Throw the walnuts on top and serve.

Scrummy side dishes

These dishes make smashing snacks, or can be added to main meals. Alternatively, put two or three of them together, and they'll make a filling main meal.

Tabouleh pyramids

The intense parsley taste makes this traditional Lebanese dish famous throughout the world. In this version, I've remained faithful to the essence of the dish, just replacing cracked wheat with sprouted quinoa. All good health food shops sell quinoa (pronounced kee-nwa).

If you soak the quinoa the previous day, just rinse and drain it in the morning and it will have sprouted enough to use in an hour or two. If you only sprout quinoa for a few hours to a day, you get a nicer taste than if you soak it for longer.

4 cups of quinoa, sprouted

1 cup of spring onions

Juice of 2 lemons

2 cups of flat leaf parsley, tightly packed

½ cup of cucumber

½ cup of plum tomatoes

Spring onions

Spring onions are also known as scallions, bunching or green onions.

If it's a frosty night and you have to use your car in the morning, use an onion! Slice it and rub it on the windscreen. This will keep the windscreen frost-free!

Rinse the quinoa. Finely chop the spring onions, cucumber, tomato and parsley. Add all the ingredients to a bowl and mix thoroughly.

Once mixed, let the flavours marry for an hour or two before serving, if you like. When ready to serve, turn out the mixture onto a plate and shape it into a pyramid with your hands. It should stay like that! Garnish with extra slices of lemon and some parsley.

Tabouleh is traditionally served with romaine lettuce. The tabouleh is scooped up onto the lettuce and then eaten like a roll. What a perfect dish to take to a party!

Sauerkraut

In just three to seven days you will be rewarded with a delicious, vinegary salad addition. There's lots of good bacteria in this, so if you have tummy problems, it might soothe you a bit. I use this in the Dolmades recipe, but why don't you try it blended with soaked sunflower seeds for a lovely pâté, or just as an addition to a salad? Sauerkraut takes about three to five days to ferment, but after that it will store in a jar in your fridge for a couple of months.

1-4 red or white or mixed (compact) cabbages

Water

Take some of the outer leaves off the cabbages and set aside. If you have a Champion juicer, roughly chop the cabbage into manageable portions and process it all using the blank blade. If you are using a food processor, chop the cabbage using the "s" blade until it's very fine (you might need to do it in batches). If you are using a blender, finely chop about half of the cabbage, and put the other half into a blender. Cover it with enough water to get it going and blend until very fine.

Put your juiced/processed/blended cabbage into a big bowl and mix thoroughly. If it doesn't seem moist, add some water, and mix again. Press the cabbage down, as far as it will go. It shouldn't be swimming in water, just moist. Put the saved cabbage leaves on top, and press it all down again. Put a layer of cling film on top and press it all down again. Now put a weight on top. I use bags of unopened lentils, as they form to the shape of the bowl really well.

Once it's all compact and weighted, cover it with a tea towel and place somewhere in the house where you don't go very often, as it will smell a little during fermentation. In three days, check it to see if you have kraut. You will know it's kraut, because it will smell pickled, and the cabbage will have a translucent appearance. If it isn't ready, check it each day. It will soon be sauerkraut.

Once it's sauerkraut, transfer it to clean jars with tight lids and again, press it down so no air is trapped. It's ready to use now, but can also be stored in the fridge for a few months and used as needed.

Variations

You can add layers of cucumber, carrots, courgettes, pepper slices, onion rings etc to the cabbage before fermentation. You will receive wonderful pickled vegetables as a result, which make lovely crisp additions to salads.

Dolmades

You can make these as big or as small as you like, but as I use seaweed instead of vine leaves, size is often dictated by the size of the strips. If you can find fresh vine leaves, you can also use those — just marinade them in the juice from Champigñónes au natural for a day or two first.

It's the sauerkraut in the stuffing which gives this variation on a Greek favourite its piquant and moreish taste. You will love eating these.

Avocados

Avocados are a good source of vitamins A, B, E, and also contain potassium and selenium.

The Aztecs believed that avocados were a sexual stimulant and so treated them as forbidden fruits. When avocados were being harvested, all the young women were made to stay indoors!

---

1 cup of **Sauerkraut**, finely chopped

1 cup of avocado, peeled and stoned

¼ cup of fresh mint

2 shallots or ¼ red onion

1 packet of wakamé

Soak the wakamé for about five or ten minutes prior to use. It becomes very soft very quickly, but won't fall apart if you leave it for longer. Use the soak water for watering plants — they love it!

Finely chop the onions and mint. In a bowl, add the onions, mint, avocado and **Sauerkraut**. Mash it all together until it becomes a paste.

Select large pieces of wakamé and lay them onto a chopping board. If there are no wide pieces, lay a few side by side and put one across the centre to strengthen it. Cut any stray or stalk pieces off.

Put about a dessertspoon of the paste in the middle of the wakamé, roll the sides of the wakamé up, and then roll the ends up, so that all the stuffing is parcelled up in the middle.

Extra sticking down isn't necessary, they will self-seal immediately. Take the next piece of wakamé from the water and continue until you have used all the mixture.

Crispy spring rolls

Serves 4.

8 chinese leaves

1 cup of beansprouts

1 cup of sprouted almonds

½ cup of chives

½ cup of spring onions

2 avocados

1 clove of garlic

1 inch of ginger

2 cups of soft dark green leaves (such as spinach or watercress)

Mince the dark leaves with the avocado, garlic, ginger and sprouted almonds, until smooth but still with pieces in it. Cut the chinese leaves so you're only using the top four-inch portion. Sliver the spring onions into thin strips. Spread the mixture onto the top of a leaf, lay on the beansprouts, chives and spring onions so they all lay lengthways. Roll up the leaf so it overlaps, and place the open side underneath on a plate. Serve with **Sweet apricot sauce**.

Fig stew

2 cups of berries such as blueberries, raspberries, strawberries, blackberries etc.

4 fresh figs (or 4 dried figs, soaked in water overnight)

1 tomato

½ red pepper

2 medjool dates, or 4 drier dates soaked overnight

1 apple, cored

A handful of raisins, gojis or sultanas

A pinch of cinnamon

Blend one cup of the berries. Finely chop the figs, dates, tomato, pepper and remaining berries. Mix all chopped and blended ingredients together, and let marinade for at least an hour. Put the mixture into your serving dish, grate the apple on top, sprinkle the raisins on top of that, and add a pinch of cinnamon. Serve with **macadamia cream**.

Onion bhajis

When I invented this for my friend's birthday meal, we were all stunned! Serve with small cauliflower florettes and Mango chutney as a starter. Serves 4 as a side dish or starter.

2 cups of walnuts, soaked for just an hour

1 cup of portabello mushrooms

4 sundried tomatoes, soaked at least 2 hours

1 dessertspoon of paprika

20-30 stalks of fresh coriander

10-20 stalks of fresh parsley

1 clove of garlic

2 cups of red onion

1 red pepper, de-seeded and destalked

1 dessertspoon of garam masala

A pinch of cayenne pepper

Finely chop the garlic, then add everything except half the onions to the food processor, and process. Then transfer to a jug and use your hand blender to achieve a finer consistency. If you have a Champion or similar juicer, then you can do the first two steps in one, by using the blank blade. Finely chop the remaining onions, add them to the mixture and mix thoroughly.

Pick up small amounts of mixture and roll into mini-2cm or bigger balls. Place them in a dehydrator for 8-24 hours, turning several times.

Basilled tomatoes

Serves 2.

1 cup of basil, tightly packed

A pinch of salt

8 juicy ripe tomatoes

4 tablespoons of olive oil

1 clove of garlic

Finely slice the tomatoes and place in a serving bowl. In a coffee mill, blend the basil with the garlic, salt and oil to create a dressing. Pour the dressing over the tomatoes and serve. This dish benefits from an hour or so for the flavours to combine.

Champiñónes au natural

You need a day or two to make this really really tasty, but it's worth it. You can store any left-over mushrooms in a jar in the fridge, and as long as they're completely covered in olive oil, they won't go off. Serves 4 as a side dish.

4 cups of button mushrooms

2 cups of raw olive oil

Juice of 4 lemons

A pinch of sea salt (optional)

4 cloves of garlic

½ cup of fresh flat leaf parsley

Wash, then finely slice the mushrooms. Place in a flat bottomed bowl.

Finely dice or crush the garlic. Finely chop the parsley.

Add all the remaining ingredients to the bowl and mix thoroughly, so that the liquid coats all sides of all the slices of mushrooms. Marinade for at least a day, stirring occasionally.

Serve with **Tabouleh**, **Dolmades** or your favourite salad.

Seeded noodles

2 cups of butternut squash

1 cup of marrow

1 teaspoon of celery seed

1 teaspoon of poppy seeds

1 tablespoon of tahini

Juice of 2 limes

Spiral slice the vegetables on the spaghetti setting to make the noodles. Mix the tahini in with lime juice until watery. Add the seeds and pour over the noodles.

"Fried" mushrooms

These mushrooms really help bring a meal alive, fill those strange gaps that you might get when detoxing, and they taste perfect! Serves 4.

4 portabello mushrooms, sliced

2 tablespoons of olive oil

1 lemon, juiced

1 teaspoon of sea salt

½ cup of water

Mix all the wet ingredients with the salt. Put the mushrooms in a glass dish and pour over the liquid. Make sure all the mushrooms are covered by the liquid. Dehydrate for 2-6 hours, mixing once to ensure all mushrooms are still coated with liquid.

You can even use the water that comes out of the mushrooms to make a quick gravy! Add the mushroom water to some carrot juice, and pour!

Lemon courgettes

This is a lovely bright side dish, which goes really well with any almond- or broccoli-based meal.

4 courgettes

2 lemons

4 sticks of celery

1 cup of flat leaf parsley, chopped

4 tablespoons of olive oil

1 clove of garlic, finely chopped

Top and tail the courgette, then slice thinly using either a mandoline or a vegetable peeler. The slices should be about 1mm thin or less. Juice the lemons and celery, and add them to a bowl with the olive oil, garlic and parsley. Scrape a few fine bits of peel from the lemon skin and also add these. Add the courgettes and mix very well, so that all the courgette surfaces are covered in the marinade. Let them marinade for 1-3 days, and stir occasionally. Once the courgettes have become slightly transparent, they are ready to eat. If you don't want to eat them immediately, transfer them to a jar with enough olive oil to cover them completely, and they will keep for a long while.

Carrot nests

This is a colourful and surprisingly tasty side dish which goes well with just about everything. Serves 4 as a side dish.

6 carrots

1 serving of **It's not really mayonnaise**

Julienne the carrots. Place equal amounts around the edges of side plates, with a hole in the middle. Fill the hole with **It's not really mayonnaise**, and serve with a touch of extra paprika on top.

Cucumber crunch

1 cucumber

4 sprigs of fresh mint

½ teaspoon of dill seeds

2 dessertspoons of **macadamia cream**

½ white onion

Finely dice the cucumber and onion. Finely chop the mint. Mix all ingredients together and serve.

Carrot crunching

Carrots have more carotene in them than any other fruit or vegetable.

Today, the most common colour for carrots is orange. However, you can still see white, yellow, red and purple ones in countries all over the world.

Coleslaw

Serves 2.

1 serving of **It's not really mayonnaise**

2 carrots

1 white onion

1 cup of white cabbage

Using the mandoline, finely shred the vegetables, then mix them into the dressing.

Japanese okra

Serves 4 as a side dish.

20 okra (ladies fingers)
1 cup of Atlantic sea salad (flakes of seaweed)
Salt to taste
1 cup of pecans

Chop the okra very finely. Mix with the sea salad and put into little dishes. Grind the salt and pecans in a coffee grinder. Add enough water to blend into a slightly runny dressing and serve this as a side dip.

Joe's chip shop chips

This is a real indulgence — so naughty, yet not! My friend Joe made these up, and I'm very grateful to him for allowing it to be shared! Serves 2 as a side dish.

2 ripe, firm avocados
A bag of poppy seeds

Slice the avocados in half and carefully remove the stone without damaging the avocado. Cut them into quarters, then eighths. Gently peel the skin off and discard. Place the poppy seeds in a flat-bottomed dish, and roll the avocados in the seeds until they're fully covered. Place on a serving plate, and put the remaining poppy seeds back in the bag for future use.

Shazzie's chip shop chips

This is my variation on the above. Serves 2 as a side dish.

2 ripe, firm avocados
A handful of Atlantic sea flakes

In a coffee mill, mill the sea flakes until very fine, then put them in a flat-bottomed bowl. Slice the avocados in half and carefully remove the stone without damaging the avocado. Cut them into quarters, then eighths. Gently peel the skin off and discard. Roll the avocados in the sea flakes until they're fully covered. Place on a serving plate, and put the remaining sea flakes in a jar for future use.

Your new dairy

Almond, hazel, hemp or sunflower milk

Always make enough milk for two days and keep it in the fridge. Drink it any time, add it to some of the recipes when it's called for, or add some to a blender with a piece of fruit for a quick and filling drink.

1 pint of water

2 cups of raw almonds, hazels, hemp or sunflower seeds, or a blend of two or all three of them, soaked for at least 6 hours

2 medjool dates, or 4 other dates, stoned

> ### Hazels
>
> A manuscript found in China from 2838 BC says that the hazelnut took its place among the five sacred nourishments that God had bestowed on humans.
>
> Mashed hazels and figs have been used on the bite of a scorpion to take the pain away.

Add half of the water to your blender, then add the other ingredients. Blend for as long as possible, to break down the solid ingredients. Pour through a strainer into a bowl. Add the solid bits back into the blender with the rest of the water and repeat the process. Store the liquid in the fridge, and use within two days. Don't worry if it separates, just shake it before use. Use the pulp in a nut burger mix (you can even freeze it if you don't want to use it immediately).

Quickest tahini milk

This is a great one for children, and can fill any hungry hole. It's very useful if you need a nut milk and haven't got any soaked nuts to make it with.

1 pint of water

½ cup of raw tahini

4 normal or 2 medjool dates, stoned

Blend all ingredients and serve. You can pop raw carob, banana, strawberries or raspberries in the blender, for a protein-rich tasty milk shake.

Macadamia cream

Add this to soups, dressings or smoothies as and when desired. It's also good served on top of your midday fruit. Make enough for two days and stir if needed before use.

10 macadamia nuts

1 orange

2 medjool or 4 other dates, stoned

Juice the orange. Add all ingredients to a coffee mill and blend until totally smooth. This might take several goes depending on the power of your mill. To make a savoury version, add coconut water or celery juice instead of orange juice.

Macadamias

The fat in these lovely white nuts is about 80% monounsaturated.

Monounsaturated fats can assist in lowering blood cholesterol levels and so reduce the risk of heart disease.

You'll also get lots of amino acids, calcium and potassium from your macadamias!

Vanilla créme

This goes well with all puddings, and is a real treat on top of the ice cream recipes!

2 oranges, juiced

1 cup of macadamia nuts

2 inches of fresh vanilla pod

Squeeze of lime

Put everything into a coffee mill grinder. If you're making a larger amount, a powerful blender such as the Vita-Mix will work. If you want it thicker: add more nuts. If you want it thinner: add more orange juice. It will keep for a couple of days in the fridge if you don't eat it all!

Savoury variation

To make a créme which goes well with savoury dishes, use a bit more lemon or lime and a bit less orange. Omit or halve the amount of vanilla.

Tropical variation

If you have a young coconut to hand, put the flesh and/or water in there, too! It gives it a completely new dimension.

Cheddary cheeze spread

Where the cheddary taste comes from is a real mystery, but you will love the versatility of this cheeze.

3 cups of pine nuts, soaked for 2 hours

4 sundried tomatoes, soaked for 2 hours

½ small orange or yellow pepper, de-seeded and destalked

1 lemon, juiced

1 clove of garlic

Chop the garlic, and blend all ingredients with a hand blender until really smooth. Serve with anything you like or make...

Cheddary cheeze squares

Using the spread above, spread it about 7mm thick onto dehydrator sheets and dehydrate for 6-24 hours, until it's peelable. Once it's peelable, cut them into squares, peel them off and turn them over. Dehydrate for another 2-4 hours, then serve with burgers, on crackers, or with your favourite meal.

It's not really mayonnaise

This has a lovely tangy feel, just like the real thing, but without the risk of salmonella and without chickens being used and abused!

2 cups of macadamia nuts

½ cucumber

5 stalks of celery

1 lemon, juiced

1 teaspoon of paprika

½ cup of olive oil

Juice the cucumber and celery, and add all the ingredients to a blender. If you're using a Vita-Mix, you can just blend until it becomes mayonnaise. If you're using a normal blender, once the nuts are broken down, transfer the mixture to a blending bowl and finish off using a hand blender for a smoother mayonnaise.

Dips, spreads, dressings, sauces and pâtés

As well as these recipes, remember good old olive oil and lemon, or avocado blended with juice, make simple dressings. Simple dressings made with oil and juice, with herbs and spices added, provide you with more variety than you can imagine.

These recipes go very well with the side dishes or salads. How about spreading some of them on marrow rounds, halved tomatoes or dehydrated crisps?

A favourite for everyone is making crudités, with these recipes. Select from: red, orange or yellow pepper, okra, asparagus, carrot, courgette, cucumber, tomatoes, celery, lettuce, radish, turnip, broccoli and cauliflower and chop into "finger food".

High vibe dressing

4 tablespoons of pumpkin seeds, dry

1 cup of water or celery juice

4 sprigs of mint, finely chopped

Grind the pumpkin seeds to a fine powder in a coffee mill. Add half the amount of water or juice and blend until smooth. Add more water to create the thickness you require (if the coffee mill is too small, you may have to transfer it to a blender, or mix in the rest of the ingredients by hand). Add the mint. If you like, you can add minced garlic, onion or other strong herbs and spices to the mixture. As time goes on, you'll want these less and less, but they're great to begin with.

Plum sauce

The plums must be sweet and ripe for this to work. It's a lovely surprise addition to Herby stir fry.

6 plums, stoned and peeled

2 medjool dates, stoned

2-4 pieces of dried papaya, soaked at least 8 hours

2 cardamom pods

Take the seeds from the cardamom pods, and discard the pods. Blend all the ingredients.

Pico de gallo

2 tomatoes

1 red pepper, de-seeded

1 red onion, peeled

1 lime

1 clove of garlic

2 stalks of celery

Skin the tomatoes and remove the seeds. Cut the remaining flesh into 1cm chunks. Place the tomatoes onto several sheets of kitchen paper, and wrap them up tightly or place a weight on top of them. Chop the onion and pepper into 1cm chunks, too.

Squeeze the last bits of juice out of the tomatoes, and add all three chopped ingredients into a bowl. Squeeze the juice of the lime into the bowl. Finely chop the garlic and celery and add to the bowl. If you want to add salt to this dish, taste it, and then decide. Mix all the ingredients together, cover and leave for a few hours to marinade before serving.

Mango chutney

Serve with onion bhajis and cauliflower florettes for a total taste sensation.

1 large mango, peeled and stoned

4 sundried tomatoes, soaked at least 2 hours

2 cardamom pods

1 teaspoon of garam marsala

A pinch of cayenne pepper

½ inch of fresh ginger

10-20 stalks of fresh coriander

Cut open the cardamom pods and scrape the seeds into a jug. Discard the pods. Finely chop the ginger, and add this to the jug. Add all other ingredients to the jug, and blend with your hand blender until smooth. If you like, you can reserve some mango, cut it into small pieces and stir it in after blending.

Guacamole

This set of guacamole recipes is taken from Detox Delights. Guacamole is the most beautiful of all processed foods and it's got so many variations I can only put a few here. Experimenting with food is such fun that you just have to do it! Oh, now I will have to get all soppy and say "Thank you, avocados, for existing and wanting me to eat you". There.

In advance

If you're making guacamole a few hours in advance, add the juice of a lemon to the ingredients before blending and place the avocado stones in the middle of the guacamole. Some say the added stones will keep it fresher, others say it's an old wives' tale.

Basic

2 avocados, peeled and stoned

1 or ½ medium red chilli, de-seeded

1 clove of garlic

2 tomatoes

Chop the garlic and chilli, then put all ingredients in a food processor and blend until smooth, but still with little bits in it. For a chunkier guacamole, don't process one of the avocados — instead, dice it and mix it in afterwards.

Fruity — Adding the juice of an orange to the ingredients before blending gives it a lovely sweet mellow taste.

Sweetie — Adding a banana to the ingredients before blending gives it a sweet and still substantial taste.

Manly — Leave out the tomatoes and add a cup of watercress or spinach. This is soooo good!

Herbie — Adding coriander, mint or basil to the ingredients before blending gives it a summery and hearty flavour.

Bertie Bassett — Mix any of the above for a different guacamole each time. Don't let this selection limit you: try adding herbs and spices or other non-sweet and sweet fruit.

Carrot and tomato spread

Spread this on romaine lettuce, top with some chopped spring onion, fold and enjoy!

2 carrots

½ avocado

1 tomato

Finely chop the carrots, and then process them in a coffee mill if you have one, or with a hand blender. The coffee mill will give the best results for this recipe. Chop the tomato, and process until everything is mixed. Chop the avocado and add that until everything is mixed. You may need to take the mill off the processor and shake it from time to time. This is a lovely light dip, but very satisfying.

Creamy herb dip

Everyone loves this wholesome flavour, which complements any spicy recipe perfectly.

1 lemon, juiced

1 dessertspoon of olive oil

2 stalks of celery

3 cloves of garlic

½ cup of fresh parsley, tightly packed

1 dessertspoon of dried dill

½ teaspoon of oregano

1 cup of cashew nuts, soaked

Juice the celery, and discard the pulp. Process all ingredients in a food processor, then transfer to a jug and blend to a creamy dip using a hand blender. If you have a Vita-Mix, you can do the above two steps together. If it's too thick: add more celery juice. If it's too thin: add more cashews.

Sunflower pâté

2 cups of sunflower seeds, soaked at least 8 hours

8 sundried tomatoes, soaked at least 8 hours

1 teaspoon of dulse, powdered

1 clove of garlic (optional)

Using a hand blender, liquidise all ingredients until the consistency of pâté. Place in a mould or on a plate. Slice or spoon your servings. Serve with **Cucumber salad**.

Tomato sauce

Perfect for Walnut burgers and Joe's chip shop chips.

6 sundried tomatoes, soaked at least 2 hours

2 cups of fresh tomatoes

10 basil leaves

4 medjool dates, soaked at least 2 hours

A pinch of paprika

1 red pepper, de-seeded and destalked

Using a hand blender, blend all ingredients until smooth. It will keep for two days in the fridge if you cover it.

Mushroom gravy

2 cups of portabello mushrooms

1 lemon, juiced

1 small onion

6 stalks of celery

1 clove of garlic

½ teaspoon of paprika

Finely chop the mushrooms, garlic and onions. Juice the celery stalks, add it all to a dish with the juice of the lemon and the paprika. Allow to marinade for 1-8 hours. Add all the ingredients to a blender and blend.

Spinach pesto

This goes perfectly with reams of Courgetti or other spiralised squashes.

1 cup of fresh basil, tightly packed

½ cup of fresh parsley, tightly packed

1 cup of chopped spinach, tightly packed

1 clove of garlic

½ teaspoon of salt

1 cup of pine nuts, not soaked

1 cup of **Mushroom gravy**

Blend all ingredients with a hand blender or food processor.

<table>
<tr><td>

Apricots

The Chinese cultivated the wild ancestor of the apricot. They believed that it had fertility enhancing properties. This fruit certainly is very sensual, with its velvety skin and delicate fragrance!

</td></tr>
</table>

Sweet apricot sauce

10 dried apricots, soaked overnight

½ teaspoon of aniseed

½ teaspoon of fennel seeds

Blend all the ingredients, and serve with **Crispy spring rolls**.

Carrot and coriander dip

2 large carrots

½ avocado, peeled and stoned

A bunch of coriander

½ mild onion, peeled

1 clove of garlic, peeled

1 lime

Dice the onion and finely chop the coriander, and set aside in a bowl with the juice of half the lime. Dice the carrots and avocado, chop the garlic and blend these three ingredients using a hand blender. The hand blender is the hardest work, but gives the best results regarding texture. Once smooth, pour into the onion and coriander bowl, and mix thoroughly. Serve with crudités of your choice and the other lime half on the side.

Very special main meals

Herby stir fry

OK, you don't actually fry this stir fry, because as you know, that'd just be too toxic for your beautiful body — but this really does come out like a stir fry. Well worth the effort. Serves 4.

1 cup of alfalfa sprouts

1 cup of broccoli

1 carrot

1 cup of cauliflower

1 bunch of chives

1 tablespoon of coconut meat

1 bunch of coriander

1 bunch of parsley

1 cup of parsnip

4 peaches, stoned and peeled

1 tablespoon of olive oil

4 spring onions

10 sundried tomatoes

2 cups of quinoa*

Broccoli

Broccoli has massive amounts of vitamin C.

It contains around 30 cancer-fighting nutrients. Broccoli sprouts are even higher in these chemicals. You can buy broccoli seeds from wholefood stores and sprout your own!

In a food processor, kibble (process until in small rice-sized pieces) the carrot, coconut meat and parsnip, and mix with the sprouted wild rice. Cut the broccoli and cauliflower into little florets, thinly slice the spring onions and mix with the alfalfa sprouts. Sliver the sundried tomatoes. Finely chop the herbs and add these to the vegetables, along with the olive oil. Mash the peaches and add all ingredients together. Serve with **Plum sauce**.

*To sprout the quinoa, soak it overnight in water. Drain and rinse it three to four times during the day and marvel at the little tails appearing! It's now ready to eat.

Double stuffed tomatoes

This filling meal is like baked tomatoes but with life force oozing out of every juicy tomato pore. Remember to soak the seeds and sundried tomatoes the day before you want to eat this dish. Serves 4 when accompanied with a side dish.

> **Basil**
>
> In addition to being used in recipes, people also use basil for toiletries and herbal remedies.
>
> Mexicans use it to stop their lovers looking at others!

4 beef (or other large) tomatoes

3 cups of sunflower seeds, soaked at least 6 hours

1 cup of sundried tomatoes, soaked at least 6 hours

½ cup of basil

½ teaspoon of paprika

5 black olives, stoned

1 clove of garlic

Cut the tops of the tomatoes off, leaving the stalk on the top of the tomato, and put them to one side. Scoop out the seeds and the middle flesh of the tomatoes. Use the discarded tomato middles in another recipe such as gazpacho soup.

Fincly chop the basil, garlic and olives, but keep some basil leaves whole for garnish. Roughly chop the sundried tomatoes. Using a hand blender, blend the sunflower seeds with the sundried tomatoes and paprika until smooth and creamy. Mix the basil, garlic and olives into this.

Stuff the tomatoes with the mixture, until they are overflowing. Top with some extra basil leaves, and place the lids of the tomatoes back on top. Serve with your favourite salad.

Variation

For a party, you can use the same filling, but stuff tiny cherry tomatoes instead. This is great finger food for monkeys in shirts!

Walnut burgers

These are well worth making as they taste great, and provide a link to the type of food you might have left behind so you don't miss it as much. Makes about 8 burgers.

6 cups of walnuts, soaked for 2 hours

2 cups of carrots, topped and tailed

1 cup of fresh herbs, such as parsley, basil and coriander, tightly packed

1½ cups of red onion

2 cups of portabello mushrooms

½ red pepper, de-seeded and destalked

6 sundried tomatoes, soaked for 2-6 hours

2 cloves of garlic

1 dessertspoon of paprika

1 teaspoon of dried pizza herbs

1 teaspoon of dried parsley

Walnuts

Walnuts are the most popular nuts in the USA. California produces 70% of the world's walnuts. They originated in ancient Persia and were traded along the Med by English merchant ships.

In the Autumn, try wet walnuts from your local grocer's. They are freshly picked and so juicy!

Set aside the fresh herbs, the pepper and half the onions. Finely chop the sundried tomatoes. Blend all other ingredients in a food processor. Transfer to a large bowl and continue blending with a hand blender until you achieve a smooth consistency.

Very finely chop the remaining ingredients by hand (you do this for the texture), and mix into the burger mix. Divide into eight or ten equal portions, form into burger shapes and dehydrate for 8-24 hours.

Here's a serving suggestion: Put 1 burger in a big romaine leaf, add your choice of **Tomato sauce**, thinly sliced onion rings, **"Fried" mushrooms**, **Mango chutney**, **Sweetcorn salsa** and mustard cress. Serve with **Joe's chip shop chips** and a smile on your face.

Super asparagus wraps

Serves 2.

Amazing asparagus
Ancient Egyptians offered asparagus to their gods. It belongs to the lily family and so is related to garlic and onions.
It was used by ancient Greeks and Romans to relieve toothache and prevent bee stings.
It is thought to be an aphrodisiac.

2 large soft cabbage leaves

1 avocado

1 teaspoon of superfood

2 spring onions

1 small hot chilli

A squeeze of lemon juice

6 stalks of young asparagus

½ cup of pumpkin seeds

2 sticks of celery

1 tomato

Finely chop the chilli. In a bowl, mash the avocado with the superfood and chilli. Cut the tips off the asparagus. Diagonally and thinly slice the celery, asparagus stalks and spring onions, and mix into the avocado. Squeeze some lemon juice into the mixture, and add the pumpkin seeds. Finely dice the tomato. Curl the cabbage leaves up into cones, so there's a big wide mouth at one end and the other end is closed. Lay the cones on a plate. Add half of the tomatoes to each one, then add half of the green mixture to each one. Then place the asparagus tips inside, so they stick out making it look pretty. Garnish with pumpkin seeds and lemon if you want.

This is a big tasty meal, and involves some lovely chewing. If you can't finish it, save some for later.

Easy sushi

Make sushi the easy way, by cutting out the need to use a rolling mat. Of course, if you want to make it the conventional way, you can still use these recipe ideas!

I haven't listed amounts at all as it really doesn't matter, and it also depends on how many wraps you make.

As well as using as a main course, the versatility of easy sushi makes it great for parties, starters, nibbles, packed lunches and side dishes. Serve with thin slices of ginger, wasabi sauce, and your favourite side dishes.

How to make Easy sushi

Take all suggested ingredients of one of the recipes below, or invent your own. Take several sheets of black nori, and fold them in half. Cut them with scissors along the half line. Cut them again so they're in strips of quarters, then cut them in the opposite direction in half. You should end up with 8 little strips per sheet. Have a glass of water handy.

Pick up one nori strip, and put about a teaspoon of the soft filling along half of the strip. Then add small slices of your other ingredients so they sit in the middle of your soft filling. Arrange them so they poke out of one end, but not the other, as you need a flat base to stand them up on. Then gently hold the fillings in place with one finger, and curl up the sheet. Roll the end with no filling over the filling end and it should all come together and overlap a little. Brush the end with a little water, and firm it down. Place it on a plate, with the newly sealed end on the bottom. Once all your sushi is made, you can turn them up on their bottoms, with all the wonderful middle ingredients sticking out the top.

If you don't feel confident doing all that, you can cheat! Just put the soft ingredient in before rolling the sushi up, and then add the other ingredients once the sushi is standing up. I call these "Sushi trees"!

So here are some suggestions, but do experiment with your own, too!

Sunflower pâté sushi
Sunflower pâté
Red pepper, de-seeded, cut into thin strips
Fresh ginger, grated

Green sushi
Manly guacamole
Sundried tomatoes, soaked and cut into thin strips
Mustard cress

Earth and fire sushi
"Fried" mushrooms, blended
Wasabi powder, mixed with water
Celery, cut into thin strips

Cheeze and onion sushi
Cheddary cheeze spread
Spring onion, cut into thin strips
Courgette, cut into thin strips

Nutter sushi
Raw almond butter
Carrot, cut into thin strips
Your favourite sprouts
Fresh coriander leaves

Super broccoli quiche
Serves 4.

1 head of broccoli florets
1 tablespoon of sunflower seeds
2 creamy avocados
1 tablespoon of superfood
1 tablespoon of seaweed flakes
1 pinch of sea salt (optional)
4 stalks of celery

Break the florets into small pieces. Mash the avocados, and mix in the seaweed flakes, superfood, broccoli and sea salt. Sprinkle sunflower seeds on top. Chop the celery up very small and place it on the same plate in the centre of the mixture. You can use this mixture as a filling in a simple pecan nut and date base if you like. Otherwise, serve in individual ramekin dishes with a light salad.

Courgetti and rawgu

This is from Detox Delights. This quick and easy meal gets the thumbs up from everyone who tries it. A spiral slicer (Saladacco) is the best tool to make the pasta successfully but if you don't have one, you can use a normal vegetable peeler.

2 courgettes

5 black olives, stoned (optional)

2 plum tomatoes

10 sundried tomatoes, soaked

1 apple, cored

1 clove of garlic

½ a lemon, juiced

2 dates, stoned

A pinch of sea salt or 1 teaspoon of seaweed flakes

6 dessertspoons of olive oil

A handful of basil

A few sprigs of oregano

Make the spaghetti by placing the courgettes on the spiral slicer (switched to pasta setting), or peel them with a vegetable peeler to get ribbons. Put them on a few layers of kitchen paper to absorb the excess moisture. It's best if you can do this for a couple of hours, but not essential.

Chop the garlic and dates. Put all the remaining ingredients (except the olives, herbs and 2 dessertspoons olive oil) into the food processor. Combine until it changes to an orangey-red colour. Add the herbs and combine for a few seconds more (you want to keep the flecks of the herbs so don't pulverise it at this point). Taste it for salt (or seaweed) and check the texture for olive oil and add more if desired.

Finely chop the olives and add them to the pasta with the remaining olive oil and an optional pinch of salt or seaweed. Place the pasta in bowls. Put the sauce on top of the pasta, and add a couple of whole olives for decoration.

For a treat, place it all in a dehydrator for about an hour before serving to allow it to warm through. Add a few basil leaves, a tiny pinch of salt and a drizzle of olive oil before serving. Whole pine nuts mixed into the sauce or pasta make a good addition.

Butternut noodles with golden curry sauce

Serves 2 as a main dish, 4 as a side dish.

1 small butternut squash, peeled

1 small handful of coriander

1 tablespoon of Madras curry powder (Or to taste. If unsure, add a small amount and taste, keep adding and blending until you have a flavour you like.)

1 large or 2 medium avocados, skinned and stoned

1 stalk of celery

2 dried apricots, soaked at least 2 hours

¼ cup of sultanas, soaked at least 2 hours

½ papaya, skinned and de-seeded

½ mango, skinned and stoned

4 baby carrots

10 baby sweetcorns

1 yellow pepper, de-seeded and topped

1 large tomato

½ lime, juiced

Set your spiral slicer onto the pasta setting and process all of the squash. You will have to do it in pieces, and cut out the seeds.

Dice the celery, papaya, mango, corn, tomato, pepper and carrots. Mix these ingredients and add half of the mixture to a blender.

Add the avocado, curry powder, sultanas, lime juice and apricots to the blender. Keep six sultanas for decoration. Blend the curry sauce until fine.

Finely chop most of the coriander and add this to the sauce.

Place the noodles on a big serving dish, pour the mixed vegetables on top, and pour the sauce on top of that. Flatten the top a little and place the six sultanas there, to make a five-petalled flower with a centre. Use the reserved coriander to make the stem.

Vegetable paella

You are about to discover how to make this yummy Mediterranean dish without cooking the life out of the food! Serves 4.

4 tablespoons of olive oil

2 lemons

4 stalks of celery

2 white onions

5 cloves of garlic

1 red pepper

1 yellow pepper

4 ripe tomatoes

4 sundried tomatoes, soaked at least 2 hours

2 cups of quinoa

1 cup of young tender asparagus

½ cup of black olives, stoned

1 teaspoon of saffron threads or half a teaspoon saffron powder

1 teaspoon of paprika

Julienne the pepper, chop the asparagus into bite-sized pieces and cut the onions into very fine rings. Crush the garlic and put these ingredients in a wide bowl. Juice the celery and the lemons, and mix with the olive oil, then pour onto the chopped vegetables. Marinade this for 1-3 days, until the vegetables become soft and juicy.

Meanwhile, sprout the quinoa as in the recipe **Herby stir fry**. After the final rinse of the quinoa, begin to add the flavours. Finely chop the fresh tomatoes along with the sundried tomatoes. Add the saffron threads and paprika to the tomatoes. Finely chop the black olives and add these to the tomatoes. Rinse the quinoa well, and put into an attractive serving dish. Pour the tomato mixture over the rice. Add the newly marinaded vegetables, and stir the whole dish well. Pour on a couple of tablespoons of the marinade, and leave the dish to stand in a non-refrigerated place for a further 12-24 hours before serving.

Serve with a generous helping of fresh chopped herbs and flowers scattered over the top.

Wild mushroom fajitas

This is a healthy and tasty variation on the Mexican favourite. For an entertaining meal, serve with guacamole, salsas and a big green salad with lots of fresh sweetcorn in it. This serves 2-4, depending on what appetite you have, and what else you eat with it!

1 yellow or orange pepper, cut into thin slices

2 cups of portabello and/or shiitake mushrooms

1 white onion, chopped

4-6 savoy cabbage leaves

1 teaspoon of cumin powder

1 teaspoon of cayenne pepper

2 tablespoons of olive oil

1 lemon

2 cloves of garlic

A handful of chives and chive flowers if you can get them

A handful of spinach

Salsa, such as **Sweetcorn salsa**

It's not really mayonnaise

Super spinach

Spinach belongs to the goosefoot family, with Swiss chard and beetroot.

It is a good source of vitamin C and beta carotene. It's high in iron.

1931 saw the start of the Popeye comic strip in the USA. Spinach consumption went up by 33%!

Julienne the pepper, finely chop the onion and the garlic, and chop the mushrooms.

Juice the lemon and mix with the olive oil. Add the chopped vegetables and the cumin and cayenne powders. Dehydrate this mixture, on dehydrator sheets or in a bowl, for four to six hours.

Once dehydrated, you can serve the fajitas: roll up the spinach leaves and finely chop them, so they end up as very thin strands.

Arrange your cabbage leaves on a big plate, and cut out any hard stems. Place equal amounts of the mushroom mixture on each, top with the spinach, and then add **Sweetcorn salsa** and **It's not really mayonnaise**. Finely chop the chives and sprinkle them on, and add flowers for decoration just before serving.

Walnut stuffed peppers

This pâté is lovely inside a juicy red pepper, but remember that you can do all sorts with it, such as spreading on vegetable rounds, using as a dip with crudités, or using as a nori stuffing. Serves 4.

8 red peppers

4 cups of walnuts, shelled

4 sundried tomatoes, soaked

2 small red onions

2 courgettes

Perky peppers

Peppers can be green, red, yellow, orange, white, chocolate and purple. Green peppers aren't ripe and so may cause indigestion.

De-seed, stalk and chop four of the peppers, and put them in a food processor. Add the walnuts and sundried tomatoes and process. Process the mixture until it's a pâté-like texture. If you have a hand blender, transfer the mixture to a bowl and finish it off with the hand blender to get a smoother finish. If you have a Champion juicer, use that with its blank blade for the above stages.

Finely chop the onion and mix this into the pâté, but don't blend it. Transfer equal amounts of pâté into each pepper. Replace the lids, and place each on a serving plate. Spiral slice the courgette and put equal amounts around the peppers. Finish off by adding some extra-finely sliced sundried tomatoes, a few fresh coriander leaves, some walnuts and a drizzle of olive oil to the courgette.

Variation

You can put the stuffed peppers into a dehydrator for around six hours which will slightly soften the pepper. Add the courgette after dehydrating.

"Roast tofu" with satay sauce

4 portabello mushrooms

2 tablespoons of olive oil

1 lemon, juiced

A pinch of sea salt

3 cloves of garlic

2 stalks of celery

4 dates, soaked

1 cup of raw peanuts

2 tablespoons of almond butter

½ teaspoon of cayenne pepper

Water

¼ cup of coconut meat

Tofu-mushrooms

The bland spongy texture of portabello mushrooms makes it an excellent substitute for tofu. I recommend that you don't eat tofu because it's a highly processed food.

The soya bean isn't nice in its natural state, and so makes it a questionable food for humans.

Skin, de-stalk and remove the gills from the mushrooms. Cut the mushrooms into 1-inch cubes to make the "tofu". Mince the garlic, juice the celery stalks, then add those to a bowl along with the lemon juice, olive oil and salt. Put the mushroom cubes into the bowl and mix around, so all sides are thoroughly coated. Allow them to soak some of the mixture for 10-20 minutes, then put them in your dehydrator. Keep the rest of the marinade for the sauce. Dehydrate for 4-6 hours.

To make the satay sauce, put the peanuts, almond butter, cayenne pepper, coconut, dates and the left-over marinade into a coffee mill and grind until sauce-like. If you need more liquid, add a little water at a time.

To serve, place the "tofu" cubes onto skewers and cover them with the sauce.

Special additions

These additions to your meals can add a whole new dimension to your new way of eating. If you sometimes miss stuff with a crunch, then this is the section for you. All dehydrated products will store for a while in sealed containers. Experiment and note the optimal storage times for when you create your next batch.

Corn tortillas

These are great to use with soups and salads. They're also a lovely snack on their own if you are really peckish.

4 cobs of sweetcorn

1 clove of garlic

1 red onion

1 bunch of coriander

1 tablespoon of flaxseed

In a spice mill, mill the flax until it becomes very fine. Crush the garlic and strip the corn. Put all the ingredients in the food processor and mix until everything is broken down. Blend more, until it becomes a dough. If it doesn't become a dough, and remains crumbly, add a tomato or two. Spread the mixture onto dehydrating trays, and flatten until about 8mm thick (they will get much flatter as they dry). Dehydrate on dehydrator sheets for four hours, then score the tortillas where you want to snap them. I like to score them into triangles. Turn them over at least once during dehydrating, and remove the dehydrator sheets. Dehydrate until crisp.

Curly crisps

Using your spiral slicer on the curly setting, slice sweet potatoes, courgettes, pumpkin, carrot, and any other usable vegetable. Lay the curls out on a dehydrator tray and dehydrate until crisp.

You can add salt or ground seaweed flakes if you like. They go really well with all dips and look beautiful on top of soups.

Variation

After slicing, marinade the vegetables overnight in a herby dressing, and then dehydrate.

Mesquite melts

This is a variation on the recipe above.

2 sweet potatoes

1 lemon, juiced

2 tablespoons of olive oil

1 teaspoon of sea salt

1 tablespoon of mesquite powder

Finely cut the sweet potatoes into crisps, a mandoline is great for this. Wash the potatoes, then put them in a wide-bottomed bowl. Add the lemon juice, the olive oil and the sea salt. Marinade for 1-2 hours, then drain the liquid from the potatoes. Add the mesquite powder to the potatoes, and mix well to make sure it's evenly spread. Place the potatoes on dehydrator trays, making sure they aren't overlapping each other. Dehydrate until crisp, turning them over once.

Savoury crisps

These are so easy to make using a dehydrator. Thinly slice vegetables such as aubergine, beetroot, carrot, tomato, turnip, swede, marrow, sweet potato and courgette, then dehydrate for a while until crisp. You can add salt or ground seaweed flakes if you like. They go really well with all dips and look beautiful on top of soups.

Variation

After slicing, marinade the vegetables overnight in a herby dressing, and then dehydrate.

Sweet crisps

As above, but with slices of apples, pineapple, pear, banana etc. Try squeezing lemon juice onto some of them before dehydrating, as you'll get a different flavour.

Flax and corn crackers

These are from Detox Delights. They are so easy to make and are a good bread substitute when first lightening your diet. These recipes can be varied so much, that I've just written a basic one and then offered a few of the many alternative ingredients.

Crackers go well with all salads, soups, cheeses — in fact most savoury recipes. They're excellent for buffets and doubting relatives alike.

2 cobs of sweetcorn

1 clove of garlic

2 cups of flax seeds

2 dessertspoons of sesame oil

Crush the garlic and strip the corn. Put the flax seeds in the mill and blend until they're broken. Put all ingredients in the food processor and blend until the mixture is fluffy. Spoon out the mixture onto dehydrating trays, and flatten until about 1cm thick (they will get much flatter as they dry). Dehydrate until crisp.

Variations

Add ingredients such as chopped herbs (chives are really good), sea salt, chopped tomatoes, peppers, chilli, onion, mushroom or mustard powder to the mixture. Try putting the mixture into different bowls and adding different flavours to each one. To identify them decorate the tops. For example, on the tomato one add a slice of tomato on the top, on the chive one add a halved chive flower bud.

Puddings and desserts

These puddings can be eaten any time of the day so don't restrict them to after a meal. They are fantastic whole meals in themselves. How exciting is detoxing? You can eat puddings galore and get healthier than ever!

Semolina pudding with figgy jam

2 bananas, peeled

1 sweet apple, peeled and cored

1 stalk of celery

4 dried figs, soaked or fresh figs, peeled

1 heaped tablespoon of raisins, soaked

1 cup of water

With a hand blender, blend the figs with the raisins to make your jam, and set aside. Chop the celery finely and put it into a blender along with the apple, bananas and water. Blend until everything is smooth. This is your semolina! Pour the semolina out into a bowl, and pour the jam in the middle. Twirl the jam so it looks beautiful!

Mousse de naranja

This is a lovely summer treat, and as it's very light you can eat lots of it! Fresh oranges from Spain are a delight most of the year round. Just eating them as they come is a thrill, but making a special pudding like this is something else... Serves 4.

4 oranges, juiced

3 cups of dried apricots, soaked at least 4 hours

A pinch of ground cinnamon

A pinch of ground cloves

Some lavender flowers or other delicate flowers of your choice

Drain and squeeze any excess moisture from the apricots. In a food processor, combine them with the orange juice and spices. If it's too watery, add some dried apricots and process again. It should end up like a very thick dollopy consistency.

Spoon the mixture into individual serving dishes and top with a sprinkling of flowers. Place in the fridge to set for about 2-4 hours or overnight.

Serve with a helping of **Vanilla créme**.

Mangoes marinaded in golden ginger syrup with lychee ice cream

This tasty pudding is so heavenly! Serves 4.

2 mangoes, stoned and peeled

6 medjool dates, soaked for 6 hours in water with 1 dessertspoon of minced ginger

Date soaking water

4 bananas, peeled, chopped and frozen at least overnight

10 lychees, peeled and stoned

Thinly slice the mangoes, and lay them in a flat bottomed dish. With your hand blender, blend the dates with the ginger, and add some of the soak water to make a syrup consistency. Pour this over mangoes and set aside to marinade for at least an hour.

In a food processor, process the frozen bananas with a few lychees until it turns into white fluff. This may take a few minutes, so stop your processor for a while if it needs to rest. Put the mango and syrup into individual bowls, and add scoops of the ice cream to serve. Decorate with mint leaves and fresh flowers for a finishing touch.

Toffee and raspberry fool

It's very important that you use fresh dates — these are white and wet inside, with shiny dark and easy-to-remove skins. If you can't find these, use plump dried dates soaked for 24 hours. Serves 4.

2 cups of sunflower seeds, soaked for about 24 hours, rinsed periodically

15 raspberries

1 inch of vanilla bean

20 dried apricots, soaked for about 36 hours, rinsed periodically

12 fresh dates, skinned and stoned

With a hand blender, blend the drained sunflower seeds and ten of the drained apricots with eleven of the raspberries until it's a smooth cream. Set aside and rinse the blender.

Scrape the seeds out of the vanilla bean into a bowl and add the remaining apricots and ten of the dates. Blend to a smooth cream. In four lovely stemmed glasses, add a layer of the date mixture, then a layer of the raspberry mixture, and repeat until you have about six layers in the glasses and all the mixture is used up. Top each pudding with a raspberry in the centre. Cut the remaining two dates into thin strips and add them around the raspberry in a sun ray pattern. You can serve it as it is or chilled on a hot day.

Christmas balls

1 cup of raisins

2 cups of dried apricots, rehydrated for 4-24 hours

½ coconut (reserve the water)

1 cup of sunflower seeds

½ teaspoon of freshly grated ginger

1 teaspoon of dried mixed spice

Using a food processor, mix all ingredients together until they form a dough ball. If this doesn't happen, slowly pour some of the coconut water in until the ball forms.

Take the ball out of the processor and pull enough mixture off to make a ball about an inch and a half or 4cm big. Continue doing this until you have no mixture left.

Variations and decorations

You can either leave the balls as they are, and serve on a plate, or press an almond, half a pecan or a mint leaf on top. Alternatively, roll some of the balls in dried coconut, raw carob powder or ground brazil nuts. This makes for a beautifully decorative Christmas treat (any time of the year!).

Multi-purpose aloe gel

To get aloe gel out of the leaf, cut down the inside of the leaf, and scrape your thumb under it, so it comes away from the gel, then just scoop the gel off.

Use the remaining gel on the inside of the leaf as an instant skin toner! Just rub it all over your face, and any problem areas such as buttocks and thighs. Lovely!

Aloe super mousse

This pudding is so filling, nutritious, and positively yummy. Serves 4.

1 avocado, peeled and stoned

2 bananas, peeled

1 mango, peeled and stoned

1-4 inches aloe gel, depending on leaf width

1 dessertspoon of superfood

1 cup of water

Lemon peel to garnish

Place everything except the lemon peel into your blender and blend. Pour into individual bowls, garnish with lemon peel and serve.

Coconut banana split

This is a really attractive dessert, and very moreish.

4 fresh bananas

4 peeled and chopped frozen bananas

½ teaspoon of cinnamon powder

½ coconut, and some of the water

4 ripe figs, or the equivalent in weight of your favourite berries

4 medjool dates, stoned

Peel the bananas and split them down the middle. Place the split side up in individual dishes.

Peel the brown layer off the coconut, and either juice the coconut (if you have a heavy duty juicer) or process it in a food processor, then set it to one side.

Blend the dates and figs or berries together in a coffee grinder, to make a drizzly fruit sauce. If it's not "saucy" enough, add some coconut water and blend again.

Make the ice cream from the frozen bananas, as in the **Whip the mister** recipe. Once it's ice cream, add the cinnamon and beat the coconut into it. If you need to add it back to the freezer for five minutes to firm up, then do that.

Put three scoops of ice cream onto the banana splits. Drizzle over the fruit sauce, and serve to a drooling waiting audience.

Whip the mister

This is another one from Detox Delights. It's a dream come true!

If you have access to a Champion juicer, then put some whole, peeled, frozen bananas through using the blank blade and then let the fake Mr Whippy take you to heaven. It doesn't taste like bananas.

Alternatively, if you have a food processor, thinly slice a couple of bananas and freeze them at least overnight. Thaw the bananas for about five minutes and process in the food processor. You might have to do it in about three or four goes, stirring it in each time, but the mixture will soon turn white and take on a different taste. Make sure you let it mix for long enough. It still doesn't taste like bananas.

Cinnamon, carob powder, chopped nuts and soft fruit all go well with this ice cream.

Smooth coconut ice cream

When you drink a lot of young coconut water, you get a lot of jelly left over! Here's an easy way to make use of it.

Jelly of 2-4 young coconuts, depending on yield

4 frozen bananas (whole if using a Champion, chopped if using a food processor)

1 vanilla bean

Put the jelly in a blender. Scrape the seeds out of the vanilla bean, and add them to the blender. Blend these until smooth.

Put the bananas through your Champion using the blank blade, adding one banana, half the jelly, another banana, the rest of the jelly, then the rest of the bananas. If you need to, mix the ice cream up afterwards to distribute the coconut mixture.

If you don't have a Champion, add the finely chopped frozen banana to a food processor. It goes like bread crumbs, then like a paste, and then it turns white, like the ice cream you got when you were a kid. At this stage, add the jelly, and process for a tiny while longer.

You can add chopped fruit or nuts, as well as a fruit or carob sauce. If you're not eating it immediately (a tough task!), put it into individual bowls and return to the freezer.

Pink porridge

2 cups of almonds, soaked at least 6 hours

2 cups of fresh or frozen raspberries

6-8 dried apricots, soaked

½ pint of water

Discard the soak water from the almonds and apricots, and put all the ingredients in your blender. Blend until a porridge consistency. You might want to add the water slowly, in case it turns out too runny.

Raspberry and physalis dream

The pungent, musky flavour of physalis makes this a very sexy pudding. Serves 4.

Pungent physalis

These are slightly smaller than cherries and come in their own paper wrapping.

They look like miniature Chinese lanterns, and that's why they are known as Chinese lanterns! They're also known as alkekengi and winter cherry.

---

20 brazil nuts, soaked at least 4 hours

60 raspberries

30 physalis

3 medjool dates

1 inch of vanilla pod

¼ avocado

In your coffee mill, blend 15 of the brazils with the avocado, dates and vanilla pod. Add water if you need to. It should resemble a very thick cream. Set aside.

Remove the paper from 26 of the physalis. With a hand blender, blend these with the remaining brazils and 20 of the raspberries.

Using four serving glasses, put equal amounts of the fruit mixture in the bottom. Then add equal amounts of the cream. Finally, add equal amounts of whole raspberries and one physalis with the paper wings spread out.

Anytime muesli

This is a great meal for when you have "nothing in"!

Choose from: dried apricots, raisins, currants, dates, prunes, figs, sultanas, pineapple, mango, papaya, etc... chopped in to various sizes for a varied texture.

Add your choice of: grated apple, carrot, courgette (yes, really!), chopped pear, banana, or any other fresh fruit that you like.

Add your choice of: soaked raw oat groats, sprouted buckwheat etc.

Add your choice of: soaked and chopped raw almonds, macadamias, hazelnuts, pecans, walnuts, sunflower, pumpkin, linseed/flax, sesame etc.

Pour on your choice of: **Almond milk** or **Sesame milk**, orange or apple juice or water.

Kumquat and nutmeg cheezecake

This cake is a dream! I made it for my friend's birthday. The next day me and another friend independently made it again! It's soooo gooood!

3 cups of almonds, dry

2 tablespoons of raw carob powder

1 cup of pecans, dry

2 cups of dates, soaked and stoned

Juice of 1 orange

1 teaspoon of nutmeg

1 vanilla pod

5 bananas, peeled, thinly chopped and frozen at least overnight

4 kumquats

1 large mango

Using a loose-based round cake tin, cover the base in cling film, and fit to the tin. Cover the sides in silver foil.

Add the almonds, carob, pecans (reserve eight for decoration), dates, an inch of the vanilla, a sprinkling of nutmeg and the juice of the orange to a food processor. Process gently to start with, and continue until you get a dough-like consistency, but still chunky. If it's not doughy enough add small quantities of water until you achieve the desired result. Place in the cake tin, and flatten down.

Clean your food processor and add the chopped frozen banana. Halve the kumquats and remove the middles, and add the skins to the processor. Slit the vanilla pod and scrape the seeds into the processor. Slice the cheeks off the mango, and remove the skin, then add those to the food processor. Add most of the rest of the nutmeg. Add a couple of chopped dates if you like, too. Process for several minutes, until the whole mixture turns to white fluff. Don't be tempted to process this for less time, it needs to go white and fluffy. Stop for a minute if your machine needs to rest. Scrape it down every now and then so everything gets processed. Add this to the cake tin, on top of the nut base. Smooth it all down so there's no trapped air, and it's level on top. Add the left-over pecans in a nice pattern and sprinkle on the rest of the nutmeg.

Return it all to the freezer for at least an hour. Once you are ready to serve it, turn out the cake by pushing the loose base out and up. Take the foil off and place on a serving plate.

Celebrate good times cake

Base

½ coconut

1 cup of soaked hazelnuts

1 cup of soaked raisins

A pinch of mixed spice or cinnamon

Finely grind the coconut. Process the other three ingredients together, then add coconut to mix. If not wet enough, add some coconut water. If too wet, add some more nuts.

Form into a cake-type circle, about one inch thick.

Middle

½ cup of raw tahini

1 dessertspoon of raw carob power

¼ cup raisins or dates or a mix of both

Water from the above coconut

Mix the first two ingredients in a bowl with a fork. It will go very stiff. Add enough coconut water to make a glossy sloppy mixture. If you run out of coconut water, add water. Process the fruit until smooth, add the mixture and process all together. Spread on top of the cake base. If it's too stiff to spread, add more water or spread with a wet knife.

Top

1 banana

½ papaya

3 dessertspoons of raw tahini

Process all ingredients. If too runny add more tahini. Spread on top of cake. Let some dribble down if you're daring!

Garnish with thinly sliced starfruit, strawberries and flowers.

If you make this cake with love it will taste all the better for it. This well-behaved cake slices well and holds its shape while being served.

Banana bites

Little easy-to-eat treats. Serves 2.

2 bananas, pecled
12 walnut halves, dry
12 raisins, dry

Cut the ends off the bananas and cut into equal rounds of six each, so you end up with twelve pieces. Stand them up on an end, and place on a serving plate. Push one raisin down into the top of each banana round, until the top of the banana is flat. Sit a walnut half on each banana round, and serve.

Entertaining meals

Many of the dishes mentioned can be enhanced to serve as meals to guests. Put your favourite ones on beautiful plates and decorate with edible flowers or herbs. If you want a traditional four course meal then the suggestions below will work well. Swap out anything you don't like with something else that you do like. These recipes are so adaptable that I never make them the same way twice. Follow your heart when making them, and love the results because you created them.

Menu 1

Onion bhajis served with **Mango chutney** and cauliflower florettes

Walnut burgers, served with **Cheddary cheeze squares**, **Tomato sauce**, **"fried" mushrooms**, **onion rings** and romaine leaves

Kumquat and nutmeg cheezecake

Walnuts and grapes

Menu 2

Cream of pepper soup with **Curly crisps**

Vegetable Paella with **"Roast tofu"** and **satay sauce**

Mousse de naranja with **Vanilla créme**

Christmas balls

Menu 3

Japanese okra

Easy sushi. **Crispy spring rolls** with **Sweet apricot sauce**

Raspberry and physalis dream

Banana bites

Buffet ideas

Buffets are a wonderfully relaxing way to eat in company, because you can eat the amount and type of food which suits you without anyone pointing and staring. All of the recipes already mentioned work well for buffets. If you want more of a pointer, try the following — but don't just stick to this, spread your recipe wings!

To dip or spread on

Flax and corn crackers

Corn tortillas

Celery sticks

Slices of pepper, de-seeded

Savoury and sweet crisps

Cherry tomatoes

Cucumbers

Courgettes

Carrots

Romaine leaves

Spring onions

Chard leaves

Dips and spreads

Guacamole

Sunflower pâté

Carrot and tomato spread

Pico de gallo

Spinach pesto

Creamy herb dip

Sweeties

Christmas balls

Banana bites

Celebrate good times cake

Plates of

Easy sushi

Walnut stuffed peppers

Wild mushroom fajitas

"Roast tofu" with satay sauce

Double stuffed tomatoes

Tomato salad

Chakra salad with High vibe dressing

Cucumber crunch

Tabouleh pyramids

Dolmades

Shazzie's chip shop chips

Romaine roll-ups

Onion bhajis with Mango salsa

Big bowls of

Olives

Nuts and seeds

Curly crisps and Mesquite melts

Fruit, arranged decoratively or simply left whole

To drink

Warm apple punch

The candy floss tart

Red whine

The best meal in the world, ever

I really did save the best until last. If you've never tried a durian before, wait until you have detoxed before doing it. Many people are put off by the smell, but when they're detoxed they often become drawn to it. Some people, no matter how detoxed they are, can't stand durian. But that's fine — it means there's more for me!

Where to get a durian
Check out The Durian Centre in London or oriental supermarkets worldwide for these fresh and creamy lovelies. Alternatively, book an expensive but well-deserved trip to Thailand and eat durians on the beach!

Duriasm

1 young coconut

1 durian

2 people

10 cushions

Cut the top off the coconut and add two straws. Break or cut open the durian. Eat the durian, until it's all gone, without fighting over it. Sip from the coconut, together. This will give you a major chakra rush! After finishing the coconut water, enjoy your post duriasmic chill by lolling about on your cushions for an hour before resuming any adult responsibilities that you may have.

Resources

Here is a list of suppliers, services and companies which may be of interest to you. As you know, web sites can go offline or move with no warning. If this happens with any of the listed resources, use a search engine such as **www.google.com** to locate alternative ones.

Mail order

Recommended products

You can find many of the items recommended in this book such as supplements, books, videos, superfoods, juicers, ionisers and toiletries at our web site:

www.detoxyourworld.com | **sales@detoxyourworld.com**

www.detoxyourworld.com also contains links to other companies which provide related goods. It is updated regularly, so keep visiting it for inspiration.

Detox Your World, Shazzie.com and The Heart Centre are all part of Rawcreation Ltd.

Rawcreation Ltd

Millennium House
Gapton Hall Road
Great Yarmouth
Norfolk, NR31 0NL
Tel: +44 (0)8700 113 119
Fax: +44 (0)8700 114 119
sales@rawcreation.com
www.rawcreation.com

If you are based in the USA, the following company offers exceptional educational resources, electrical goods, supplements, superfoods and hard to find foods such as raw tahini, nut butters, raw carob and wheatberries for growing wheatgrass. If you buy these items in bulk, it saves re-ordering time as well as postage and transportation costs. This company operates under extremely high ethical standards and delivers worldwide. In addition to supplying mail order goods, it hosts motivating, health-related events and retreats.

Nature's First Law / Sunfood Nutrition

PO Box 900202
San Diego, CA 92190 USA
Tel: +1 (619) 596-7979
Tel orders: +1 (800) 205-2350
Fax: +1 (619) 596-7997
nature@rawfood.com
www.rawfood.com

Further support

Email support

www.rawfoodsupport.com — many of your questions and concerns can be answered by joining this forum. People from all over the world share their experiences here. Best of all, it's a free service given with love!

Web sites of interest

www.detoxyourworld.com — a great place to shop! We sell superfoods, books, videos, enema kits, supplements, magnotherapy, lots of different juicers and much more! You can also find some of the recipes from the book of the same name on there! We're based in the UK, and serve the whole world.

www.shazzie.com — my personal web site. Amongst other things, read inspiring articles, my seven year long journals and guides then take a peek at my photo album and art gallery. There are lots more raw food links here: www.shazzie.com/raw/links.

www.nakedchocolate.com — my little web site that has some great and unique raw chocolate recipes on it.

www.rawliving.co.uk — my ever present friend Kate Wood's online shop, selling superfoods, equipment and magic!

www.totalrawfood.com — my friend and The Raw Lifestyle Coach, Jess' online shop. She's the best UK raw food and detox coach, and she's a total love, too!

www.livinglifealive.com — Ruth Allen is a wholistic lifestyle counsellor. Her consultations opens doors to living, making conscious choices and drawing towards us what we need by way of support and listening.

www.karunaretreats.com — wonderful UK-based holistic detox retreats, run by my wonderfully loving friends Shoshanna and Dao.

Magazines

Funky Raw Magazine — UK based, sold worldwide, groovy and happening raw food magazine. It's a radical earth-based spiritual magazine, dedicated to restoring connection and recreating paradise on earth.

Credits

Without the reference of many books, web sites and lectures, I would still be drowning in ill-health. For this reason, I thank all contributors of this book, all information-givers, and all light-bearers from the bottom of my heart.

Thanks

Special thanks go to:

My proofreaders: Debbie Garcia, Karen Jessett, Ruth Allen, Jatinder Daniels.

My editor: David Smith.

The success stories folks: Arlyn Grant, Jatinder Daniels, Jay Banks, Michele Déradune and Tony Thorpe.

To David Wolfe again for writing the foreword to this book.

To Karen Jessett again for taking the Tibetan Rejuvenation Rites photos.

And to you, for begging me to write this, for stumbling upon it, or just for holding it in your hands right now.

References and bibliography

I have scoured, referenced and cross-referenced resources all over the world to bring you the information in this book. Here is a list of books which I believe is representative of the information delivered. However, if you feel you should be credited here, please email **sales@detoxyourworld.com** with your reasons, and I'll add you to the next edition.

Astanga Yoga — Liz Lark
Carlton Books, 2000

Blatant Raw-Foodist Propaganda — Joe Alexander
Blue Dolphin Press, 1990

Carol Vorderman's Detox For Life — Carol Vorderman
Virgin Books, 2001

Detox — Carol Morley and Liz Wilde
MQP Publications, 2001

Eating for Beauty — David Wolfe
Maul Bros, 2002

Essene Gospel Of Peace — Translated by Edmond Szekely
The CW Daniel Company Ltd

Fast Food Nation — Eric Schlosser
The Penguin Press, 2001

Fats That Heal, Fats That Kill — Udo Erasmus
Alive Books, 1993

Eat Smart Eat Raw — Kate Wood
Grub Street, 2002

Food For Free — Richard Mabey
HarperCollins, 1992

Nature's First Law: The Raw-Food Diet — Arlin, Dini, Wolfe
Maul Bros, 1999

Raw Perfection — Mike Nash
Raw Perfection, 2002

Recipes for Natural Beauty — Katie Spiers
Quarto Publishing, 1998

Detox Delights — Shazzie
Rawcreation Ltd, 2001

Survival into the 21st Century — Viktoras Kulvinskas
21st Century Publications, 2002

The Complete Raw Juice Therapy — Thorsons Editorial Board
Thorsons, 1989

The Healing Miracles of Coconut Oil — Bruce Fife
Piccadilly Books, 2000

The Healing Power of Papaya — Barbara Simonsohn
Lotus Press, 2000

The Optimum Nutrition Bible — Patrick Holford
Judy Piatkus, 1998

The New Raw Energy — Leslie Kenton
Vermilion, 1994

The Sunfood Diet Success System — David Wolfe
Maul Bros, 2000

Wild Health — Cindy Engal
Phoenix, 2003

Yoga Mind, Body & Spirit — Donna Farhi
Newleaf, 2000

Your Body's Many Cries For Water — Dr Batmanghelidj
Global Health Solutions, 1997

The last bits

I've separated the index into two categories, so the food doesn't get lost amongst the mercury fillings! First, you'll see the recipe index, and then afterwards you'll see the full index.

Recipe index

African spicy sesame soup 293

Almond, hazel or sunflower milk 309

Aloe super mousse 335

Anytime muesli 338

Apple and orange juice 281

Banana bites 341

Basilled tomatoes 304

Big green smoothie 278

Bottoms up juice 279

Brutus is scared juice 280

Buffet ideas **343**

Butternut noodles with golden curry sauce 325

Cabbage and carrot juice 283

Cardamom cooler drink 286

Carrot and coriander dip 317

Carrot and tomato spread 315

Carrot nests 307

Carrot top-up juice 284

Celebrate good times cake 340

Chakra Salad 295

Champiñónes au natural 305

Cheddary cheeze spread 311

Cheddary cheeze squares 311

Cheeze and onion sushi 323

Cherry chaser 282

Chockie milkshake drink 286

Chocolate orange smoothie 278
Christmas balls 335
Coconut banana split 336
Coconut drink 277
Coleslaw 307
Corn tortillas 330
Courgetti and rawgu 324
Cream of orange soup 290
Cream of pepper soup 289
Cream of shiitake soup 291
Creamy herb dip 315
Crispy spring rolls 303
Cucumber and apple juice 283
Cucumber crunch 307
Cucumber number juice 281
Cucumber salad 296
Curly crisps 330
Dips, spreads, dressings, sauces and pâtés **312**
Dolmades 302
Double stuffed tomatoes 319
Drinks **285**
Duriasm 344
Earth and fire sushi 323
Easy sushi 322
Entertaining meals **342**
Fig stew 303
Flax and corn crackers 332
Fractal fortnight juice 280
"Fried" mushrooms 306

Golden gazpacho soup 294

Green hemp milk drink 288

Green sushi 323

Guacamole 314

Herby stir fry 318

High vibe dressing 312

Hopping wild juice 280

Hot orange juice 283

I can't believe it's not Waldorf salad 299

It's not really mayonnaise 311

Japanese okra 308

Jessie's tropical soup 292

Joe's chip shop chips 308

Juices **279**

Kumquat and nutmeg cheezecake 339

Lemon courgettes 306

Macadamia cream 310

Mango chutney 313

Mangoes marinaded in golden ginger syrup with lychee ice cream 334

Melonlemon drink 285

Mesquite melts 331

Mousse de naranja 333

Mushroom gravy 316

Nutter sushi 323

Onion bhajis 304

Puddings and desserts **333**

Pico de gallo 313

Pink porridge 337

Plum sauce 312

Quick chockie thickshake drink 287

Quickest tahini milk 309

Raspberry and physalis dream 338

Red whine drink 286

"Roast tofu" with satay sauce 329

Rocket fuel juice 282

Romaine roll-ups 296

Runny romaine juice 284

Salads **295**

Sangria Maria juice 282

Savoury crisps 331

Sauerkraut 301

Scrummy side dishes **300**

Seaside smoothie 277

Seeded noodles 305

Semolina pudding with figgy jam 333

Shazzie's chip shop chips 308

Smooth coconut ice cream 337

Smoothies **277**

Soups **289**

Special additions **330**

Spicy pear juice 281

Spinach pesto 316

Squash and kumquat soup 290

Strawberry patch juice 283

Sunflower pâté 315

Sunflower pâté sushi 322

Sunrise drink 287

Super asparagus wraps 321

Super broccoli quiche 323

Supercharged celery juice 281

Sweet apricot sauce 317

Sweet beet soup 289

Sweet crisps 331

Sweet grapefruit juice 284

Tabouleh pyramids 300

Thai salad 297

The best meal in the world, ever **344**

The candy floss tart juice 279

The gratest salad in the world 298

The lady juiced her fingers juice 282

This is where the sun got to smoothie 278

Toffee and raspberry fool 334

Tomato salad 298

Tomato sauce 316

Vanilla créme 310

Vegetable paella 326

Very special main meals **318**

Wake up, ginger juice 279

Walnut burgers 320

Walnut stuffed peppers 328

Warm apple punch drink 285

Whip the mister ice cream 336

Wild mushroom fajitas 327

Yellow pepper and almond soup 291

Your new dairy **309**

Index

A

Abhva 133
Aborigine 100
Absorption 108
Abundance 22, 30, 166, 167, 182, 208
Acetone 66
Aches and pains 16, 18, 24, 45, 181, 185, 233
Acid 83, 121, 140, 145, 174, 235
Acne 8, 20, 50
Acorn squash 202
Acquired Immune Deficiency Syndrome 94
Acrylamide 9, 161
Active
Activity 14, 204, 232
Addiction 35, 45
  cigarette 63, 70
  coffee 44
  drug 85, 224
  food 19, 21, 22, 23, 24, 35, 83, 139, 144
  grain 146-147
  television 75, 115
Additive 138
Adenoid 142
Aduki 169, 175
Adult onset diabetes 17. See also Diabetes
Affirmation 115-116
Aflatoxin 175
Ageing 11
Ageless 127
Aggression 44
Agrochemical 152, 156, 157. See also Chemical
Ahara 133
AHT. See Autohaemotherapy
AIDS 94
Air 51-55
  fresh 47, 93, 112, 221, 224
  freshener 51

oxygen and 92
purifier 53, 232
quality 54
Alarm clock 73, 192, 193, 201
Alcohol 40-43, 51, 120, 182, 221, 224, 234, 286
  babies and 42
  brain and 42
  cancer and 41
  depression and 43
  family history 42
  fat and 41
  Foetal Alcohol Syndrome 42
  freedom from 117
  guidelines on 40
  liver damage 41
  units of 40
  your body and 41
Alert 17, 19
Alfalfa 169, 190, 230
Algae 109, 170
Alkaline 121, 168
Allergen 54
Allergy 56, 87, 94, 140
Alligator, environmental damage to 46
Almond 173, 190, 202, 211, 213
  milk 230
Aloe 52, 335
Aluminium 56, 77, 79
Alzheimer's 87
Amalgam 85, 86, 87
Amino acid 121, 145, 151, 168, 170, 293, 310
Ammonia 51, 66
Amphetamine 44
Anaemia 56, 145, 162
Anaerobic 95, 121
Anal 123
Anatomy 21
Anger 113
Animal 79, 154, 161, 180
  eating and 21, 138
  exercise and 102

experiment 80
fat. See Fat, animal
flesh and pesticides 158
kingdom 21
meditation and 111
mud eating and 109
plants and 52
sexless 46
Ankle 36, 125
Antibiotic 121, 154
Antifreeze 77
Anti-neoplastic 95
Antioxidant 95, 168, 170, 278
Antisocial 40
Anxiety 45, 146. See also Stress
Apathy 86
Aphrodisiac 321
Appetite 20, 96
Apple 22, 30, 138, 152, 159, 166, 191, 202, 221, 224, 225, 229, 299
  pesticides and 156
Apricot 156, 167, 173, 190, 202, 317
Aquatic greens 170
Areca palm 51
Arm 125, 209
Aromatherapy 108
Arsenic 67
Artery 11
Arthritis 8, 10, 11, 15, 17, 18, 57, 76, 80, 94, 103
  rheumatoid 88
Arugula 273
Asexual 46
Ashtanga. See Astanga
Asia 144
Asparagus 321
Astanga 133
Asthma 11, 15, 17, 53, 57, 143
  children and 11, 46
  Ioniser and 53
  Smoking and 65, 68
Atherosclerosis 56, 299

Atkins Diet 27
Atlantic sea salad 202, 273
Atmosphere 53, 92, 95, 154
Atmospheric ozone 94
Autism 76
Autohaemotherapy 95
Avocado 138, 140, 156, 166, 187, 191, 202, 226, 229, 230, 235, **302**
Awareness 206
Azalea 52

B

B17 173
Baby 42, 121, 158
  alcohol and 42
  mercury and 85
  organic food and **158**
  products 49
  vaccines and 76
Back 125, 195
  ache 99
  banana 206
Bacteria 53, 56, 76, 95, 98, 109
  bad 100, 121
  E. coli 0157:H7 144
  good 100, 123, 152, 301
  spirochete 122
  streptococcus mutans 89
Balance 31, **32**, 209
Bamboo 52
Banana 156, 166, 167, 174, 187, 191, 202, 229
Baron Justus von Leibig 156
Basil 175, 202, 230, 233, **319**
Bass, environmental damage to 46
Bath 56, 60
Bayleaf 176
Bean 139
  green 156
  kidney 175
Beautiful 213, 231
Beauty 46, 139, 157, 213
  natural **49**
Bed 232
Bedroom 47, 52

Beet 273
Beetroot 191
Behaviour 181
  problems 42
Bell pepper 273
Benzene 51, **67**
Benzethonium chloride 77
Bergamot 108
Berry 149, 166, 191
Beta carotene 151, 278, 327
Betty 179
Beyond detoxing 33-34
Bhakti 133
Bikram 133
Binge 141, 146
Bird 155
Birth 180
Biscuit 146, 235
Black pepper 108
Blackberry 211
Blender **275**
  hand **275**
Bliss 93, **111-112**
Bloat 12, 19, 37, 99, 185, 187
Blood 12, 41, 58, 64, 84, 85, 92, 95, 124, 208, 224
  alcohol 41
  bloodstream 11, 41, 54, 65, 84, 98
  blue 122
  cancer 65
  cells 67, 95, 160
  circulation 125
  loss 18
  lymphocytes 85
  massage 108
  oxygen 92, 95
  plant 168
  pressure 57, 66, 105, 113, 154, 277
  sugar 187
  test 145
  transfusion 58, 162
  type 27
  vessels 283, 299
Blood Type Diet 27
Blue, the colour 209

Blueberry 166, 202, 221
Body 84, 133, 134, 154, 181, 185, 188, 195, 203, 211, 217, 224, 232
  odour 19, 99
  scrub 210
Body brushing. See Skin, brushing
Boil 20
Bone 142
Bone marrow 67
Book 112
Boston fern 52
Bovine serum albumin 143
Bowel 11, 99
Bra 231
Brace 79
Bradford, Colonel. See Colonel Bradford
Brain 41, 62, 84, 211, 213
  alcohol and **42**
  caffeine and 44
  damage 42
  fog 9
  left 115
  mercury and 87
  right 116
  spatial 116
Brazil 173
Bread 166, 178, 182, 189, 190, **200**, 201, 226, 235
  cancer and 161
  eczema and 11
  replacement 146, 169
Breakfast 229
Breath 84, 132, 134, 153, 192, 193, 208
  bad 17, 19
  bad breath 99
  conscious **92**
Breathe 85, 92, 105, 142, 225
Broccoli 156, 169, 191, **318**
Bronchitis 53
Brushing, body. See Skin, brushing
BSA. See Bovine Serum Albumin
BSE 154

Buckwheat 169
Buddha 131
Buddhi 133
Burdock 151
Burger 179
Burrito 230
Butter 174, 178, 190, 200
Butterfly 33, 155
Butternut squash 202
Buttock 125

C

Cabbage 27, 138, 191, 202, 221
The Cabbage Soup Diet 27
Cacao 176
Cadmium 67-68
Caffeine 44, 182
Cake 190, 201
Calcium 142, 150, 151, 277, 293, 310, 331
Calf 125
Calm 92, 132
Calorie 28, 29, 120, 168
Cancer 9, 10, 11, 15, 17, 18, 40, 44, 49, 61, 94
  acrylamide and 161
  alcohol and 41
  allergy 56
  ammonia and 66
  anti- 95, 105, 109, 318
  awareness 64
  B17 173
  bladder 56, 65, 67, 68
  breast 41, 108
  cervix 65, 170
  colon 56, 64, 99
  cure 105, 163, 170
  dairy 142
  deaths 63, 64
  fluoride 80
  food 161
  green food 170
  kidney 65, 67
  leukaemia 65
  liver 41, 56, 67
  lung 41, 64, 65, 67, 72
  mobile phones and 62
  mouth 41, 65, 170

non-organic food 153, 156
oesophagus 65, 146
oral 62
ovarian 49
pancreas 65
prostate 64, 67
rectum 56
skin 67
smoking 63, 69
statistic 68
stomach 56, 65
tar 66
therapy 109
throat 65
treatment 168
woman 68
Candida 94
Cantaloupe 138, 222
Car 62, 67, 231
Carbohydrate 139, 157
  complex 160
Carbon dioxide 51, 162
Carbon monoxide 51, 52, 65-66, 68, 162
Carcinogen 65, 67, 68, 147, 161, 168
Cardamom 173, 202
Carob 175, 202, 272
Carotene 307
Carpet 53, 60
Carrot 21, 152, 191, 202, 221, 230, 307
Cashew 173, 202
Cat 54, 79
Catarrh 53
Cauliflower 156
Cavity 89
Celery 138, 153, 169, 191, 207, 218, 221, 225, 230, 277
  seed 202
Celibate 129
Cell 14, 56, 95, 96, 103, 105, 121, 141, 157
  B-cell 105
  damage 162
  detox 190, 225
  emotional release 18, 217
  fat. See Fat, cells

killer 105, 109
liver 41
membrane 96
red blood 67
renew 126
T-cell 105
tumour 105
white blood 67, 80, 95, 160, 161
Cellulite 17, 126
Central Nervous System. See CNS
Ceramic 60
Cereal 146, 178
Chakra 134, 200, 210
  base 203
  brow 211
  crown 213
  heart 208
  sacral 204
  solar plexus 206
  third eye 211
  throat 209
Challenge 37, 181
Change 36
Chant 134, 225
Chard 169
Charity work 232
Cheese 23, 178, 189, 190, 200, 201
Chemical 30, 149, 158, 160, 168, 218, 231. See also Agrochemical. See also Phytochemical.
  bond 87
  lung 122
Cherimoya 153, 166
Cherry 141, 156, 166
Chest 125, 208
Chew 83, 141, 194, 197, 225, 275
Chick pea 169, 175
Chickweed 151
Child 47, 79, 144, 154
  fasting a 47
Chilli 202, 222
Chin, double. See Double chin
China 118, 124, 317
Chip 139, 190, 201, 273

Chive 202

Chlordane 158

Chlorine **56**

Chlorophyll **168**

Chocolate 25, 187

Choice 34

Cholesterol 41, 57, 120, 162, 168, 299, 310
  coffee and 44

Chorella 170

Chrysanthemum 52

Cigarette 54, 63, **64**, 230. See also Nicotine. See also Smoking. See also Tobacco.

Cilantro 273

Cinnamon 176, 191, 221

Circulation 104, 118, 185

Circulatory system 105

Cirrhosis 41

Citrus 175

Clarity 206, 217

Clay 49, 108, 195, 215
  Fuller's earth 109
  green 109
  white 109

Clean 28, 36, 178, 182, 185
  teeth 79-82

Cleanse 138, 183, 217, 223
  colon 101
  juice 217
  skin 120

Clear 206

Clothing 46, 51, **54-55**, 231, 234
  children and 47
  dry-clean 51
  therapeutic 47

Clover 169

Cloves 176

Clutter 36

CNS 211, 213
  disorder 94

Cobalt 151

Cocaine 44

Coconut 141, 173, 191, 202
  water 143

Coffee 13, 24, **44-45**, 178, 221, 224, 228, 234

Coffee/spice mill **276**

Cold turkey 179

Cold, feelings of 19, 20, 30, 194, 196

Cold, virus 10, 12, 18, 19, 64, 88, 122
  dealing with 184

Colitis 94

Colon 124, 206
  cancer. See Cancer, colon
  cleaning **98-101**
  function 152
  impacted 108
  irrigation 98
  skin and 98
  wall 99

Colonel Bradford 127

Colonic hydrotherapy 99

Colour consultation 234

Comedy 106

Comfort zone 179

Communicate 210

Communication 209

Compassion 131, 197

Compost 46

Computer 62, 88, 102

Concentration 86

Condom 49

Confidence 204

Confident 37

Confusion 16, 19, 66, 88, 99

Connected 88

Conscious 116

Constipation 17, 99, 100, 143, 185

Control 29, 213

Cook 57, 62, 147, **160-163**, 166, 233

Cookie 190, 201, 235

Co-ordination 104

Copper 151

Coriander 173, 191, 202, 230, 233

Corn 273

Corn Palm 52

Cortisol 105

Cot death 65

Cotton 55, 153, 231

Couch potato 75, 102

Cough 64

Counsellor 217

Countryside 47

Courage 203

Courgette 138, 166, 191, 202

Cow 21, 142, 143, 154

Cracker 146, 179, 190, 201, 235

Cramp 187

Craving 19, 25, 146, 161, 178, 187

Cream 21, 178

Create 212

Creative 96, 201, 235

Creativity 93, 116, 209, 211

Cress 169

Crisps 190, 201

Crohn's disease 76, 94

Crown 79, 84

Crudité 230

Crystal 58, 118
  soda. See Soda crystal

Crystal Manna 170

Cucumber 138, 156, 166, 202, 207, 222, 224, 225, 296

Cumin 173, 202

Curiosity 206

Currant 167

Cystic fibrosis 103

Cystitis 17

D

Dairy 154, 158, 178, 189, 235

Dancing 102

Dandelion 150, 169

Date 191

DDT 156

Decay 82

Decision 33

Defecation. See Elimination

Deformed 46

Degenerative diseases. See Disease

Dehydration 57, 58, 228

Dehydrator 276
Dementia 42
Dental dam 87
Dentine 84
Dentist 85, 88
Deodorant 124
Depression 8, 21, 45, 116, 227
  alcohol and 43
  mercury and 88
Dessertspoon 273
Detergent 67
Detoxification 105, 181, 186, 189, 192, 231
Diabetes 10, 12, 15, 18, 44, 57, 76, 143, 217
  adult onset 17
Diarrhoea 19, 99, 143
Dieldrin 158
Diet 15, 19, 24, 25, **27-29**, 95, 161, 232, 233
  Atkins 27
  Cabbage Soup 27
  calorie restriction 186
  children and 47
  detox 11, 13, 14, 139, 151, 175
  Egg 27
  grain-based 146
  green 145, 168
  high fruit 166
  juice 140
  low-sodium 277
  natural 21, 145
  organic 228, 273
  pre-menstrual 187
  raw plant 145, 161, 163
  simple 139
  toxic 24, 25, 178
  vegetarian 144, 145
  western 8, 10, 13, 168, 186, 224
  wild food 149
Digest 28, 83, 140, 157, 173, 175, 184
  digestion 126, 141, 142, 183, 185, 187, 299
Dill 176, 202
Dinner 183
Dioxin 46

Dip 169, 174, 230
Discover 112, 201
Disease 15, 16, 18, 34, 41, 113, 149, 153, 162. **See also** Illness
  childhood **46-47**
  contagious 162
  mind 106
  resistance 92
  respiratory tract 106
  smoking-related 64
Disinfectant 77
Dizzy 19, 58, 66, 67, 128, 197
Documentary 21
Dog 79, 168
Dopac 105
Double chin 28
Doubleday, Jock. See Jock Doubleday
Dr Norman Walker 140
Dracaena Marginata 52
Dreams 18, 33, 198, 215
Drink 24, 174, 223, 230, **234**
  fizzy 57, 82, 83, 228
  vaccine 76
  water. **See** Water
Drinking culture 40
Drug 10, 40, 44, 45, 132, 154, 230
  hard 24
Dry cleaning 51
Dulse 202
Durian 166, 235, **344**
Dust 53, 125
Dust mite 53-54

E

E. coli 0157:H7 144
E3Live 170, 202, 222, 229, 230
Ear 19, 118, 122, 211
  infections 142
Earth 9, 21
Ecosystem 100
Eczema 11, 15, 17
  bread and 11
  children and **11, 46**
Egg 27, 108, 189, 190, 200, 201, 235
The Egg Diet 27

Eggplant 273
Ego 206
Egypt 118
Ejuva 180
Electricity 170
Elimination 185
  organs 11, 18, 96, 122, 218
  pollution 11
  skin 124
Emotion 15, 18, 19, 27, 35, 105, 116, 131, 134, 179, 194, 217, 227
Enamel 82
Endive 169
Endocrine 156
Endorphin 105
Enema 99, 100
  chew 221
  kit 221, 224
Energy 120, 203, 205, 220, 221
  chakra 206, 208, 209, 212, 214
  conservation 102, 209, 225
  creative 234
  digestive 13, 185, 187, 206
  food and 29, 41, 96, 160, 161, 166
  kundalini 133, 134
  levels 8, 17-19, 31, 37, 43, 95, 104, 122, 152, 181, 183, 189, 190, 213, 231, 233
  life force. See Life force
  nuclear 80
  pathways 92
  sexual 129
  shaktipat 133
Enervate 180
English ivy 52
Enlightenment 112, 133, 144
Environment 9, 46, 49, 65, 95, 109, 154, 166, 227, 231
  arsenic in the 67
  care of 154
  colon 100
  friendly 9, 54, 231
  germs and 146
  pollution 12, 46
  responsibility 71
Enzyme 95, 121, 122, 154, 168
Epinephrine 105

Epsom salts **193**, 204, 213
Equilibrium 113, 134
Eric Schlosser 144
Esoteric 232
Essential fatty acids 168, 288
Ethylene glycol 77
Eucalyptus 108
Evening **183-184**
Exercise 92, 98, **102-104**, 127, 182, 218, 232
  breathing 93
Exhilarating 210
Exorphin 146
Expression 209
Extinct 155
Extraction 84
Eye 49, 68, 206, 211
  dark circle 185
  irritation 56

F

Face 125
  treat 212
Faeces 98, 138
Farmer 228
Farmer's markets 153
Farming 121, 155
Fasting 5, 100, 139, 141, **217-220, 224-226**
  children and 47
  shivambu 131
Fat 95, 96, 121, 138, 226
  alcohol 41
  animal 198, 215
  cells 11, 18, 36
  cooked 178
  eating 140
  eliminating 120, 168
  liver 41
  monounsaturated 310
  plant 173
  ratio 41
Fatigue 11, 19, 30, 45, 99, 143. See also Lethargy
Fear 113
Fennel 108
Ferment 145

Fibre, dietary 27, 100, 101, 168, 278, 299
Fibre, material 54, 181, 231
Fig 138, 166, 174, 191, 213
Filbert 173
Filter 56
  cigarette 63
Fish 46, 67, 139, 158, 189, 190, 200, 201, 235. See also Meat
Flavouring 138
Flax 174, 179
Flexibility 17, 168
Floor 73
Flour 138, 198, 215
Flow 232
Flower 108, 149, 151
Fluid 108
Fluoride 49, 79, **80-82**
  poisoning 122. See also Tooth
Flush 18
Focus 12, 111
Foetal Alcohol Syndrome 42
Foetus 87
Food 8, 11-15, 88, 95, 204, 233
  addictive 139
  bad 24, 102
  best 24
  cancer and 161, 170
  chemical 182
  comfort 23
  digest 35
  disorder 146
  fresh 21, 25, 83, 182, 185
  fried 235
  health 149
  lovely 14
  modern 25, 170
  mood 23
  natural 13, 15, 31, 33, 82, 143
  raw 83, 170, 198, 216, 221, 224, 233, 235
  symbol 23
  toxic 9
  unnatural 9, 11, 15, 30, 82
  waste 46
  whole 30
  wild and organic **149-159**
Food combining **139-140**

Food processor 276
Foot 36, 118, 125
Forehead 211
Formaldehyde 51, **68**, 77
Formic acid 68
F-Plan Diet 27
Fractal 170
Frankincense 108
Free radical 95
Fresh air. See Air, fresh
Fries 273
Frog 155
Frugivorous 160
Fruit 14, 21, 58, 101, 138, 140, 149, **166-167**, 183, 184, 198, 211, 221, 224, 225, 228, 229, 233
Fruity water **191**
Fulfil 209
Fulfilment 209
Full 31
Fuller's earth clay 109
Fungicide 157
Fungus 54, 95, 121, 157, 162
Furniture 54

G

Galactose 142
Galangal 202
Gamma-interferon 105
Garbanzo 273
Gardening 190
Garlic 176, 191, 202, 230
Gas 19, 68, 99, 109, 139
Gastrointestinal 86
Gastrointestinal tract 84
Gazelle 21
Gender 46
Generation 149
Generosity 197
Genetic modification 149, **155**
Genital 46, 49
Gerbera daisy 52
Germs and environment 146
Ginger 108, 109, 202, 207, 222, 283
gingko biloba 173

Glass ionomer 87
Glaucoma 94
Glow 37
Gluten 235
GM. See Genetic modification
Goals 204
God 133, 309
Goji berry 45, 176
Golden pathos 52
Gonorrhea 121
Gotama Buddha. See Buddha
GP 30
Grain 145-147, 178, 221, 235
Grandma 60
Grape 138, 156, 166, 213
Grapefruit 108, 202, 222, 284
The Grapefruit Diet 27
Grass 21, 150, 168
Greek 122
Green, the colour 194, 197, 208, 229, 231
Green bean 156
Green onion 273
Green Power/Kempo 156
Greens 168-171, 175, 228, 229, 230, 235
    aquatic 170
    sunflower 169
Gristle 180
Grounded 96
Groundnut 175
Guacamole 229, 230
Guideline 33, 183, 184
    alcohol 40
Guinea pig 155
Gum chewing 88
Guru 112
Gut 138
Gynaecologist 142

H

Haemoglobin 162
Haemorrhoid 11, 17, 139
Hair 17, 185
    chlorine and 56
    deficient 30

loss 30, 49
Halitosis. See Breath, bad
Hand 118, 125, 209
Hand blender 275
Happiness. See Happy
Happy 12, 13, 15, 16, 22, 33, 52, 53, 96, 102, 107, 119, 131, 160, 179, 227, 231
    colour 204
    mantra 205
Hard drug 24
Harmony 113, 208
Hate 113
Hatha 133
Hatter 85
Hay fever 53
Hazel 173, 309
HDL. See also Cholesterol
Head 213
Headache 11, 17, 18, 19, 45, 66, 99, 286
Healing 101, 122, 131, 133, 134, 170, 203, 208
Healing crisis 20
Health 15, 29, 41, 43, 52, 94, 144, 160, 168, 173, 179, 181, 186, 217
    optimal 15
    warning 60
Healthcare 153
Heart 35, 154, 208, 234
    patients 95
    rate 120
Heart disease 8, 10, 11, 15, 17, 18, 41, 44, 56, 64, 71, 94, 103, 162, 283, 299, 310
    coffee and 44
Heavy metal 56, 120
Hedgerow 155
Hemp 55, 202, 231, 288
    seed 173
HEPA filter 53, 54
Hepatitis 94
Heptachlor 158
Herb 175, 179-180, 191, 229
High fruit diet 166
Herpes 94

Higher purpose 154
The Hippocrates Health Institute 170
HIV 94
Holistic 49, 89
Home 230
Homeopath 77
Hormone 24, 51, 105, 154, 158, 187
House 231. See also Home
Human potential 34
Humour therapy 105
Hunger 22, 29, 139, 160, 183, 225
    apple 218
    fasting and 218
    fruit 218
    greens 218
    melon 218
    organic 218
Hydrogen 51
Hydrogen peroxide 95, 162

I

IBS 87, 94
Ice cream 141
Ice cube 197
Ideal 213
IgA. See Immunoglobulin A
Ill 21, 224
Illness 15, 17, 89, 234. See also Disease
Imagination 211, 225
Imagine 212
Immune function 86, 104, 108
Immune system 90, 105, 109, 116, 126, 142, 163
Immunity 9, 111, 113, 143, 160, 161, 168, 197
Immunoglobulin A 106
Immunological system 85
Impacted colon 108
Incense 112
India 118
Indigo, the colour 211
Infection 85, 123
    ear 142

Infertile 46
Information 232
Infra-red 157
  sauna. See Sauna, infra-red
Inner child 198
InnerTalk 43, 48, 72, 102, 104, 114, **115-117**, 146, 148, 228, 232
Insect 145, 157
Insecticide 157
Insight 131
Insomnia 19
Inspiration 213
Inspire 213
Instinct 21-22, 31, 180, 183
Insufflation 95
Insulin 143
Intellectual 133
Intelligence 206
Interferon 95
Interleuken-2 95
Intestinal 204
Intuition 133, 160, 211, 212
Intuitive 25, 113
Iodine 296
Ion 53
Ionic minerals 1, 121, 123, 157, 153
Ioniser 53-54
  therapeutic 47, 54
Iron 145, 150, 151, 293, 327, 331
Irritability 99
Irritable Bowel Syndrome. See IBS
Itch 20
Iyengar 134

J

Jacuzzi 197
Jaw 84
Jealousy 113
Jesus 99
Jock Doubleday 76
Jog 103, 120, 195, 207, 209, 210
Joint 19
Journal 36, 112, 179, 187, 188, 189, 194, 197, **200,** 203, 210,

211, 227, 233, 234
Journey 235
  inward 225
Joy 111, 139
Juice 58, 82, 101, **140-141**, 143, 187, 224, 225, 226, 234
  celery 58
  cleanse 100, 217
  craving 141
  dandelion 150
  detox **221-223**
  diet. See Diet, juice
  green 70, 83, 141, 159, 184, 218, 229
  how to eat 221
  lemon 60
  orange 83, 167
  watermelon 163
  wheatgrass 168
Juicer 140, **275. See also** Green Power/Kempo
  centrifugal 141
  masticating 141
Jungle 51
Juniper 108
Justus von Leibig, Baron 156

K

Kale 138, 202, 207, 222
Karma 133, 144
Kidney 35, 49, 68, 118
  cancer. See Cancer, kidney
  mercury and 86, 87
Kidney bean 175
Kind 132
Kitchen 56
Knowledge 180
Kumquat 202, 290
Kundalini 134

L

Lactose 142
Lambsquarter 151
Laughing 105-107
Layer 36
Leach 30
Lead 56
Leaf 58, 83, 149, 151, 157, 168,

222, 229
Learning 206
Learning difficulties 42
Lecture 232
Left brain 115
Legs 36
Legume 175
Lemon 191, 202, 222, 228
Lemon grass 176, 202
Lentil 169
Lesions 46
Lethargy 8, 19, 234
Lettuce 30, 138, 150, 151, 153, 225, 226, 230
  Batavia 169
  butterhead 169
  frise 169
  iceberg 169
  lamb's 169
  Little gem 202, 222, 273
  lollo rosso 169
  oakleaf 169
  radicchio 169
  romaine 169, 191, 202, 222, 225, 229
  Sesame 202
Leukaemia 67
Leukocyte 162
Leukosytosis 161, 162
Liberty 160
Life 6, 8, 11, 14, 15, 16, 28, 29, 32, 33, 34, 178, 179, 185, 186, 216
Life force 92, 134, 149, 150
Lifestyle 12, 15, 16, 17, 25, 28, 29, 41, 50, 62, 63, 79, 92, 95, 99, 102, 154, 178, 181, 185, 186, 199, 216, 231
Lime 191, 202
  ripe 292
Lindane 156
Linen 55, 231
Lino 231
Lion 21, 150
Liver 18, 35, 41, 49, 179, 206
  cancer. **See** Cancer, liver
Locust bean 175
Lonely 35

Longevity 18
Loofah 124
Loss of blood 18
Lotion 124
Lotus 111, 194, 196
Love 35, 40, 113, 131, 132, 133, 161, 187, 197, 203, 208, 232
Low-sodium diet 277
Lunch 183
Lung 49, 67 68, 84
  cancer. **See** Cancer, lung
  disease 64
Lupus 88
Lycopene 160, 298
Lyme 122
Lymph 103, 122, **124**, 134, 189, 195, **200**, 209, 211
  node 108
  stimulant 151
Lymphocytes 85
Lymphatic drainage massage 108
Lysine 331

M

Maca 176, 187
Macadamia 138, 173, 191, 202, **310**
Mace 176
Magnesium 151, 331
Maha 133
Maize 273
Mammal 155
Mandoline 275
Mango 30, 138, 153, 166, 167, 187, 191, 202, 209, 222, 223, **278**
Manifest 209, 217
Manifestation 209
Mantra 112, 133, 195, 203, 206, 210, 214
Market 228
Marrow 202
Massage 105, **108-110**, 182, 187, 189, 195, **200**, 218, 225, 232
Mastery 132
ME 17, 76
Meat 21, 24, **144-145**, 154, 158,

160, 189, 190, 200, 201, 226, 235
  killing 144
Medical ozone. See Ozone
Medical practitioner 15, 19, 186, 217
Medication 15, 120, 123
Medicine 154, 168
Meditation 111-114, 181, 217, 232
  chakra rejuvenation and 203-216
  meditate 189, 200, 225
  vipassana 131-132
  yoga and 133-134
Mediterranean 175
Melon 140, 166, 184, 187, 191, 206, 222, 223, 224
Membrane 96
Memory 86
Meningitis 76
Menstruation 18, 20, 67, 187-188
  pain 8, 11
  pre-menstrual symptoms 18, 107, 185, 187
Mental disorder 17, 18, 28
Mercury 77, 233
  baby and 85
  brain and 87
  depression and 88
  filling 79, **84-87**, 233
  hazardous 86
  ionic 85
  leak 86
  poison 85
  removal 89
  vapour 84
  waste 86
Mesquite 331
Metabolise 41
Metal 60
Metal, heavy. See Heavy metal
Methane 51
Methanol 68
Methylaldehyde 68
Methylene oxide 68
Microleakage 87
Micro-organism 162

Microwave 62, **162**
Midday 183
Middle East 175
Midnight 182-183
Migraine 11, 17, 53, 57, 74
Mildew 54
Milk 24, **142-143**, 178, 189, 190, 200, 201
  allergy 143
  almond 230
  breast 87, 143, 152, 158
  calcium 142
  children and 47
  formula 158
  immunity 142
  nut 143, **272**
  pesticide 142
Mill 276
Mind 18, 34, 92, 111, 132, 133, 134, 181, 185, 186, 211, 224, 225, **232**
  subconscious 115
Mineral 30, 98, 121, 151, 157, 168, 170, 230
  ionic. See ionic minerals
Mint 191, 202, 222
Miracle 30
Miscarriage 44, 65
Mizuna 169
Mobile phone 62
Mobility 104
Modern diet. See Diet, western
Molars 82
Molecule 162
Monastery 127
Monk 127
Monkey 21, 42, 150
  nut 175
Mono eating 138
Monounsaturated fat 310
Mood 17, 40, 54
Moon 230
  full 10
  new 10
Morning 183
Mother-in-law's tongue 52
Motivate 102

Mould 54
Mouth 49, 84, 86, 123, 141, **233**
 cancer. **See** Cancer, mouth
MS 17, 87, 94, 103
MSM 47, 50, 58, 140
Mucous 17, 98, 126, 169
 producer 142
Mud 108, 205, 215
Mud wrap 214-215. See also
Wraps
Multiple sclerosis. See MS
Mung 169, 175
Muscle 103, 105, 120
 tone 104
Mushroom 152, 202
Music 103, 195
Mustard gas burn 94
Mutate 86
Mysticism 211

N

Nadi shodhana 92
Nail 17, 185
Natural 180
 beauty 49
 diet. **See** Diet, natural
 hygiene 100, 140
 law 33
 world 12
Nature 12, 30, 31, 34, 53, 96, 160
 lesson 21
Nature's First Food 170
Nature's Living Superfood 170
Nausea 19
Neck 209
Nervous system 161, 206
Nettle 151
Niacin 293
Nicotine 65, 120, 182. **See also**
Cigarette. See also Smoking.
See also Tobacco.
Nipple 125
Nitrogen 156
Norman Walker. See Dr
Norman Walker
Nose 211
Nuclear energy 80
NPK 156

Nut 140, 149, **173-174**, 175, 187,
221, 226, 235
Nutmeg 173
Nutrient 22, 31, 79, 100, 154,
158, 166, 170, 182
 deficient 29
 lies 29
Nutrition 14, 180
Nutritionist 30, 56, 160, 183

O

Oat groat 191
Obese 11, 28, 57
Octopus 144
Odour, body 19, 99
Oesophagus cancer. See Cancer,
oesophagus
Oil 108, 109, 167, 175, 195, 202,
272
Okra 202, 222
Olive 166, 202, 226, 230, **272**
 leaf 45
Omega 3 288
Omega 6 288
Omega 9 288
One 113
Onion 156, 169, 176, 191, 202
 bunching 300
 spring. **See** Spring onion
Opioid 146
Opportunity 18, 34
Oral cancer 62
Orange 83, 138, 140, 166, 191,
202, 222, 228
 peel 60
Orange, the colour 204
Orchid 52, 287
Oregano 202
Organ 9, 18, 35, 103, 118, 179,
204, 224, 231
Organic
 clothing 47, 55, 231
 diet. **See** Diet, organic
 farm 228
 food 47, 145, **149-159**, 168,
 170, 185, 201, 235, 273
 toothpaste 82
Organism, single-celled. See

Single-celled organism
Osteoporosis 17
Outgass 54
Ovarian cancer 49
Overdose 49
Overnight 25
Overweight 21, 27, 28, 29, 35,
146, 227
Oxidise 96
Oxomethane 68
Oxygen 41, 51, 52, 54, 92, 95,
105, 120, 168, 225, 231
Oxymethyline 68
Ozone 89, 94
 therapy **94-96**

P

Pain 104, 105, 113, 119, 188, 227
 rheumatic 109. **See also** Aches
 and pains
Painkiller 105, 188
Paint 60, 67, 190
Pamper 187
Pancreas 12, 143
 cancer. **See** Cancer, pancreas
Pants 231
Papaya 166, 202, 207, 223
Paprika 176, 191, 202
Parasite 94, 98, 154, 160, 180
Parkinson's 87, 103
Parsley 202
Particle 53
Passion 203
Pasta 146, 166, 178, 190, 201,
226
Pasteurise 142
Pâté 141, 174, 229, 230
Patent 94
Pathogen 95, 96, 109, 121, 122,
144, 190
Pau d'Arco 45
PCB. See Polychlorinated
biphenyl
Pea 169
Peace 131, 208
Peace lily 52
Peach 156, 166, 222
Peanut 175, 202

Pear 166, 191, 202, 218
Pears 222
Pecan 173, 191, 202
Pectin 299
Peer-pressure 63
Pepper 138, 156, 166, 191, 202, 222, 328
Pepper, black. See Black pepper
Peptic ulcer 57
Peptide 146
Perception 33
Peristalsis 138
Persimmon 166, 273
Personality 206
Perspective 232
Pesticide 154, 156, 158
Petrochemicals 95
Petrol 67
Pharmaceutical 123
   industry 12, 77
Phenol 77
Phosphorous 142, 150, 156
Photograph 36
Physalis 338
Phytochemical 168, 298. See also Chemical
Pie 146
Piel de sapo 222
Pili 173
Pine nut 173
Pineapple 166, 191
Pistachio 173
Pituitary gland 211
Placebo 89
Placenta 79
Plant 51-53, 76, 108, 157, 173, 231
Plastic 60
Play 14, 102
Pleasure 204
Plum 156, 211
Pod 175
Poinsettia 52
Poison 161
Pollutant 218
Pollution 12, 46

sensory 74-75
Polychlorinated biphenyl 158
Polychlorinated dibenzodiozin 158
Poo 100, 101, 138, 139
Poppy seed 202
Porous 230
Positive thinking 116
Potassium 151, 156, 302, 310, 331
Potato 160, 161, 166, 189, 190, 200, 201, 226
Potato, sweet. See Sweet potato
Poultry 189, 200
Power 203
Prana 134
Pranayama 92, 93
   lesson 93
Prayer 133
Preconception 30
Pre-menstrual diet. See Diet, pre-menustrual
Pre-menstrual symptoms. See Symptoms, pre-menstrual
Pregnant 14, 44, 85, 87, 88, 108, 109, 120, 123, 186, 217
   fasting 224
Preventative 94
Primate 57, 145
Priority 33
Process 235
Prognosis 15
Propylene glycol 49
Prostate cancer. See Cancer, prostate
Protection 208
Protein 27, 56, 96, 145, 151, 170, 175, 331
   milk 142
Protoplast 122
Psychic 211, 212
Pumpkin 173, 191, 202
Punnet 273
Pure 178, 213
Purge 36
Purifier. See Air, purifier

Purify 134
Purity 213
Purselane 151
Pyramid 118

Q

Quinoa 169

R

Radiation 62, 76
Radish 169
Radon 56
Rainbow 200
Raisin 167
Ramie 55, 231
Rash 20, 49
Raspberry 166
Raw plant diet. See Diet, raw plant
Read 189, 232
Reality 139
   Renew 208
Red blood cell. See Cell, red blood
Reasons to detox 8-14
Rebounder 102-104, 195, 204, 207, 210
Rectal cancer 56
Recycle 46, 53
Red, the colour 203
Reflex 17, 104, 118
Reflexology 118-119, 187
Rehydrate 57
Rejuvenate 10, 12, 13, 28, 95, 120, 127, 203, 218, 225
Relationship 113
Relax 120, 192, 193, 209, 232
Relaxation 209
Release 179
Religion 111
Renew 196
Repair 13, 28, 161, 185
Repetitive strain injury 75
Reproductive 204
   disorder 87
Resourceful 204

Respiratory 65, 106, 204
Restaurant 233
Restructure 28
Result 33
Rheumatoid arthritis 88
Retox 32
Rice 161, 166, **200**, 226
Right brain 116
Ripe 83, 201
River 86
Rocket 202, 218, 222
Roman 122
Root 151, 157
Root canal 79, 84
Rosemary 108, 176
RSI. See Repetitive strain injury
Rule 33
Rye 169, 235

S

Sad 53
Saddle-bags 28
Sage 176
Salad 145, 169, 229, 230, 233
  dressing 174
Saliva 141
Salt 109, 138, 147, 156, 202, **273**
  pepper and **147**
Sandalwood 108
Sandwich 146, 229, 230
Sankharas 131
Sauna 182, 197, 214, 218, 232
  infra-red 14, 120
Sausage 146
Scallion 300
Schlosser, Eric. See Eric
Schlosser
Scientist 30
Scorpion 309
Scrub,body. See Body, scrub
Sea 53
  lettuce 202
  salad 202, 273
Season 10
Seasonal 31
Seaweed 233, **273**

Seed 173-174, 221, 226, 235
Selenium 302
Self 210, 211, 213
  assurance 213
  confidence 203
  esteem 206
  observation 132
  respect 29
Selfless 133
Senile 18
Sense of direction 88
Sensitive 230
Senza, the 188
Serene 55
Sesame 173, 293
Sew 190
Sex 132
  celibacy 129
  energy 129
  stimulant 302
Sexless 46
Sheep 55
Shepherd's purse 151
Shiga 144
Shirt 231
Shivambu fasting 131
Shoe 231, 234
Shoot 151
Shopping list 186, 190, 201, 221
Shower 53, 56
Sickness. See Nausea
Side-effect 123
  dealing with **179**
  of detox **18-20**, 126
Silver 79, **121-123**
  colloidal 121
Simplicity 139
Single-celled organism 170
Sinusitis 53, 142, 143
Skin 11, 35, 36, 120, 296
  alcohol and 43
  brushing122, **124-126**
  burn 109
  cancer. See Cancer, skin
  care **49-50**
  chlorine and 56
  clear 17, 180

cleanse 120
clothing and 54, 231
colon and **98-99**
colour 17
damage 66-69
dead 109
dry 30
irritant 55
itchy 56
problem **185**
smooth 108
texture 20
tone 108
wrinkled 80
younger **185**
Sleep 17, 18, 24, 36, 37, 96, 189, 232
  disturbance 86
Slim-Fast 27
Slimming Club 27
Slipper 196
SLS. See Sodium Lauryl
Sulphate
Smell 141
Smoke 24, 41, 67
  removal of 53
Smoking 63-72. See also
Cigarette. **See also** Cancer,
smoking and. **See also** Smoke,
cancer and. **See also** Smoking.
See also Tobacco.
  quitting 69
Smoothie 140, 143, 167, 169, 174, 178, 187, 223, 229
Snack bag 167, 186, 187, **191**, 192, 193, 202
Snake 155
Soap 124
Social conditioning 21
Sock 196, 221
Soda crystal 60
Sodium 277
Sodium Lauryl Sulphate 49, 82
Soil erosion 155
Soup 169, 174, 182, 187, 223, 225, 229
Soya 155, 189, 190, 200, 201
Spain 153, 175

Spice 173, 175, 230
Spice/coffee mill 276
Spider plant 52
Spinach 138, 151, 156, 207, 222, 327
Spine 203
Spiral slicer 275
Spirit 133, 134, 181, 185, 211, 224
Spiritual 131, 133, 134, 213, 217. See also Spirituality
Spirituality 9, 213
Spirulina 170
Sport 232
Spots. See Acne
Spring 12, 150
Spring onion 156, 191, 202, 300
Sprouts 169-170, 175, 235, 273, 318
Squash, acorn 202
Squirrel 21
Stagnant 124
Stalk 151
Stamina 17, 19, 225
Starch 160, 175
Starve 29
Steam room 182
Still 194
Stillbirth 65
Stimulant 44
Stimulate 124, 126
Stomach 41, 141, 168, 206, 226
    cancer. See Cancer, stomach
Straw 83
Strawberry 156, 191, 202, 222
Strength 168, 181, 186, 203
Stress 33, 62, 92, 104, 105, 111, 113, 187. See also Anxiety
Stretch mark 17
Striped dracaena 52
Subconscious 33, 116
Success 204
Suck 140
Suffer 18
Sugar 83, 121, 138, 160, 175, 182, 198, 215
Suicide 85, 154

Sulphur 167
Sultana 167
Sunflower 169, 173, 191, 202
Sunshine 157, 190
Suntan 17
Superfood 170, 191, 202, 229, 230
Supplement 30
Sweet breath 92
    practising 93
    teacher 93
Sweet potato 156
Sweet tooth 166
Sweets 82, 190, 201
Swim 14, 102, 197, 214
Symbiosis 53
Symbiotic 157
Symmetry 79
Symptom 10, 54, 184
    detox 18, 19, 168, 178, 179, 194
    drugs 179
    -free 188
    hard 224, 228
    milk 143
    relief of 53
    teeth 83, 89
    thirst 58
    toxic 10, 185
    vaccine-related 76
    withdrawal 25, 44, 45, 70, 146
Syphilis 86, 122

T

Tahini 191, 202
Talc 49
Talent 213
Tan. See Suntan
Tar 66
Taste 22, 152, 167
Taste bud 230
Tea 13, 44, 178, 221, 224, 228, 234
Teetotal 42
Telephone 112, 190
Television 62, 75-76, 102, 111, 115, 189, 193, 196, 201, 232

Temperate 166
Temple 211
Tension 104
Therapy 153
Thiamin 293
Thigh 125
Thimerosal 77
Thirst 58, 139
Throat 209
    cancer 65
Thrush 17
Thunderstorm 53
Thyme 176
Tibet 127
Tibetan Rejuvenation Rites 127-130, 192, 194, 196, 198, 203, 204, 206, 207, 209, 211, 213, 215
Tie 231
Tights 231
Time 127
Tired. See Lethargy/Fatigue
Tissue 84, 95, 124
    cellular 98
Toast 146
Tobacco 63, 69
Toilet 101
    habit 100
Toiletry 49
    toxins 49
Tomato 57, 138, 153, 160, 166, 191, 202, 222, 230, 233, 298
Tongue 123, 185
Tonsil 142
Tooth 79-90
    brush 82
    grind 88
    paste 49, 82, 233
Topical 95
Touch 108
Town 47
Toxic 39, 40, 46, 124, 153, 168, 175, 188, 232
    body 185
    fumes 60
    waste 46
Toxin 103, 108, 109, 120, 133,

153, 158, 160, 162, 179, 184, 230, 234
  Shiga 144
Trampoline 102
Tranquil 232
Transfusion 162
Tree 47, 57, 138
Tremor 67
Tropical 166
Tuberculosis 76
Tummy 36, 125, 235
  ache 139
Tumour 95
Turmeric 202

U

Ulcer, peptic. See Peptic ulcer
Ulcerative colitis 17
Ultraviolet light 190
Unbleached 55
Undernourish 29
Understand 212
Understanding 211
Units, alcohol 40
Unity 134
Universal law 33
Universe 111
Upholstery 60
Urine 18
Utensils 60

V

Vaccination 76-77
Vagina 123
Vanilla 191, 287
Varicose vein 103
Vegan 158, 170
Vegetable 101, 139, 150, 152, 182, 189, 198, **200,** 221
  sea 235
Vegetarian 109, 132, 144, 158
  diet. **See** Diet, vegetarian
Veneer 79
Verruca 122
Vibration 231
Vinegar 60
Violet, the colour 213

Vipassana 131-132
Virus 76, 95, 121, 162
  infected 105
Vitality 29, 55, 203
Vitamin 30, 98, 121, 154, 168, 170
Vitamin A 150, 151, 278, 302
Vitamin B 98, 150, 151, 302
Vitamin B12 152
Vitamin B17 173
Vitamin C 151, 278, 318, 327
Vitamin E 151, 296, 302
Vitamin K 98
Vitamineral Green 170
Vomit 168

W

Walk 190, 195, 210
Walker, Norman. See Dr Norman Walker
Walnut 138, 173, 179, **320**
Wardrobe 231, 234
Warming 182
Wart 67, 122
Water 56-59, 100, 138, 143, 162, 191, 217, 227, 228, 232, 234, 274
  allergy 57
  chlorine 56
  coconut. **See** Coconut water
  dehydration 56, 57
  drink 45, 57, 101
  live 58
  retention 28
  tap 56
Watercress 207
Waterfall 53
Watermelon 57-58, 138, 156, 187, 298
Weak 157
Weed 149
Weight 17, 24, 27, 28, 34, 185, 234
  control 213
  loss 93, 104
Weight Watchers 27
Western diet. See Diet, western
Western society 15
Wheat 24, 47, 169, 178, 190, 201
  children and 47

Wheatgrass 168, 170
White blood cell. See Cell, white blood
Wild food 149-151
Wildcraft 170
Willpower 24
Wind 139
Window 54, 181, 201, 224
Wine 24, 40, 43, 234
Winter 94
Wisdom 31, 113, 206, 224
Wise 206
Withdrawal 24
Woman 187, 188
  cancer and 68
Womb 44, 79, 118
Wood 231
Wool 55
Workshop 232
World 39
World War I 94
Worm 98
Wraps 108-110
Wrinkles 17, 49

X

X-ray 57

Y

Yeast 95
Yeast infection. See Thrush
Yellow, the colour 206
Yoga 14, 92, 113, 129, 131, **133-136,** 200, 232
Yoghurt 142, 178
Yogi 92
Yogini 92
Younger 17, 95, 185
Yo-yo 15, 17, 27

Z

Zebra 21
Zeolites 79, **90**
Zinc 151, 331
The Zone Diet 27
Zucchini 273

Further copies and other products

To order this book and any of Shazzie's other products:

www.detoxyourworld.com — worldwide easy online ordering
Tel: 08700 113 119 (international: +44 (0)8700 113 119)

Detox Delights — There are over a hundred tasty unique recipes in this book to add even more variety to your life!

"I bought Detox Delights about a month ago and I have to say the recipes are great. The raw pizza recipe is amazing and tastes better than cooked pizza. The Italian soup is one of my new favorites also. After trying many of the recipes in her book, going back to cooked food would be so boring. This is a must have book for anyone who thinks eating raw is limiting."— **Allen, USA**

Shazzie's raw food delights — A series of three raw food preparation DVDs, offering you a total of 22 recipes to keep your taste buds dancing all week long.

"I have had so much fun watching your video! I found it all very easy to follow and your instructions on how to use various pieces of kitchen machinery was invaluable as I have never used a Champion, Vita-Mix or dehydrator and have often wondered what they looked like and did! All of your dishes looked so amazingly delicious and were really pleasing to the eye. I especially loved the look of the crudités and tahini dips, the ratatouille, the seed-style bread, and the soup! Gosh — I learned so much! I have always preferred visual aids and I so wish something like this video had been around three years ago when I first heard about raw foodism!"— **Janey, UK**

Naked Chocolate — co-authored with **David Wolfe**, 248 pages, full colour. Over 60 photographed raw vegan cacao recipes. Thanks to authors David Wolfe and Shazzie, we can finally live by chocolate! We get right under the skin of the chocolate industry, the cacao tree, the cacao fruit and finally, we find the raw bean — full of nutrients and full of life.

"Naked Chocolate is fantastic! I love it very much. Thank you. Thank you. Thank you a million times."— **Dr Patrick Flanagan**, USA (voted one of America's top 10 scientists at the age of 17!)

What they say about Detox Your World

Detox Your World brings forth a calm, holistic understanding of health, healing, detoxification, transformation, and raw-food nutrition. This book is filled with clever insights by the United Kingdom's most inspiring health author and speaker. Shazzie has made the impossible probable as she describes how she rejuvenated her mind, body, and spirit. Certainly, this is one of the best books in the entire health field.

David Wolfe, USA
Author of **Eating For Beauty**, **Naked Chocolate** *(with Shazzie)* and **The Sunfood Diet Success System**
CEO of **www.rawfood.com**
Founder of **The Fruit Tree Planting Foundation**

Detox Your World is the most comprehensive book I've seen on the raw/living foods lifestyle since **The Sunfood Diet Success System** and **Conscious Eating**.

Stephen Arlin, USA
Author of **Raw Power!**

Dear Shazzie

I had been high raw for about 18 months before doing the three day detox in **Detox Your World**. I felt much lighter for it and it made me realise that I was further along the raw road than I thought I was. I didn't struggle with it, it seemed really natural to do. I've been able to incorporate a lot of the ideas that you suggested into my everyday life now. The book is very clear, easy to use, a practical step-by-step approach and everybody will get something out of it in their raw life.

Frances, UK

Hi Shaz

What a book!!!!! I knew it was gonna be good but it's *phew* the best! You've done an absolutely flipping(!) good job!! Well done, it's a classic. And I ain't saying that just because I love you!

Jatinder, Spain

Shazzie, you blessed creature!

Thank you so much for writing that book. It was such a joy to read your book that I gulped it down very quickly.

Everything you said made such perfect sense. I loved reading the other testimonials in the book. It's always great to read them and know how much a sane way of eating can make you feel so much better in all ways.

One of my friends here where I teach saw the cover of your book and asked what it was. I told her and she said: "Well we all should look so good as her. She's a model, right?" I told her the picture was of the author of the book, showed her the before and after picture of you, and she kinda got silent and didn't say any more. Made her think maybe?

Thank you ever so much for the book **Detox Your World**. The world wouldn't have been quite the same without your sunshine in it!

Namaste, dear sister

Nerissa, USA

Dear Shazzie

Through reading your journal and seeing your transformation pictures it has helped me to stay on the path. Every time I am tempted to eat cooked food I just read from your journal and it helps me to stay on the path. Your honesty and sense of humor are truly gifts, although obviously not the only gifts you possess.

I would just like to thank you from the bottom of my heart for helping me to stay on this path. After my daughter saw your transformation photos all she could say was, "Oh my gosh, oh my gosh. I'm going raw this summer." She wants to help me try new recipes so there are more that she enjoys. As she told me, "Mom I can't just live on guacamole and hummus." Everyone keeps telling me that my skin is glowing and how great I look. Thanks, and don't stop sharing.

Doreen, Delaware, USA

Your new book is so brilliant that I even took it to the theatre with me last night and in between performances I was busy reading away. I really cannot put it down — literally!

Janey, UK

Dear Shazzie,

Thanks so much for the time and energy you invested in writing this wonderful book. It is fantastic to read a book that approaches detox from so many directions. And your encouraging recommendation for your readers to take the steps they are ready for and not to judge themselves so harshly has really touched me! You've once again inspired me with your style and personality. I feel like you are my friend, although we have never met or spoken. I look forward to reading your next book!

Thanks for all you do!

Julie Disser, USA
Art of Living Well, **www.artoflivingwell.com**

Dear, sweet Shazzie,

Reading your book was like having a wonderful, inspiring chat with a friend... a friend who shares my world. Your book is such a relaxing read and I learned so much. I felt like I was reading a novel. I couldn't put it down.

Keep writing and teaching Shazzie. The raw world is blessed to have an angel like you guiding and teaching us.

Much love,

Jeannie Curtis, Scottsdale, Arizona, USA

As soon as I got your book I began it and couldn't put it down. Really, it was as gripping as a novel though this was and is real life. I think this is because you put so much of yourself in there, there is no hiding behind the words. I honour your courage in being so real always in all ways. The information inspired me to go even further in detoxing my world — I have had my (amalgam) fillings removed since I read the book!!!! As always, your recipes are delicious yet simple.

Thank you for all you are.

Jood, UK

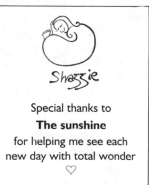

Special thanks to
The sunshine
for helping me see each
new day with total wonder
♡

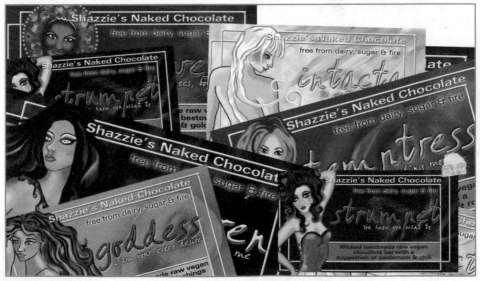